TRADITIONAL CHINESE MEDICINE ATLAS

中药图册（下卷）

VOLUME 2

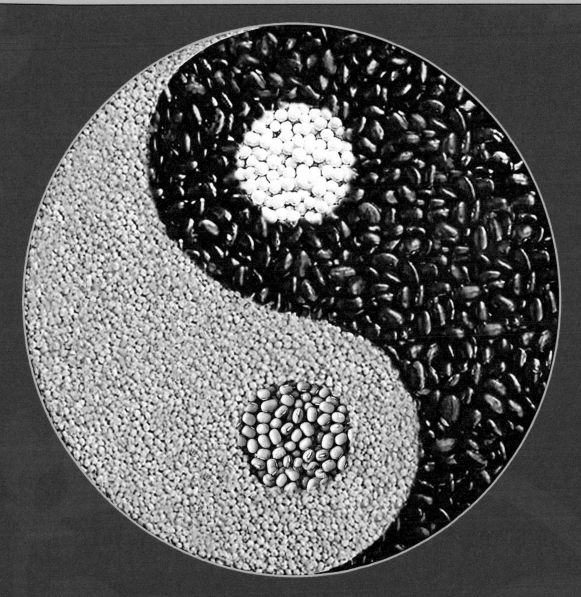

CHEN RUI

Traditional Chinese Medicine Atlas
Volume 2

iUniverse books may be ordered through booksellers or by contacting:

iUniverse
1663 Liberty Drive
Bloomington, IN 47403
www.iuniverse.com
1-800-Authors (1-800-288-4677)

Because of the dynamic nature of the Internet, any web addresses or links contained in this book may have changed since publication and may no longer be valid. The views expressed in this work are solely those of the author and do not necessarily reflect the views of the publisher, and the publisher hereby disclaims any responsibility for them.

Any people depicted in stock imagery provided by Getty Images are models, and such images are being used for illustrative purposes only.
Certain stock imagery © Getty Images.

ISBN: 978-1-5320-8136-1 (sc)
ISBN: 978-1-5320-8137-8 (e)

Library of Congress Control Number: 2019912741

Print information available on the last page.

iUniverse rev. date: 10/11/2019

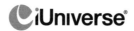

Traditional Chinese Medicine Atlas

中药图册（下卷）

(volume II)

Menu

Attention

The Earth is the home of us and other creatures. Do not use the herb get from rare wildlife and rare wild plant. Use the herb abide by local laws.

Use with caution in people who are allergy to the component of the herb.

By
Chen Rui
(Qinghai Province Institute for Food Control, China)
Shu Tong
(Qinghai Province Institute for Food Control, China)
Zeng Yang
(Qinghai Normal University, China)
Yan Peiying
(Qinghai Normal University, China)
Yao Yilei
(OKAYAMA University, Japan)
Hongping Han
(Qinghai Normal University, China)
Luo Qiaoyu
(Qinghai Normal University, China)

Part Ⅰ Chinese Matera Medica and Prepared Slice of Traditional Chinese Drugs

Huo Xue Yao(活血药)-herbs for invigorating blood circulation and eliminating stasis

Huo Xue Yao is a kind of herbs which's the major functions are to stimulate the circulation of blood and disperse blood stasis.

Szechwan Lovage Rhizome (Chuanxiong)

Chinese phonetic alphabet/pin yin: chuān xiōng

Chinese characters simplified/traditional:川芎/川芎

Chinese nickname's alphabet (Nickname's Chinese characters): Jingxiong/ Guanxiong(京芎/贯芎)

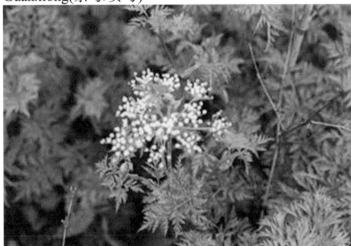

Latin: Chuanxiong Rhizoma (Common name: Szechwan Lovage Rhizome)
Plant: *Ligusticum chuanxiong* Hort.

TCM prepared in ready-to-use forms (medicinal parts): it's dried rhizome which harvested in summer.
Property and flavor: warm; pungent.
Main and collateral channels: liver, gallbladder and pericardium meridians.
Administration and dosage: 3-10 g.

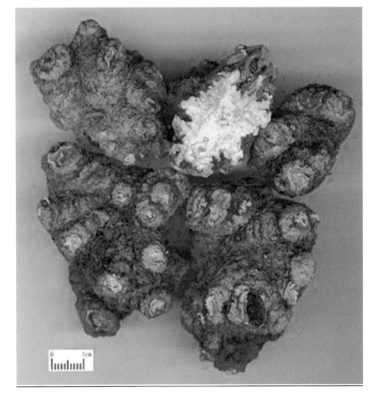

Indication: irregular menstruation, dysmenorrhea, amenorrhea, chest and abdominal pain, swelling with pain or flutter, headache and painful *bi* disorder.

It is key herb to treat headache, amenorrhea and dystocia.

(The picture is only for learning and identification the herb; the specific use of the herb please consult the herbalist or health professionals)

Yanhusuo (Yanhusuo)

Chinese phonetic alphabet/pin yin: yán hú suǒ

Chinese characters simplified/traditional:延胡索/延胡索

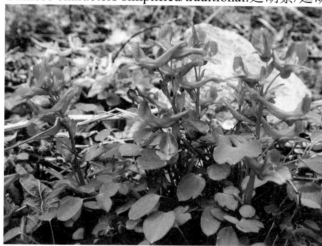

Chinese nickname's alphabet (Nickname's Chinese characters): Xuanhusuo/ Yuanhu (玄胡索/元胡)

Latin: Corydalis Rhizoma (Common name: Yanhusuo)

Plant: *Corydalis yanhusuo* W. T. Wang ex Z. Y. Su et C. Y. Wu

TCM prepared in ready-to-use forms (medicinal parts): it's dried tuber root which harvested in summer. Property and flavor: warm; pungent, bitter. Main and collateral channels: spleen and liver meridians. Administration and dosage: 3-10 g. Ground into powder for oral administration:1.5-3 g per time.

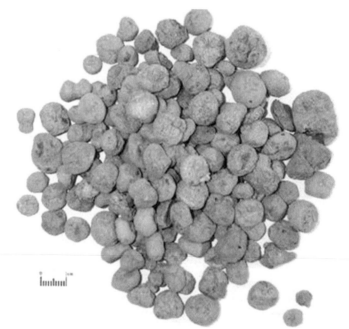

Indication: heart and abdominal pain, amenorrhea, dysmenorrhea, blood stasis, postpartum stasis resistance, swelling or flutter and traumatic injuries.

It is key herb to treat acute heart pain.

(The picture is only for learning and identification the herb; the specific use of the herb please consult the herbalist or health professionals)

Turmeric Root Tuber (Yujin)

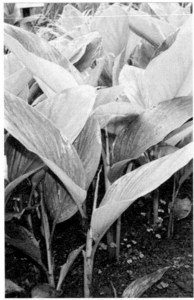

Chinese phonetic alphabet/pin yin: yù jīn
Chinese characters simplified/traditional:郁金/鬱金
Chinese nickname's alphabet (Nickname's Chinese characters): Chuanyujin/ Huangyu(川郁金/黄郁)
Latin: Curcumae Radix
(Common name: Turmeric Root Tuber)
Plant: *Curcuma wenyujin* Y. H. Chen et C. Ling. (or *Curcuma kwangsiensis* S. G. Lee et C. F. Liang.*, Curcuma phaeocaulis* Val.)

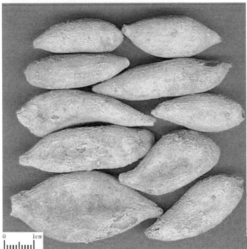

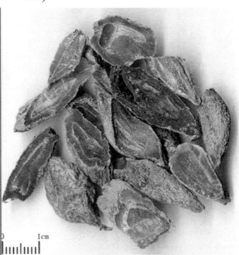

TCM prepared in ready-to-use forms (medicinal parts): it's dried tuber root which harvested in winter.
Property and flavor: cold; pungent, bitter.
Main and collateral channels: liver and heart meridians.
Administration and dosage: 3-10 g.
Indication: amenorrhea, dysmenorrhea, heart and abdominal pain, epilepsy and jaundice.
It is key herb to treat heart pain, irregular menstruation.
Precaution and warning: Incompatible with Clove and Clove Fruit.
Attachment: Wenyujin Concise Rhizome is rhizome of *CuFrcuma wenyujin* Y. H. Chen et C. Ling. which heavested in autumn when stem and leaf withered. It is known as "Pianjianghuang(片姜黄)"
(The picture is only for learning and identification the herb; the specific use of the herb please consult the herbalist or health professionals)

Zedoray Rhizome (Ezhu)

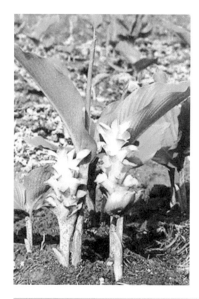

Chinese phonetic alphabet/pin yin: é zhù
Chinese characters simplified/traditional:莪术/
莪術
Chinese nickname's alphabet (Nickname's
Chinese characters): Peng'ezhu(蓬莪术)
Latin: Curcumae Rhizoma (Common name:
Zedoray Rhizome)
Plant: *Curcuma phaeocaulis* Valeton. (or
Curcuma kwangsiensis S. G. Lee et C. F.
Liang., *Curcuma wenyujin* Y. H. Chen et C.
Ling., *Curcuma zedoaria* (Christm.) Rosc.)

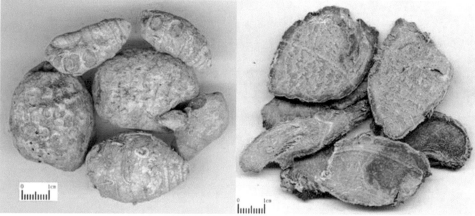

TCM prepared in ready-to-use forms (medicinal parts): it's dried rhizome which
harvested in winter.
Property and flavor: warm; pungent, bitter.
Main and collateral channels: liver and spleen meridians.
Administration and dosage: 6-9 g.
Indication: lump, mass, blood stasis, amenorrhea, dyspeptic, abdominal pain and
glomus.
It is commonly used in expelling abdominal mass and lump.
Precaution and warning: contraindicated during pregnancy.
Attachment: Zedoray Furmeric Oil is volatile oil obtained by steam distillation from
Zedoray Rhizome.
(The picture is only for learning and identification the herb; the specific use of the
herb please consult the herbalist or health professionals)

Danshen Root (Danshen)
Chinese phonetic alphabet/pin yin: dān shēn
Chinese characters simplified/traditional:丹参/丹参
Chinese nickname's alphabet (Nickname's Chinese characters): Chishen/ Hongshen
(赤参/红参)

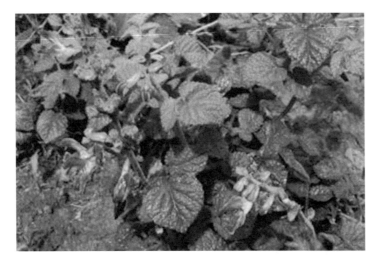

Latin: Salviae Miltiorrhizae Radix et Rhizoma (Common name: Danshen Root)
Plant: *Salvia miltiorrhiza* Bge.

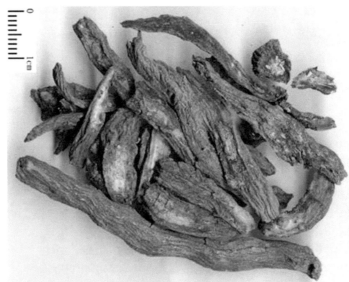

TCM prepared in ready-to-use forms (medicinal parts): it's dried root and rhizome which harvested in spring or autumn. Property and flavor: mild cold; bitter.

Main and collateral channels: heart and liver meridians.
Administration and dosage: 10-15 g.
Indication: irregular menstruation, amenorrhea, dysmenorrhea, malignant masses in the abdomen, heart and abdominal pain, sore throat, insomnia by vexation, sore, ulcer, swelling and pain.
It is key herb to treat blood stasis, pain, dysmenorrheal and amenorrhea.
Precaution and warning: incompatible with Black False Hellebore.
(The picture is only for learning and identification the herb; the specific use of the herb please consult the herbalist or health professionals)

Giant Knotweed Rhizome (Huzhang)
Chinese phonetic alphabet/pin yin: hǔ zhàng
Chinese characters simplified/traditional:虎杖/虎杖
Chinese nickname's alphabet (Nickname's Chinese characters): Dachongzhang/ Kuzhang (大虫杖/苦杖)
Latin: Polygoni Cuspidati Rhizoma et Radix (Common name: Giant Knotweed Rhizome)

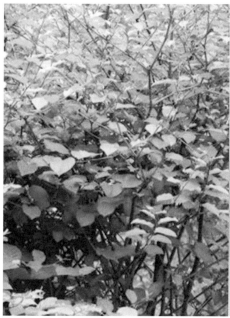
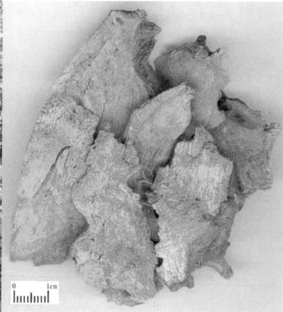

Plant: *Polygonum cuspidatum* Sieb. et Zucc.

TCM prepared in ready-to-use forms (medicinal parts): it's dried root and rhizome which harvested in spring or autumn.

Property and flavor: mild cold; mild bitter.

Main and collateral channels: liver, gallbladder and lung meridians.

Administration and dosage: 9-15 g. Appropriate amount for topical application, made into decoction or oil paste for applyment.

Indication: joint pain, jaundice, turbid strangury, amenorrhea, abdominal mass, scald and burn, painful *bi* disorder, traumatic injury, carbuncle sore, cough and excessive phlegm.

It is key herb to treat burn and scald, insect and snake bites.

Precaution and warning: use with caution during pregnancy.

(The picture is only for learning and identification the herb; the specific use of the herb please consult the herbalist or health professionals)

Motherwort Herb (Yimucao)
Chinese phonetic alphabet/pin yin: yì mǔ cǎo
Chinese characters simplified/traditional:益母草/益母草

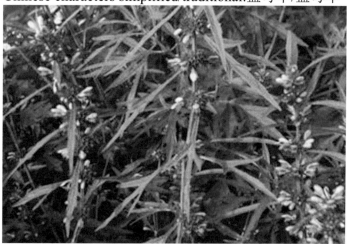

Chinese nickname's alphabet (Nickname's Chinese characters): Chongwei/ Kuncao(茺蔚/坤草)
Latin: Leonuri Herba (Common name: Motherwort Herb)

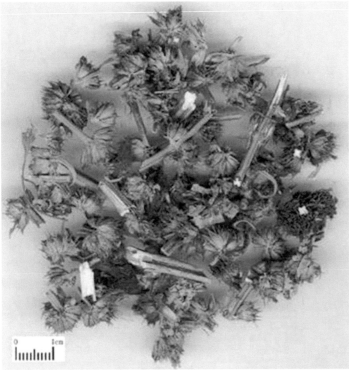

TCM prepared in ready-to-use forms (medicinal parts): it's dried above-ground part which harvested in summer when it is just to bloom. Property and flavor: mild cold; bitter, pungent. Main and collateral channels: liver, pericardium and bladder meridians.

Plant: *Leonurus japonicus* Houtt. (or *Leonurus artemisia* (Laur.) S. Y. Hu. F)
Administration and dosage: 9-30 g. 12-40 g for unprocessed one.
Indication: irregular menstruation, dysmenorrhea, amenorrhea, lochia, edema, oliguria, acute nephritis, sore, ulcer swelling and toxin.
It is key herb to treat persistent lochia, induce diuresis to reduce edema.
Precaution and warning: use with caution during pregnancy.
(The picture is only for learning and identification the herb; the specific use of the herb please consult the herbalist or health professionals)

Peach Seed (Taoren)

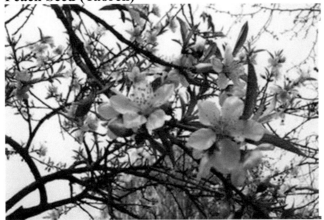

Chinese phonetic alphabet/pin yin: táo rén
Chinese characters simplified/traditional:桃仁/桃仁
Chinese nickname's alphabet (Nickname's Chinese characters): Taoheren(桃核仁)

Latin: Persicae Semen (Common name: Peach Seed or Peach Kernel)
Plant: *Prunus persica* (L.) Batsch (or *Prunus davidiana* (Carr.) Franch.)
TCM prepared in ready-to-use forms (medicinal parts): it's dried mature seed.

Property and flavor:
neutral; sweet, bitter.
Main and collateral
channels: heart, liver and
large intestine meridians.
Administration and
dosage: 5-10 g.
Indication: dysmenorrhea,
amenorrhea, abdominal
mass lump, traumatic
injury, constipation,
cough and wheezing.
It is taken as food in some
part of China.

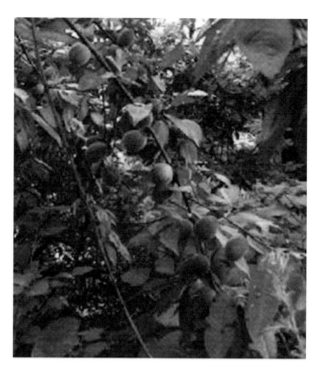

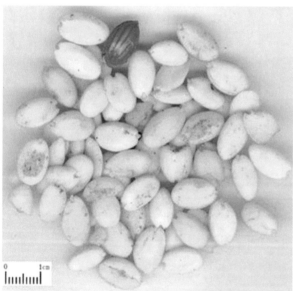

Caution: this peach is
the *Prunus persica* (*or
davidiana*), not
Amygdalus persica.
**Precaution and
warning:** use with
caution during
pregnancy.
(The picture is only for
learning and
identification the herb;
the specific use of the
herb please consult the
herbalist or health
professionals)

Safflower (Honghua)

Chinese phonetic
alphabet/pin yin: hóng huā
Chinese characters
simplified/traditional:红花/
红花
Chinese nickname's
alphabet (Nickname's
Chinese characters):
Honglanhua/ Cihonghua (红
蓝花/刺红花)

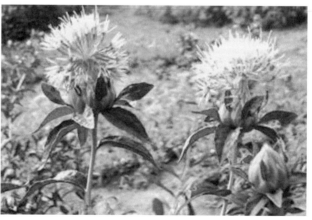

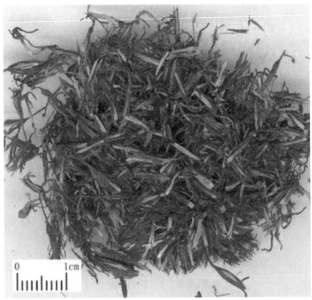

Latin: Carthami Flos
(Common name:
Safflower)
Plant: *Carthamus tinctorius* L.
TCM prepared in
ready-to-use forms
(medicinal parts):
it's dried flower.
Property and flavor:
warm; pungent.
Main and collateral
channels: heart and
liver meridians.

Administration and dosage: 3-10 g.
Indication: amenorrhea, dysmenorrhea, lochia, abdominal lump, traumatic injury, sore throat, carbuncle, sore, ulcer, swelling and pain.
Precaution and warning: use with caution during pregnancy.
(The picture is only for learning and identification the herb; the specific use of the herb please consult the herbalist or health professionals)

Twotoothed Achyranthes Root (Niuxi)
Chinese phonetic alphabet/pin yin: niú xī
Chinese characters simplified/traditional:牛膝/牛膝
Chinese nickname's alphabet (Nickname's Chinese characters): Huainiuxi(怀牛膝)

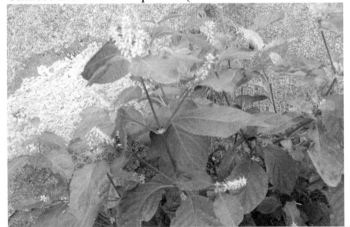

Latin: Achyranthis
Bidentatae Radix
(Common name:
Twotoothed
Achyranthes Root)
Plant: *Achyranthes bidentata* Blume.

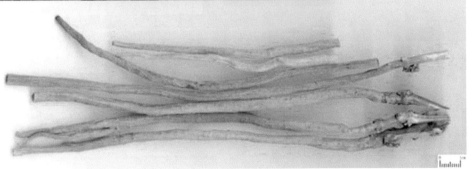

TCM prepared in ready-to-use forms (medicinal parts): it's dried root which harvested in winter. Property and flavor: neutral; bitter, sweet and acidity.

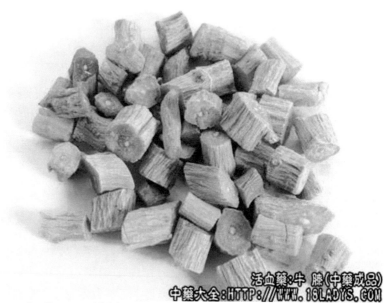

活血藥：牛 膝(中藥成品)
中藥大全：HTTP://WWW.16LADYS.COM

Main and collateral channels: liver and kidney meridians.
Administration and dosage: 5-12 g.
Indication: waist and knee pain, muscles weakness, amenorrhea, dysmenorrhea, abdominal mass, edema, headache, dizziness, toothache, hematemesis and epistaxis. It is key herb to treat amenorrhea and dysmenorrheal.
Precaution and warning: use with caution during pregnancy.
(The picture is only for learning and identification the herb; the specific use of the herb please consult the herbalist or health professionals)

Leech (Shuizhi)
Chinese phonetic alphabet/pin yin: shuǐ zhì
Chinese characters simplified/traditional:水蛭/水蛭
Chinese nickname's alphabet (Nickname's Chinese characters): Mahuang(蚂蟥)
Latin: Hirudo (Common name: Leech)

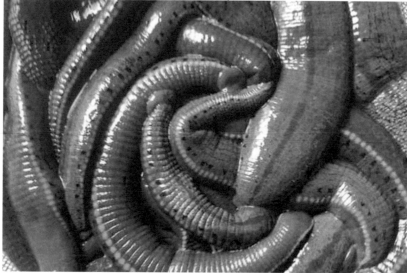

Animal: *Whitmania pigra* Whitman. (or *Hirudo nipponica* Whitman., *Whitmania acranulata* Whitman.)

TCM prepared in ready-to-use forms (medicinal parts): it is dried body get in summer or autumn and boiled to dead. Property and flavor: neutral; bitter, salty. Main and collateral channels: liver meridian.

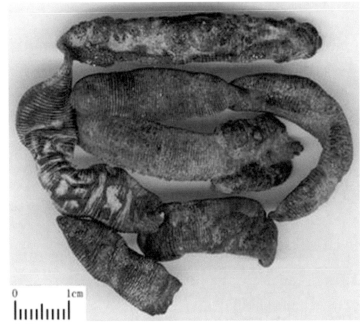

Administration and dosage: 1-3 g.

Indication: blood stasis, lump, amenorrhea, hemiplegia and traumatic injury.

Precaution and warning: slightly toxic. Contraindicated during pregnancy.

(The picture is only for learning and identification the herb; the specific use of the herb please consult the herbalist or health professionals)

Olibanum (Ruxiang)

Chinese phonetic alphabet/pin yin: rǔ xiāng

Chinese characters simplified/traditional:乳香/乳香

Chinese nickname's alphabet (Nickname's Chinese characters): Rutouxiang/ Tianzexiang(乳头香/天泽香)

Latin: Olibanum (Common name: Olibanum or Frankincense)

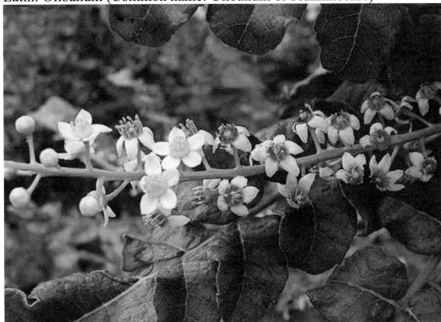

Plant: *Boswellia carterii* Birdw. (or *Boswellia bhawdajiana* Birdw.)

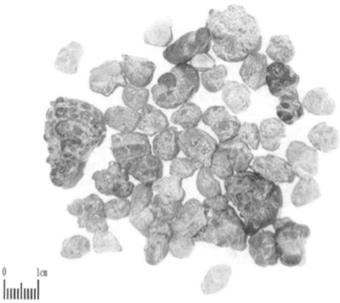

TCM prepared in ready-to-use forms (medicinal parts): it's dried resin exuding form the bark which harvested in spring or summer.

Property and flavor: warm; bitter, pungent.

Main and collateral channels: heart, liver and spleen meridians.

Administration and dosage: decocted or used in pill or powder, 3-5g. Topical application in appropriate amount, ground into powder and apply to the *pars affecta*.

Indication: heart pain, amenorrhea, dysmenorrhea, painful *bi* disorder, carbuncle sore, blood stasis, traumatic injury, sore and ulcer.

It is key herb for relieving the pain, dispersing blood stasis, detumescence and promoting tissue regeneration.

Precaution and warning: use with caution during pregnancy and in patients with weak stomach.

(The picture is only for learning and identification the herb; the specific use of the herb please consult the herbalist or health professionals)

Myrrh (Moyao)

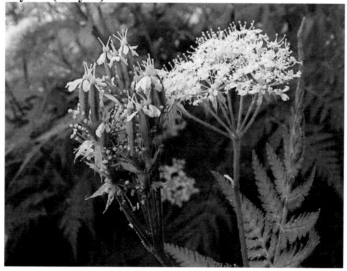

Chinese phonetic alphabet/pin yin: mó yào
Chinese characters simplified/traditional: 没药/沒藥
Chinese nickname's alphabet (Nickname's Chinese characters): Moyao/ Mingmeiyao (末药/明没药)

Latin: Myrrha (Common name: Myrrh)
Plant: *Commiphora myrrha* Engl. (or *Commiphora molmol* Engl.)
TCM prepared in ready-to-use forms (medicinal parts): it is dried resin collected form truck which harvested from December to February.
Property and flavor: neutral; bitter, pungent.
Main and collateral channels: heart, liver and spleen meridians.
Administration and dosage: 3-5 g, processed to remove oil, usually used in pill or powder.

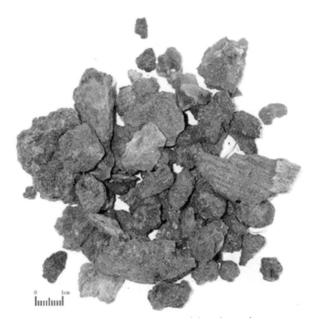

Indication: heart pain, amenorrhea, dysmenorrhea, carbuncle sore, blood stasis, traumatic injury, sore and ulcer.
It is key herb for relieving the pain, dispersing blood stasis, detumescence and promoting tissue regeneration.
Precaution and warning: use with caution during pregnancy and in patients with weak stomach.
(The picture is only for learning and identification the herb; the specific use of the herb please consult the herbalist or health professionals)

Turmeric (Jianghuang)
Chinese phonetic alphabet/pin yin: jiāng huáng
Chinese characters simplified/traditional:姜黄/薑黃
Chinese nickname's alphabet (Nickname's Chinese characters): Baodingxiang/ Huangjiang (宝鼎香/黄姜)
Latin: Curcumae Longae Rhizoma (Common name: Turmeric)

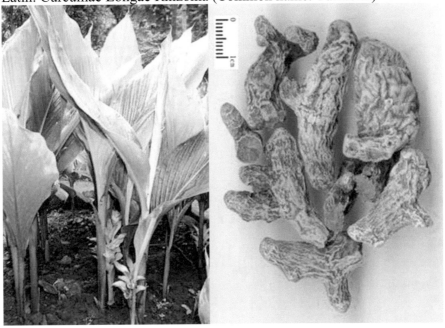

Plant: *Curcuma longa* L.

TCM prepared in ready-to-use forms (medicinal parts): it's dried rhizome which harvested in winter.

Property and flavor: warm; pungent, bitter.

Main and collateral channels: spleen and liver meridians.

Administration and dosage: 3-10 g. Topical application in appropriate amount.

Indication: angina, amenorrhea, dysmenorrhea, shoulder and arm pain, swelling or flutter and traumatic injuries.

It is taken as seasoning in some part of China.

(The picture is only for learning and identification the herb; the specific use of the herb please consult the herbalist or health professionals)

Common Burreed Tuber (Sanleng)

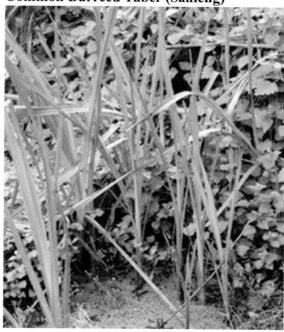

Chinese phonetic alphabet/pin yin: sān léng
Chinese characters simplified/traditional: 三棱/三棱
Chinese nickname's alphabet (Nickname's Chinese characters): Jingsanleng/ Heisanlen(京三棱/黑三棱)

Latin: Sparganii Rhizoma (Common name: Common Burreed Tuber)
Plant: *Sparganium stoloniferum* Buch.-Ham.
TCM prepared in ready-to-use forms (medicinal parts): it's dried tuber rhizome which harvested in winter or spring.
Property and flavor: neutral; bitter, pungent.

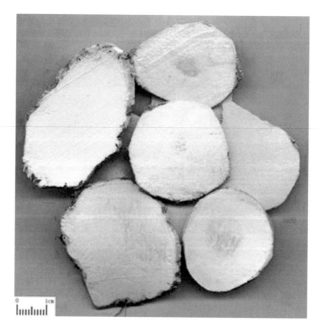

Main and collateral channels: liver and spleen meridians.
Administration and dosage: 5-10 g.
Indication: abdominal mass, amenorrhea, blood stasis, indigestion and heart pain.
It is commonly used in expelling abdominal mass and lump.
Precaution and warning: contraindicate during pregnancy. Incompatible with Sodium Sulfate and Exsiccated Sodium Sulfate.
(The picture is only for learning and identification the herb; the specific use of the herb please consult the herbalist or health professionals)

Suberect Spatholobus Stem (Jixueteng)
Chinese phonetic alphabet/pin yin: jī xuě téng
Chinese characters simplified/traditional:鸡血藤/雞血藤
Chinese nickname's alphabet (Nickname's Chinese characters): Xuefengteng(血风藤)

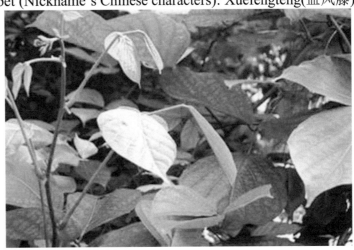

Latin: Spatholobi Caulis (Common name: Suberect Spatholobus Stem)
Plant: *Spatholobus suberetus* Dunn. (or *Millettia reticuiata*)

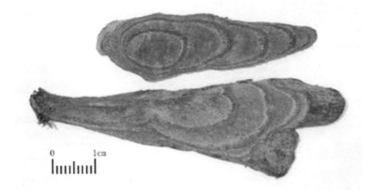

TCM prepared in ready-to-use forms (medicinal parts): it's dried lianoid cane which harvested in autumn or winter.

Property and flavor: warm; bitter, sweet.
Main and collateral channels: liver and kidney meridians.
Administration and dosage: 9-15 g.
Indication: irregular menstruation, dysmenorrhea, amenorrhea, blood deficiency, numbness, paralysis and painful *bi* disorder.
It is commonly used in treating painful *bi* disorder and numbness of limb.
(The picture is only for learning and identification the herb; the specific use of the herb please consult the herbalist or health professionals)

Kadsura Stem (Dianjixueteng)
Chinese phonetic alphabet/pin yin: diān jī xuě téng

Chinese characters simplified/traditional:滇鸡血藤/滇雞血藤
Chinese nickname's alphabet (Nickname's Chinese characters): Neinanwuweizi(内南五味子)

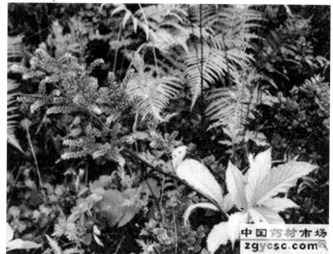

Latin: Kadsurae Caulis (Common name: Kadsura Stem)
Plant: *Kadsura interior* A. C. Smith.

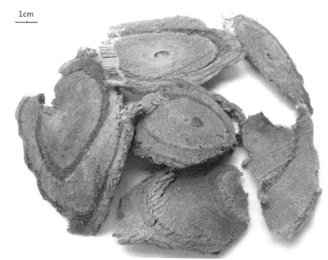

TCM prepared in ready-to-use forms (medicinal parts): it's dried lianoid stem which harvested in autumn.
Property and flavor: warm; bitter, sweet.

Main and collateral channels: liver and kidney meridians.
Administration and dosage: 15-30 g.
Indication: menstrual irregularities, dysmenorrhea, numbness, paralysis and pain caused by rheumatic arthralgia.
(The picture is only for learning and identification the herb; the specific use of the herb please consult the herbalist or health professionals)

Medicinal Cyathula Root (Chuanniuxi)
Chinese phonetic alphabet/pin yin: chuān niú xī
Chinese characters simplified/traditional:川牛膝/川牛膝
Chinese nickname's alphabet (Nickname's Chinese characters): Maniuxi/ Rouniuxi (麻牛膝/肉牛膝)

Latin: Cyathulae Radix (Common name: Medicinal Cyathula Root) Plant: *Cyathula officinalis* Kuan.

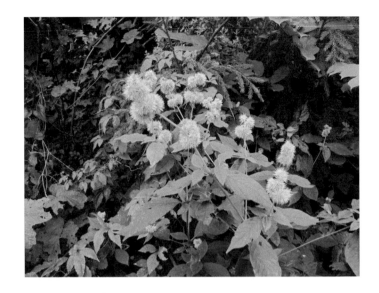

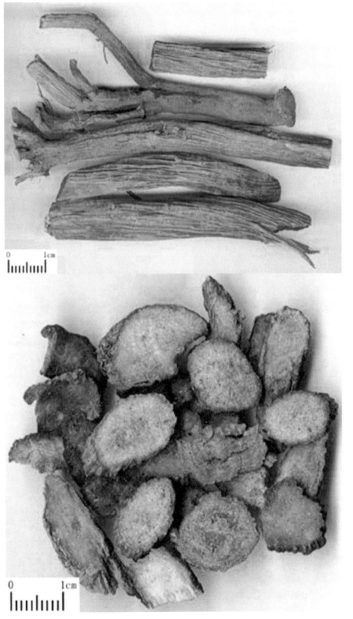

TCM prepared in ready-to-use forms (medicinal parts): it's dried root which harvested between autumn or winter. Property and flavor: neutral; sweet, mild bitter. Main and collateral channels: liver and kidney meridians. Administration and dosage: 5-10 g. Indication: amenorrhea, painful *bi* disorder, blood stasis, joint pain, paralysis foot cramps, hematuria, blood strangury and traumatic injury. **Precaution and warning:** use with caution during pregnancy. (The picture is only for learning and identification the herb; the specific use of the herb please consult the herbalist or health professionals)

Sappan Wood (Sumu)

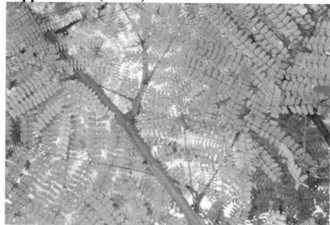

Chinese phonetic alphabet/pin yin: sū mù
Chinese characters simplified/traditional :苏木/蘇木

Chinese nickname's alphabet (Nickname's Chinese characters): Sufang/ Zongmu(苏方/棕木)
Latin: Sappan Lignum (Common name: Sappan Wood or Hematoxylon Wood)
Plant: *Caesalpinia sappan* L.

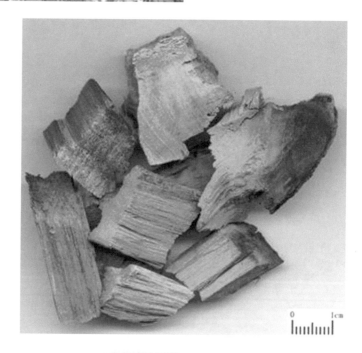

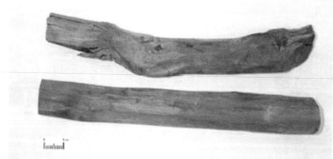

TCM prepared in ready-to-use forms (medicinal parts): it's dried heartwood which harvested in autumn.

Property and flavor: neutral; sweet, salty.
Main and collateral channels: heart, liver and spleen meridians.
Administration and dosage: 3-9 g.
Indication: amenorrhea, dysmenorrhea, blood stasis, stabbing pain in the chest and abdomen, trauma, swelling and pain, traumatic injuries, fracture and sinew injury.
Precaution and warning: use with caution during pregnancy.

(The picture is only for learning and identification the herb; the specific use of the herb please consult the herbalist or health professionals)

Saffron (Xihonghua)
Chinese phonetic alphabet/pin yin: xī hóng huā
Chinese characters simplified/traditional:西红花/西紅花

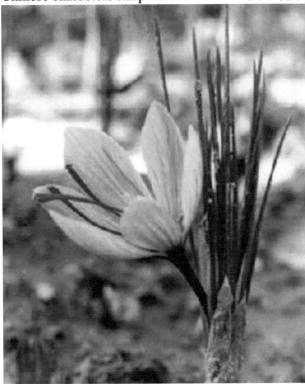

Chinese nickname's alphabet (Nickname's Chinese characters): Zanghonghua/Fanhonghua(藏红花/番红花)
Latin: Croci Stigma (Common name: Saffron)
Plant: *Crocus sativus* L.
TCM prepared in ready-to-use forms (medicinal parts): it's dried flower stigma.
Property and flavor: neutral; sweet.

Main and collateral channels: liver and heart meridians. Administration and dosage: 1-3 g, decocted or soaked in boiling water.

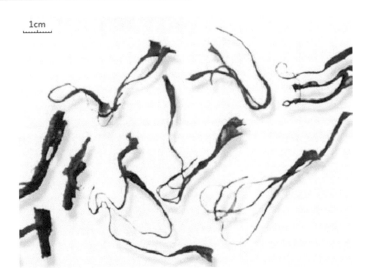

1cm

Indication: amenorrhea, dysmenorrhea, postpartum blood stasis, macule and papule caused warm toxin, melancholy, palpitation, delirium.
It is key herb to treat blood stasis, amenorrhea and dysmenorrheal.
It is taken as seasoning in some part of China.
Precaution and warning: use with caution during pregnancy.
(The picture is only for learning and identification the herb; the specific use of the herb please consult the herbalist or health professionals)

Flying Squirrel's Faeces (Wulingzhi)
Chinese phonetic alphabet/pin yin: wǔ líng zhǐ
Chinese characters simplified/traditional:五灵脂/五靈脂
Chinese nickname's alphabet (Nickname's Chinese characters): Hanquefen(寒雀粪)
Latin: Trogopterori Faecas (Common name: Flying Squirrel's Faeces)

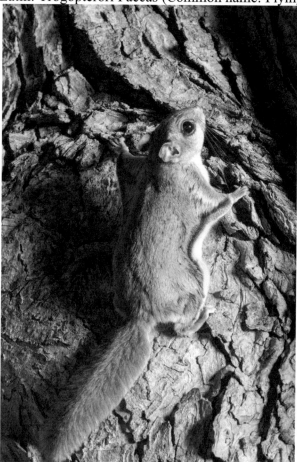

Animal: *Trogopterus xanthipes* Milne. et Edwards. (or *Aeretes melanopterus* Smith.)
TCM prepared in ready-to-use forms (medicinal parts): it's dried faeces.
Property and flavor: warm; sweet.
Administration and dosage: 3-10 g, wrap-boiled.
Indication: blood stasis, the pain caused blood stasis, amenorrhea, dysmenorrhea, insect and snake bites.
It is key herb to treat the pain caused by blood stasis.

Precaution and warning: used with caution for puerperal woman, incompatible with Ginseng.
(The picture is only for learning and identification the herb; the specific use of the herb please consult the herbalist or health professionals)

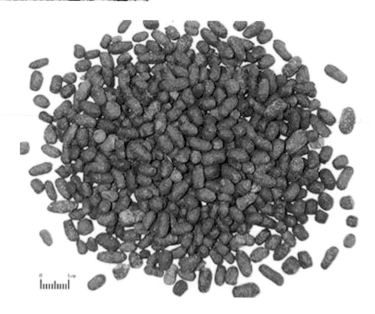

Ground Beetle (Tubiechong)

Chinese phonetic alphabet/pin yin: tǔ biē chóng
Chinese characters simplified/traditional:土鳖虫/土鱉蟲
Chinese nickname's alphabet (Nickname's Chinese characters): Tuyuan/ Diwugui/ Dibie/ Zhechong(土元/地乌龟/地鳖/廑虫)
Latin: Eupolyphaga seu Steleophaga (Common name: Ground Beetle or Woodlouse)

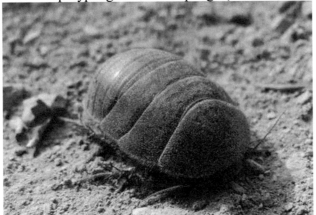

Animal:
Eupolyphaga sinensis Walker. (or *Steleophaga planc yi* (Boleny.))
TCM prepared in ready-to-use forms (medicinal parts): it's dried female insect scorpion.

Property and flavor: cold; salty.
Main and collateral channels: liver meridian.
Administration and dosage: 3-10 g.
Indication: fracture, muscle strain, blood stasis, amenorrhea, abdominal lump and traumatic injuries.

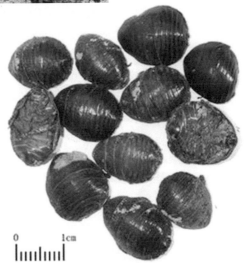

Precaution and warning: slightly toxic, contraindicated during pregnancy.
(The picture is only for learning and identification the herb; the specific use of the herb please consult the herbalist or health professionals)

Dragon's Blood (Xuejie)

Chinese phonetic alphabet/pin yin: xuě jié
Chinese characters simplified/traditional:血竭/血竭
Chinese nickname's alphabet (Nickname's Chinese characters): Qilinxue/ Haila(麒麟血/海蜡)
Latin: Draconis Sanguis (Common name: Dragon's Blood)

Plant:
Daemonorops draco Bl.
TCM prepared in ready-to-use forms (medicinal parts): it's dried resin get from the fruit which harvested in winter.

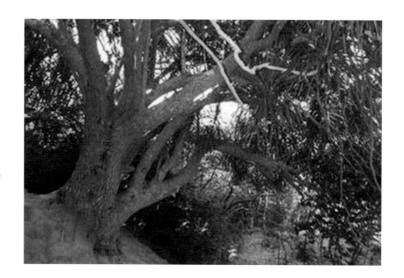

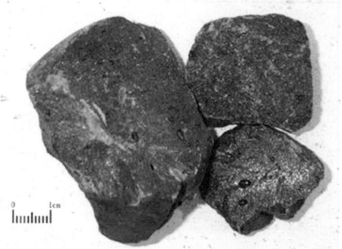

Property and flavor: neutral; sweet, salty.
Main and collateral channels: heart and liver meridians.
Administration and dosage: ground into powder, 1-2 g, or used in pill. Appropriate amount for topical application: ground into powder for spreading or used in paste.

Indication: traumatic injury, internal injury, blood stasis, trauma, heart pain and hemorrhage.
It is key herb to treat bleeding and disperse blood stasis.
(The picture is only for learning and identification the herb; the specific use of the herb please consult the herbalist or health professionals)

Diverse Wormwood Herb (Liujinu)

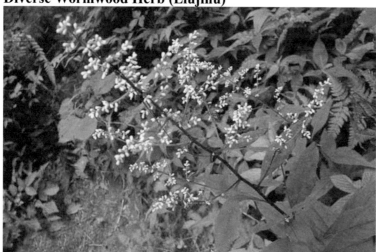

Chinese phonetic alphabet/pin yin: liú jì nú
Chinese characters simplified/ traditional:刘寄奴/劉寄奴
Chinese nickname's alphabet (Nickname's Chinese characters): Jinjinu/ Jiuliguang/ Jiuniucao(金寄奴/九里光/九牛草)

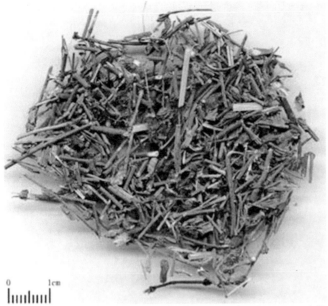

Latin: Artemisiae Anomalae Herba (Common name: Diverse Wormwood Herb or Siphonostegia Herb)
Plant: *Artemisia anomala* S. Moore.
TCM prepared in ready-to-use forms (medicinal parts): it's dried whole herb which harvested in August or September.
Property and flavor: warm; bitter.

0   1cm

Main and collateral channels: heart and spleen meridians.
Administration and dosage: 3-10 g.
Indication: traumatic injury, swelling and bleeding, blood stasis, postpartum abdominal pain, dyspepsia, amenorrhea and dysmenorrhea.
Precaution and warning: used with caution for pregnant woman.
(The picture is only for learning and identification the herb; the specific use of the herb please consult the herbalist or health professionals)

Chinese Siphonostegia Herb (Beiliujinu)
Chinese phonetic alphabet/pin yin: běi liú jì nú
Chinese characters simplified/traditional:北刘寄奴/北劉寄奴
Chinese nickname's alphabet (Nickname's Chinese characters): Lingyincao/Yinxingcao(灵茵草/阴行草)

Latin: Siphonostegiae Herba (Common name: Chinese Siphonostegia Herb)
Plant: *Siphonostegia chinensis* Benth.

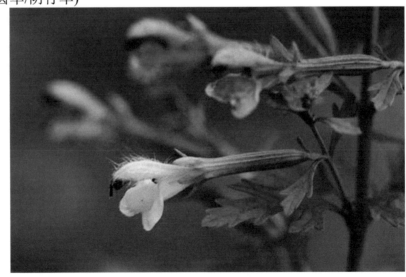

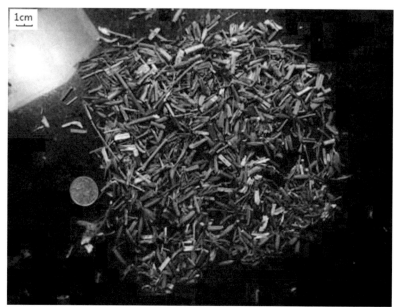

TCM prepared in ready-to-use forms (medicinal parts): it's dried whole herb which harvested in autumn.

Property and flavor: cold; bitter.

Main and collateral channels: spleen, stomach, liver and gallbladder meridians.

Administration and dosage: 6-9 g.

Indication: traumatic injury and bleeding, blood stasis, amenorrhea, irregular menstruation, hematuria, blood dysentery, jaundice, edema, abdominal distension, leucorrhea excessive.

(The picture is only for learning and identification the herb; the specific use of the herb please consult the herbalist or health professionals)

Pangolin Scales (Chuanshanjia)

Chinese phonetic alphabet/pin yin: chuān shān jiǎ

Chinese characters simplified/traditional:穿山甲/穿山甲

Chinese nickname's alphabet (Nickname's Chinese characters): Linglijia(鲮鲤甲)

Latin: Manis Squama (Common name: Pangolin Scales) Animal: *Manis pentadactyla* L.

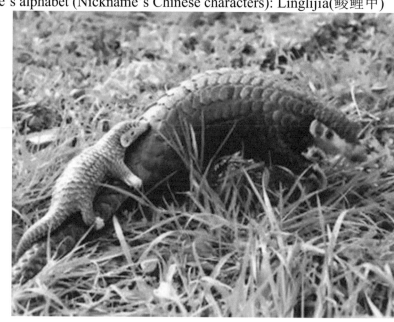

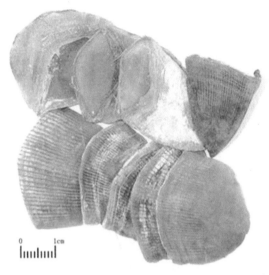

TCM prepared in ready-to-use forms (medicinal parts): it's scale.
Property and flavor: mild cold; salty.
Main and collateral channels: liver and stomach meridians.
Administration and dosage: 5-10 g.
Usually used after being fired with sand.

Indication: amenorrhea, abdominal mass, carbuncle sore, arthralgra, numbness and spasm; lactagogue.
It is key herb to promote lactation.
Precaution and warning: use with caution during pregnancy.
Attention: to protect the rare wild animals, don't use it from wild animal.
(The picture is only for learning and identification the herb; the specific use of the herb please consult the herbalist or health professionals)

Cowherb Seed (Wangbuliuxing)
Chinese phonetic alphabet/pin yin: wáng bù liú xíng
Chinese characters simplified/traditional:王不留行/王不留行
Chinese nickname's alphabet (Nickname's Chinese characters): Wangbuliu/ Buliuxing/ Liuxingzi(王不留/不留行/留行子)

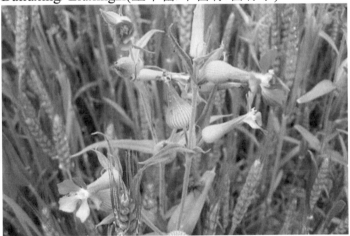

Latin: Vaccariae Semen (Common name: Cowherb Seed)
Plant: *Vaccaria segetalis* (Neck.) Garcke.

Property and flavor: neutral; bitter.
Main and collateral channels: liver and stomach meridians.
Administration and dosage: 5-10 g.
Indication: amenorrhea, dysmenorrhea, mastitis, chronic and painful strangury; lactagogue.
It is key herb to promote lactation.

TCM prepared in ready-to-use forms (medicinal parts): it's dried mature seed.
Precaution and warning: use with caution during pregnancy.
(The picture is only for learning and identification the herb; the specific use of the herb please consult the herbalist or health professionals)

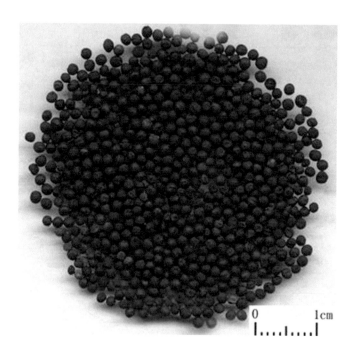

Chinese Rose Flower (Yuejihua)
Chinese phonetic alphabet/pin yin: yuè jì huā
Chinese characters simplified/traditional:月季花/月季花

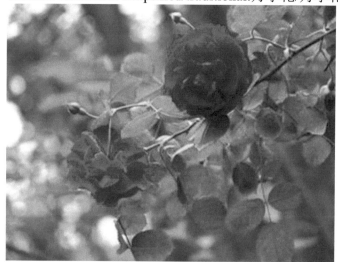

Chinese nickname's alphabet (Nickname's Chinese characters): Sijihua/ Yueyuehong/ Changchunhua(四季花/月月红/长春花)
Latin: Rosae Chinensis Flos (Common name: Chinese Rose Flower)
Plant: *Rosa chinensis* Jacq.

TCM prepared in ready-to-use forms (medicinal parts): it's dried flower.
Property and flavor: warm; sweet.
Main and collateral channels: liver meridian.
Administration and dosage: 3-6 g.

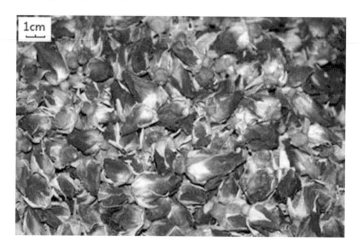

Indication: irregular menstruation, dysmenorrhea, amenorrhea and blood stasis.
(The picture is only for learning and identification the herb; the specific useof the herb please consult the herbalist or health professionals)

Dried Lacquer (Ganqi)
Chinese phonetic alphabet/pin yin: gān qī
Chinese characters simplified/traditional:干漆/干漆

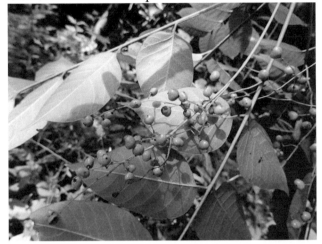

Chinese nickname's alphabet (Nickname's Chinese characters): Xumingtong/ Heiqi/ Qidi(续命筒/黑漆/漆底)
Latin: Toxicodendri Resina (Common name: Dried Lacquer)
Plant: *Toxicodendron vernicifluum* (Stokes) F. A. Barkl.

TCM prepared in ready-to-use forms (medicinal parts): it's dried purified resin.
Property and flavor: warm; pungent.
Main and collateral channels: liver and spleen meridians.
Administration and dosage: 2-5 g.

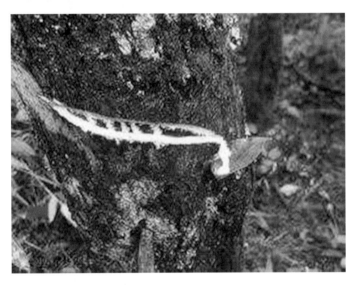

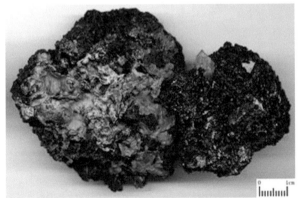

Indication: blood stasis, amenorrhea, abdominal lump; expel intestinal parasites.
Precaution and warning: toxic. Contraindicated for pregnant women and those who are allergic to lacquer.

(The picture is only for learning and identification the herb; the specific use of the herb please consult the herbalist or health professionals)

Pyrite (Zirantong)
Chinese phonetic alphabet/pin yin: zì rán tóng
Chinese characters simplified/traditional:自然铜/自然銅
Chinese nickname's alphabet (Nickname's Chinese characters): Shisuiqian/
Huangtiekuang (石髓铅/黄铁矿)

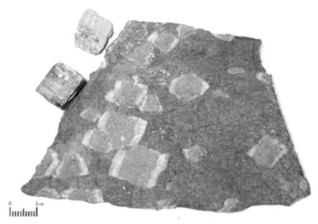

Latin: Pyritum
(Common name:
Pyrite)
Mineral: main
component FeS_2
TCM prepared in
ready-to-use
forms (medicinal
parts): it's
cleaned mineral.

Property and flavor: neutral; pungent.
Main and collateral channels: liver meridian.
Administration and dosage: 3-9 g, usually used in pills or powder, and should be
decocted first for decoction. Appropriate amount for topical application.
Indication: traumatic injury, fracture of bones and muscles, blood stasis, swelling and
pain.
It is key herb to set a broken bone and disperse blood stasis.
(The picture is only for learning and identification the herb; the specific use of the
herb please consult the herbalist or health professionals)

Snow Lotus Flower (Xuelianhua)
Chinese phonetic alphabet/pin yin: xuě lián huā
Chinese characters simplified/traditional:雪莲花/雪蓮花
Chinese nickname's alphabet (Nickname's Chinese characters): Tianshan Xuelian/
Xuelian/ Damuhua(天山雪莲/雪莲/大木花)

Latin:
Saussureae
Involucratae
Flos (Common
name:
Snow Lotus
Flower)
Plant: *Saussurea
involucrata* (Kar
. et Kir.)
Sch.-Bip

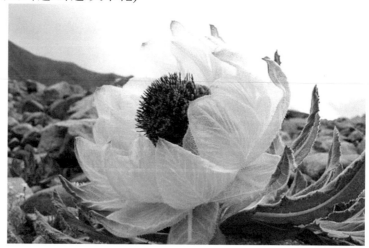

TCM prepared in ready-to-use forms (medicinal parts): it's dried aerial part which harvested in summer or autumn. Property and flavor: warm; mild bitter.

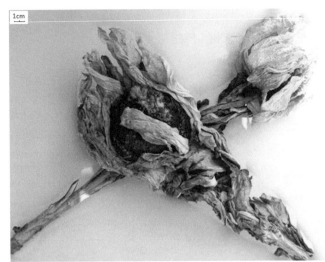

Administration and dosage: 3-6 g, decocted with water or soaked in or liquor. Appropriate amount for topical application.

Indication: impotence, waist weakness, irregular menstruation, joint pain, rheumatoid and arthritis. It is especially suitable for painful *bi* disorder.

Precaution and warning: contraindicated for pregnant women.

Attention: to protect the rare wild plant, please don't use the herb from wild plant.

(The picture is only for learning and identification the herb; the specific use of the herb please consult the herbalist or health professionals)

Pyrolusite (Wumingyi)
Chinese phonetic alphabet/pin yin: wú míng yì
Chinese characters simplified/traditional:无名异/無名異
Chinese nickname's alphabet (Nickname's Chinese characters): Tuzi/
Ruanmengkuang(土子/软锰矿)

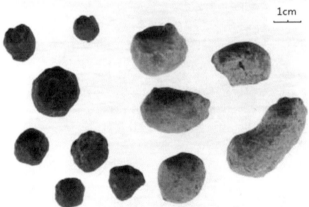

Latin: Pyrolusitum (Common name: Pyrolusite)
Mineral: main component MnO_2
TCM prepared in ready-to-use forms (medicinal parts): it's cleaned mineral.

Property and flavor: neutral; salty, sweet.
Main and collateral channels: spleen and liver meridians.
Administration and dosage: 4-7.5 g, usually used in pill or powder. Appropriate amount for topical application, ground into powder and mixed oil apply for *pars affecta*.
Indication: traumatic injury, sore and carbuncle.
Precaution and warning: long-term applying is inadvisable.
(The picture is only for learning and identification the herb; the specific use of the herb please consult the herbalist or health professionals)

Cochinchina Momordica Seed (Mubiezi)

Chinese phonetic alphabet/pin yin: mù biē zǐ

Chinese characters simplified/traditional:木鳖子/木鱉子

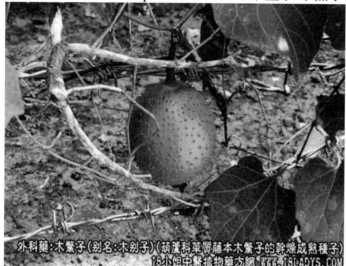

Chinese nickname's alphabet (Nickname's Chinese characters): Mubieteng/ Tumubie (木鳖藤/土木鳖)

Latin: Momordicae Semen (Common name: Cochinchina Momordica Seed)

Plant: *Momordica cochinchinensis* (Lour.) Spreng.

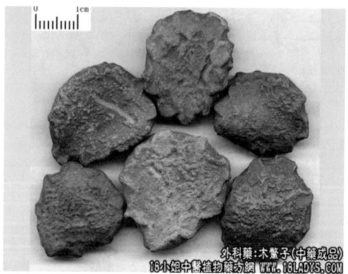

TCM prepared in ready-to-use forms (medicinal parts): it's dried mature seed.

Property and flavor: cool; bitter, mild sweet.

Main and collateral channels: liver, spleen and stomach meridians.

Administration and dosage: 0.9-1.2 g. topical application in appropriate amount, ground into powder, apply it with oil or vinegar.

Indication: scrofula, sores, ulcer, carbuncles, hemorrhoids, fistula, dry ringworm and favus; external use can detumescence.

Precaution and warning: toxic. Contraindicated for pregnant women.

(The picture is only for learning and identification the herb; the specific use of the herb please consult the herbalist or health professionals)

Coral Ardisia Root (Zhushagen)

Chinese phonetic alphabet/pin yin: zhū shā gēn

Chinese characters simplified/traditional:朱砂根/朱砂根

Chinese nickname's alphabet (Nickname's Chinese characters): Dalousan/ Pingdimu(大罗伞/平地木)

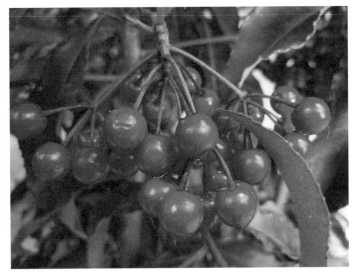

Latin: Ardisiae Crenatae Radix (Common name: Coral Ardisia Root or A. Bicolor)
Plant: *Aridisia crenata* Sims.
TCM prepared in ready-to-use forms (medicinal parts): it's dried root which harvested in autumn or winter.

Property and flavor: neutral; mild bitter, pungent.
Main and collateral channels: lung and liver meridians.
Administration and dosage: 3-9 g.
Indication: sore throat, swelling, traumatic injuries, painful *bi* disorder.

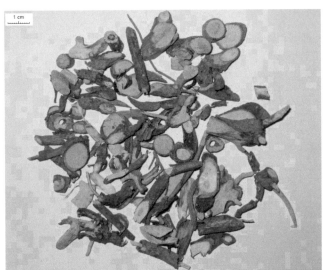

(The picture is only for learning and identification the herb; the specific use of the herb please consult the herbalist or health professionals)

Trumpetcreeper Flower (Lingxiaohua)

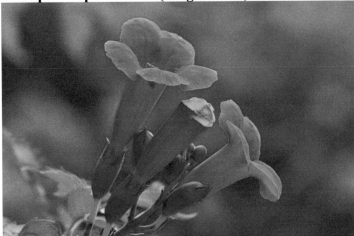

Chinese phonetic alphabet/pin yin: líng xiāo huā
Chinese characters simplified/traditional:凌霄花/凌霄花
Chinese nickname's alphabet (Nickname's Chinese characters): Ziwei(紫葳)
Latin: Campsis Flos (Common name: Trumpetcreeper Flower)

Plant: *Campsis grandiflora* (Thunb.) K. Schum. (or *Campsis radicans* (L.) Seem.)

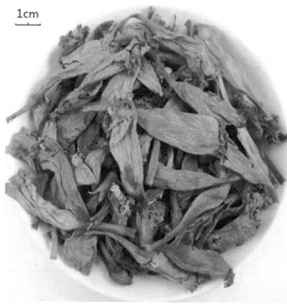

1cm

TCM prepared in ready-to-use forms (medicinal parts): it's dried flower.
Property and flavor: cold; sweet, acidity.
Main and collateral channels: liver and pericardium meridians.
Administration and dosage: 5-9 g.
Indication: menstrual irregularities, amenorrhea, abdominal mass, postpartum mammary swelling, red rubella, skin pruritus and acne.

Precaution and warning: use with caution during pregnancy.
(The picture is only for learning and identification the herb; the specific use of the herb please consult the herbalist or health professionals)

Hawthorn Leaf (Shanzhaye)

Chinese phonetic alphabet/pin yin: shān zhā yè

Chinese characters simplified/traditional:山楂叶/山楂葉

Chinese nickname's alphabet (Nickname's Chinese characters): Shanlihongye(山里红叶)

Latin: Crataegi Folium (Common name: Hawthorn Leaf)

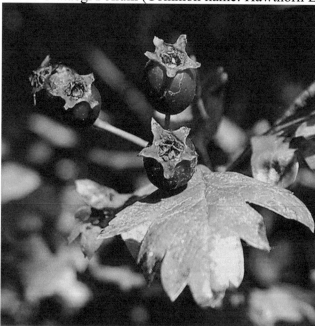

Plant: *Crataegus pinnatifida* Bge. var. *major* N. E. Br. (or *Crataegus pinnatifida* Bge.)
TCM prepared in ready-to-use forms (medicinal parts): it's dried leaf which harvested in summer or autumn.
Property and flavor: neutral; acidity.
Main and collateral channels: liver meridian.

Administration and dosage: 3-10 g or served as tea drink.

Indication: chest and heart pain, palpitation, forgetfulness, dizziness, tinnitus, hyperlipidemia. (The picture is only for learning and identification the herb; the specific use of the herb please consult the herbalist or health professionals)

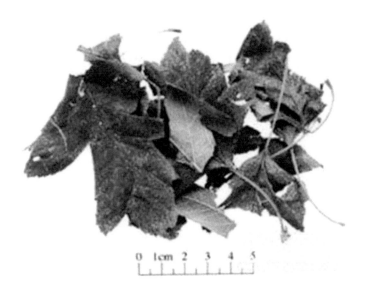

Creeping Euphorbia (Dijincao)
Chinese phonetic alphabet/pin yin: dì jǐn cǎo
Chinese characters simplified/traditional:地锦草/地錦草

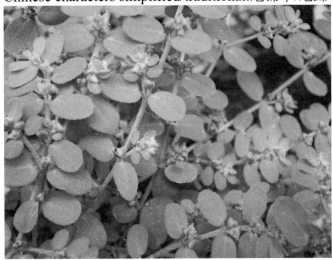

Chinese nickname's alphabet (Nickname's Chinese characters): Xuejianchou/ Hongsicao/ Naijiangcao(血见愁/红丝草/奶浆草)
Latin: Euphorbiae Humifusae Herba (Common name: Creeping Euphorbia)
Plant: *Euphorbia humifusa* Willd. (or *Euphorbia maculata* L.)

TCM prepared in ready-to-use forms (medicinal parts): it's dried whole herb which harvested in summer or autumn.
Property and flavor: neutral; pungent.
Main and collateral channels: liver and large intestine meridians.

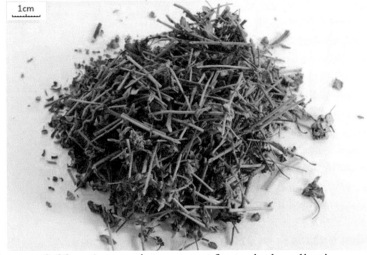

Administration and dosage: 9-20 g. Appropriate amount for topical application.

Indication: dysentery, diarrhea, hemoptysis, hematuria, hematochezia, menstrual flooding and spotting, sore and boil, abscess and jaundice.
(The picture is only for learning and identification the herb; the specific use of the herb please consult the herbalist or health professionals)

Common Gendarussa Herb (Xiaobogu)

Chinese phonetic alphabet/pin yin: xiǎo bó gǔ
Chinese characters simplified/traditional:小驳骨/小駁骨
Chinese nickname's alphabet (Nickname's Chinese characters): Jiegumu/Xiaojiegu(接骨木/小接骨)
Latin: Gendarussae Herba (Common name: Common Gendarussa Herb)

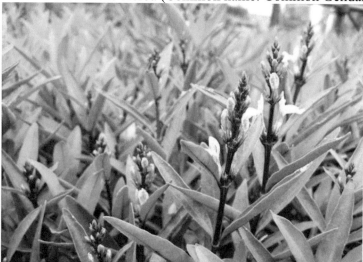

Plant: *Gendarussa vulgaris* Nees. TCM prepared in ready-to-use forms (medicinal parts): it's dried aerial part which harvested all year round. Property and flavor: warm; pungent.

Main and collateral channels: liver and kidney meridians. Administration and dosage: 9-15 g. Topical application in appropriate amount. Indication: traumatic injuries, sinew injury and fracture, bone pain, blood-stasis amenorrhea and postpartum abdominal pain.

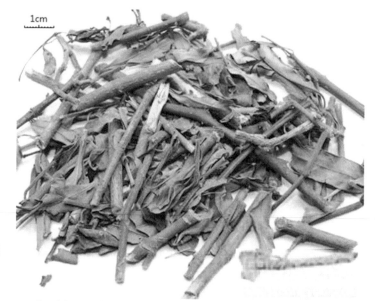

Precaution and warning: used with caution during pregnancy.
(The picture is only for learning and identification the herb; the specific use of the herb please consult the herbalist or health professionals)

Garden Balsam Seed (Jixingzi)

Chinese phonetic alphabet/pin yin: jí xìng zī

Chinese characters simplified/traditional:急性子/急性子
Chinese nickname's alphabet (Nickname's Chinese characters): Fengxianhuazi(凤仙花子)

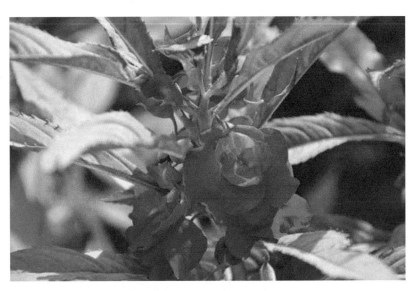

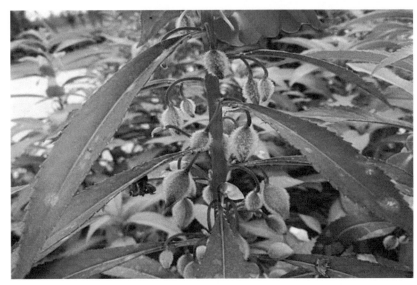

Latin: Impatientis Semen (Common name: Garden Balsam Seed)
Plant: *Impatiens balsamina* L.

TCM prepared in ready-to-use forms (medicinal parts): it's dried ripe seed.
Property and flavor: warm; mild bitter and pungent.
Main and collateral channels: lung and liver meridians.
Administration and dosage: 3-5 g.

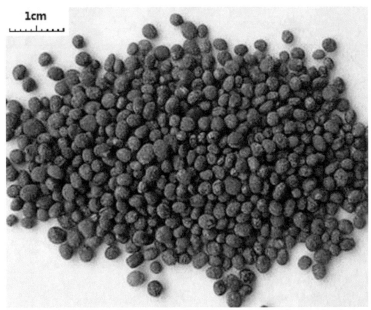

Indication: abdominal masses, glomus, lump, amenorrhea and dysphagia-occlusion.

Precaution and warning: slightly toxic. Used with caution during pregnancy.
(The picture is only for learning and identification the herb; the specific use of the herb please consult the herbalist or health professionals)

Common Lamiophlomis Herb (Duyiwei)
Chinese phonetic alphabet/pin yin: dú yí wèi
Chinese characters simplified/traditional:独一味/獨一味
Chinese nickname's alphabet (Nickname's Chinese characters): Daba/ Dabuba(大巴/
打布巴)

Latin:
Lamiophlomis
Herba
(Common
name:
Common
Lamiophlomis
Herb)
Plant:
*Lamiophlomis
rotata*
(Benth.)
Kudo.

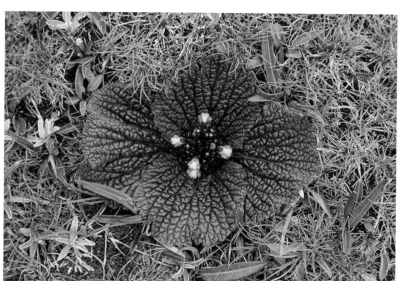

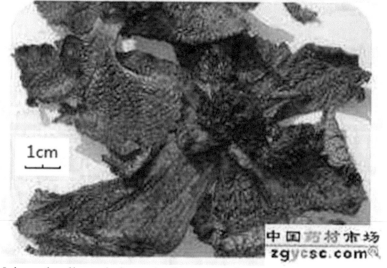

TCM prepared in ready-to-use forms (medicinal parts): it's dried aerial part which harvested in autumn. Property and flavor: neutral; sweet, bitter.

Main and collateral channels: liver meridian.
Administration and dosage: 2-3 g.
Indication: traumatic injuries, external bleeding, arthralgia and urticaria.
(The picture is only for learning and identification the herb; the specific use of the herb please consult the herbalist or health professionals)

Motherwort Fruit (Chongweizi)
Chinese phonetic alphabet/pin yin: chōng wèi zǐ
Chinese characters simplified/traditional:茺蔚子/茺蔚子

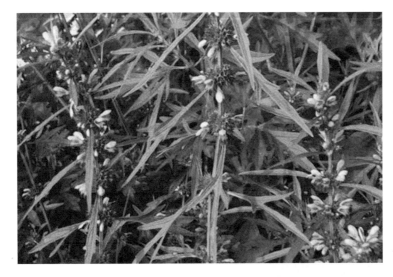

Chinese nickname's alphabet (Nickname's Chinese characters): Kucaozi/ Yimucaozi(苦草子/ 益母草子)
Latin: Leonuri Fructus (Common name: Motherwort Fruit)
Plant: *Leonurus japonicus* Houtt.

TCM prepared in ready-to-use forms (medicinal parts): it's dried ripe fruit.
Property and flavor: mild cold; bitter, pungent.
Main and collateral channels: pericardium and liver meridians.
Administration and dosage: 5-10 g.

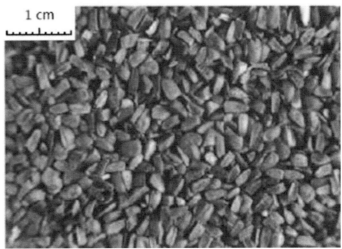

Indication: menstrual irregularities, amenorrhea and dysmenorrhea, nebula, blurring vision, dizziness and headache.
Precaution and warning: use with caution in patients with mydriasis.
(The picture is only for learning and identification the herb; the specific use of the herb please consult the herbalist or health professionals)

Beautiful Sweetgum Resin (Fengxiangzhi)

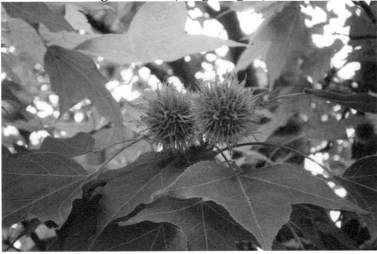

Chinese phonetic alphabet/pin yin: fēng xiāng zhǐ
Chinese characters simplified/traditional:枫香脂/楓香脂
Chinese nickname's alphabet (Nickname's Chinese characters): Fengzhi/ Baijiao(枫脂/白胶)

Latin: Liquidambaris Resina (Common name: Beautiful Sweetgum Resin)
Plant: *Liquidambar formosana* Hance.

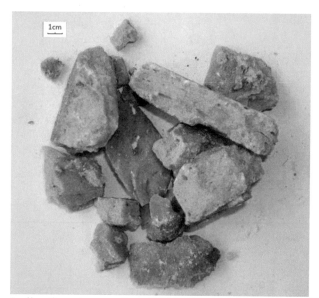

TCM prepared in ready-to-use forms (medicinal parts): it's dried resin.
Property and flavor: neutral; mild bitter, pungent.
Main and collateral channels: lung and spleen meridians.
Administration and dosage: 1-3 g, usually used in pill or powder. Appropriate amount for topical application.

Indication: traumatic injuries, abscess, cellulitis, swelling and pain, hematemesis and epistaxis.
(The picture is only for learning and identification the herb; the specific use of the herb please consult the herbalist or health professionals)

Hirsute Shiny Bugleweed Herb (Zelan)
Chinese phonetic alphabet/pin yin: zé lán
Chinese characters simplified/traditional:泽兰/澤蘭

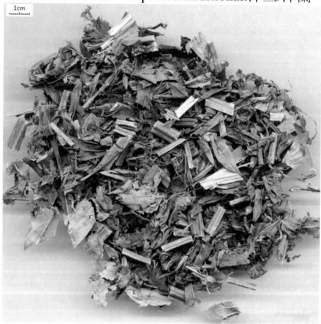

Chinese nickname's alphabet (Nickname's Chinese characters): Diguamiao/ Disun(地瓜苗/地笋)
Latin: Lycopi Herba (Common name: Hirsute Shiny Bugleweed Herb)
Plant: *Lycopus lucidus* Turcz. var. *hirtus* Regel.
TCM prepared in ready-to-use forms (medicinal parts): it's dried aerial part which harvested in summer or autumn.
Property and flavor: mild warm; bitter, pungent.

Main and collateral channels: liver and spleen meridians.
Administration and dosage: 6-12 g.
Indication: menstrual irregularities, amenorrhea, dysmenorrhea, postpartum blood static with abdominal pain, sore, abscess, swelling, edema and ascites; remove toxin.

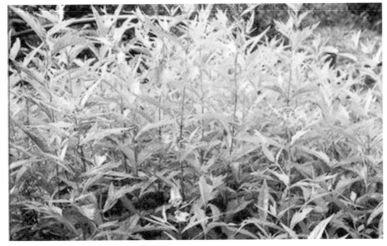

(The picture is only for learning and identification the herb; the specific use of the herb please consult the herbalist or health professionals)

Prince's-feather Fruit (Shuihonghuazi)
Chinese phonetic alphabet/pin yin: shuǐ hóng huā zǐ

Chinese characters simplified/traditional:水红花子/水紅花子
Chinese nickname's alphabet (Nickname's Chinese characters): Shuihongzi/ Hongcaoshi/ Heliaozi(水荭子/荭草实/河蓼子)
Latin: Polygoni Orientalis Fructus (Common name: Prince's-feather Fruit)
Plant: *Polygonum orientale* L.

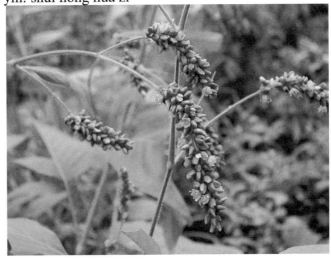

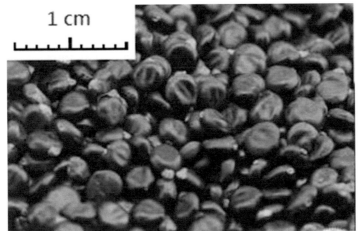

TCM prepared in ready-to-use forms (medicinal parts): it's dried ripe fruit.
Property and flavor: mild cold; salty.
Main and collateral channels: liver and stomach meridians. edema and ascites.

Administration and dosage: 15-30 g. Topical application in appropriate amount, boiled into paste for applying to the *pars affecta*.
Indication: abdominal masses, glomus, goiter, stomach distend and pain, indigesting,
(The picture is only for learning and identification the herb; the specific use of the herb please consult the herbalist or health professionals)

Common Sinopodophyllum Fruit (Xiaoyelian)
Chinese phonetic alphabet/pin yin: xiǎo yè lián
Chinese characters simplified/traditional:小叶莲/小葉蓮
Chinese nickname's alphabet (Nickname's Chinese characters): Tao'erqi(桃儿七)

Latin:
Sinopodophylli
Fructus (Common
name: Common
Sinopodophyllum
Fruit)
Plant:
*Podophyllum
hexandrum* Royle
Ying.

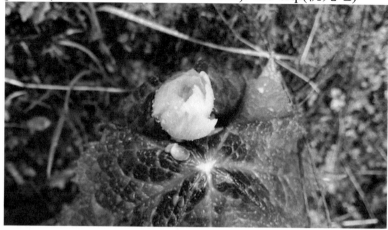

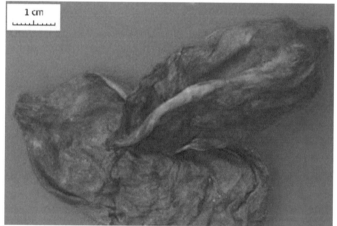

TCM prepared in
ready-to-use forms
(medicinal parts): it's
dried ripe fruit.
Property and flavor:
neutral; sweet.
Administration and
dosage: 3-9 g, usually
used in pills or powder.

Indication: blood-stasis, amenorrhea, dead fetus, placenta retention.
Precaution and warning: slightly toxic.
(The picture is only for learning and identification the herb; the specific use of the herb please consult the herbalist or health professionals)

European Verbena Herb (Mabiancao)

Chinese
phonetic
alphabet/pin yin:
mǎ biān cǎo
Chinese
characters
simplified/traditi
onal:马鞭草/馬
鞭草

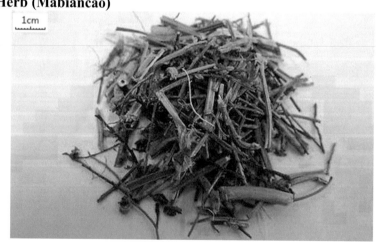

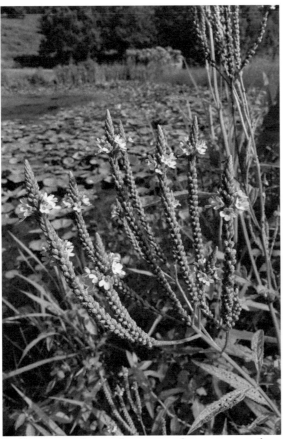

Chinese nickname's alphabet (Nickname's Chinese characters): Tiemabian/ Yejingjie(铁马鞭/野荆芥)
Latin: Verbenae Herba (Common name: European Verbena Herb)
Plant: *Verbena officinalis* L.
TCM prepared in ready-to-use forms (medicinal parts): it's dried aerial part which harvested from June to August
Property and flavor: cool; bitter.
Main and collateral channels: liver and spleen meridians.
Administration and dosage: 5-10 g.

Indication: edema, dysmenorrhea, amenorrhea, swelling, abscess, jaundice and malaria.
(The picture is only for learning and identification the herb; the specific use of the herb please consult the herbalist or health professionals)

Gadfly (Mengchong)
Chinese phonetic alphabet/pin yin: méng chóng
Chinese characters simplified/traditional:虻虫/虻蟲
Chinese nickname's alphabet (Nickname's Chinese characters): Niumeng(牛蝱)

Latin: Tabanus (Common name: Gadfly)
Animal: *Tabanus bivittatus* Mats.

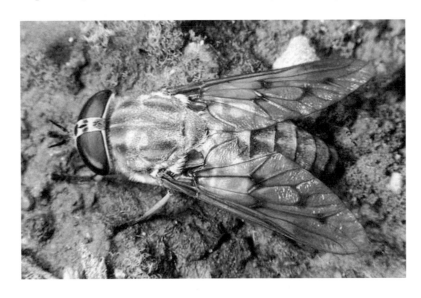

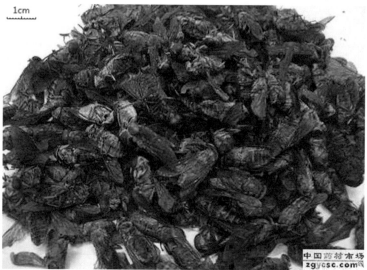

1cm

TCM prepared in ready-to-use forms (medicinal parts): it's dried female body which harvested from May to June after boiled. Property and flavor: mild cold; bitter.

Main and collateral channels: liver meridian.
Administration and dosage: 1-1.5 g. For baked powder: 0.3 g.
Indication: amenorrhea or abdominal, epigastric masses and external injury.
Precaution and warning: slightly toxic. Contraindicated during pregnancy.
(The picture is only for learning and identification the herb; the specific use of the herb please consult the herbalist or health professionals)

Gynura Root and Leaf (Juyesanqi)

Chinese phonetic alphabet/pin yin: jú yè sān qī
Chinese characters simplified/traditional:菊叶三七/菊葉三七
Chinese nickname's alphabet (Nickname's Chinese characters): Tusanqi(土三七)
Latin: Gynurae Radix et Folium (Common name: Gynura Root)

Plant: *Gynura segetum* (Lour.) Merr.
Property and flavor: warm; sweet, mild bitter.
Administration and dosage: 6-10 g.
Indication: epistaxis, carbuncles and mastitis; stop bleeding; dispel toxin.
Precaution and warning: use with caution during pregnancy.
(The picture is only for learning and identification the herb; the specific use of the herb please consult the herbalist or health professionals)

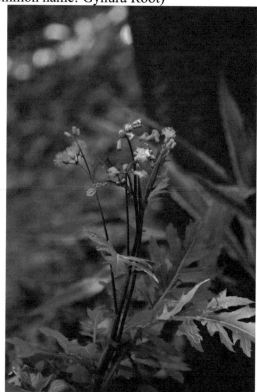

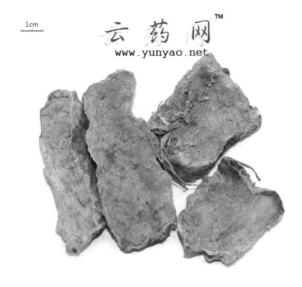

TCM prepared in ready-to-use forms (medicinal parts): it's fresh or dried root or leaf which harvested in summer.

Zhi Ke Hua Tan Yao(止咳化痰药)-herbs for relieving cough and resolving phlegm

Zhi Ke Hua Tan Yao is a kind of herbs which's the major functions are to relieve cough with asthma and reduce phlegm.

Pinellia Tuber (Banxia)

Chinese phonetic alphabet/pin yin: bàn xià

Chinese characters simplified/traditional:半夏/半夏

Chinese nickname's alphabet (Nickname's Chinese characters): Diwen/ Shuiyu/ Shouyu(地文 /水玉/守玉)

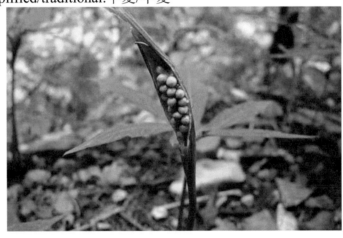

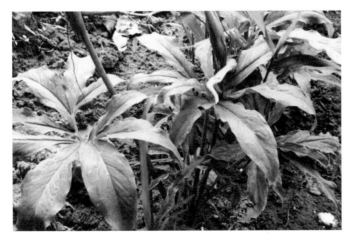

Latin: Pinelliae Rhizoma (Common name: Pinellia Tuber)
Plant: *Pinellia ternata* (Thunb.) Breit.

TCM prepared in ready-to-use forms (medicinal parts): it's dried tuber root which harvested in summer or autumn. Property and flavor: warm; pungent. Main and collateral channels: spleen, stomach and lung meridians.

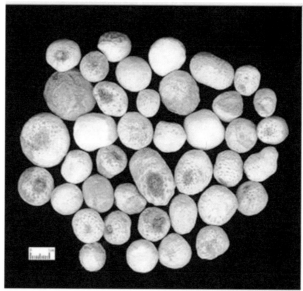

Administration and dosage: generally processed before oral administration, 3-9 g. Appropriate amount for topical application, ground into powder or squeezed out the juice mixed with liquor and applied for *pars affecta*.

Indication: excessive phlegm, cough, throb, dizziness, headache, nausea and vomiting; external use for carbuncle.

It is key herb to treat cold-phlegm.

Precaution and warning: toxic. Incompatible with Common Monkshood Mother Root, Short-pedicel Aconite Root, Kusnezoff Monkshood Root, Common Monkshood Daughter Root ant their prepared one. Unprocessed one should be used cautiously for oral administration.

(The picture is only for learning and identification the herb; the specific use of the herb please consult the herbalist or health professionals)

Prepared Pinellia Tuber (Fabanxia)

Chinese phonetic alphabet/pin yin: fǎ bàn xià

Chinese characters simplified/traditional:法半夏/法半夏

Latin: Pinelliae Praeparatum Rhizoma (Common name: Prepared Pinellia Tuber)

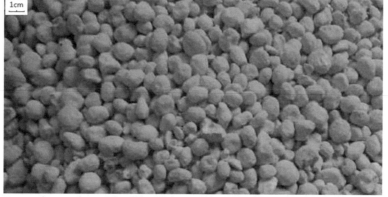

Plant: *Pinellia ternata* (Thunb.) Breit (See Pinellia Tuber).
TCM prepared in ready-to-use forms (medicinal parts): It is processed Pinellia Rhizome.

Procedure: chop Pinellia Rhizome in suitable size, immerse in water until the center of the herb is devoid of a dry core, and take out. Decoct liquorice (15kg/100kg herb) with a quantity of water twice, combine the decoctions and pour into the lime (10kg quick lime/100kg herb) solution prepared with suitable amount water, stir well, add the soaked Pinellia Rhizome, soak, stir 1-2 times per day until the surface in uniform yellow color and slight numbing taste, take out and dry.

Administration and dosage: 3-9 g.

Indication: wheezing and cough with profuse sputum, headache, dizziness and palpitation.

Precaution and warning: toxic. Incompatible with Common Monkshood Mother Root, Short-pedicel Aconite Root, Kusnezoff Monkshood Root, Common Monkshood Daughter Root ant their prepared one.

(The picture is only for learning and identification the herb; the specific use of the herb please consult the herbalist or health professionals)

Jackinthepulpit Tuber (Tiannanxing)
Chinese phonetic alphabet/pin yin: tiān nán xīng
Chinese characters simplified/traditional:天南星/天南星

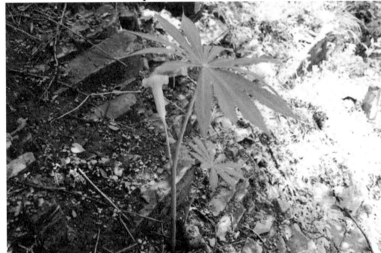

Chinese nickname's alphabet (Nickname's Chinese characters): Nanxing/ Sanbangzi/ Shanbangzi(南星/三棒子/山棒子)
Latin: Arisaematis Rhizoma (Common name: Jackinthepulpit Tuber)

Plant: *Arisaema heterophyllum* Blume. (or *Arisaema erubescens* (Wall.) Schott., *Arisaema amurense* Maxim.)
Property and flavor: warm; pungent, bitter. Main and collateral channels: lung, liver and spleen meridians.

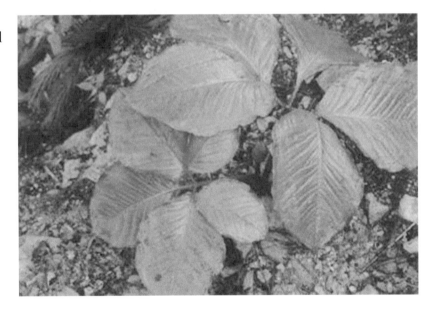

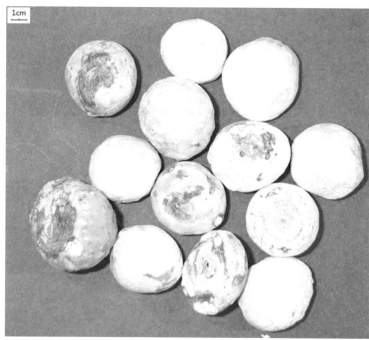

TCM prepared in ready-to-use forms (medicinal parts): it's dried tuber root which harvested in autumn or winter. Administration and dosage: generally processed before oral administration. Appropriate amount for topical application, ground into powder and mixed with liquor, wine or vinegar cautious.

Indication: cough with phlegm, dizziness, apoplexy, hemiplegia, epilepsy, convulsion and tetanus; external use to treat carbuncle, insect and snake bites.

Precaution and warning: toxic. Use with caution during pregnancy. Unprocessed drug for oral administration should be cautious.

(The picture is only for learning and identification the herb; the specific use of the herb please consult the herbalist or health professionals)

Prepared Jackinthepulpit Tuber (Zhitiannanxing)
Chinese phonetic alphabet/pin yin: zhì tiān nán xīng

Chinese characters simplified/traditional:制天南星/制天南星
Latin: Arisaematis Rhizoma Preparatum (Common name: Prepared Jackinthepulpit Tuber)
TCM prepared in ready-to-use forms (medicinal parts): it is processed Jackinthepulpit Tuber
Plant: See Jackinthepulpit Tuber

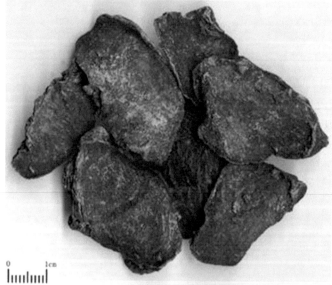

Procedure: chop Jackinthepulpit Tuber in suitable size, immerse in water, change water 3 times a day, add alum (2kg/100kg herb) after change water if the white foam appears, change water per day until herb with a slight tongue-numbing taste, takes it out. Boil the slice of fresh ginger and alum (both of ginger and alum 12.5kg/100kg herb), then add the Jackinthepulpit Tuber boil to no dry part at center; take out cut into slice, dry.

Administration and dosage: 3-9 g.

Indication: chronic cough, phlegm congestion, hemiplegia, epilepsy, dizziness, convulsion, tetanus; external use for swelling abscess, insect or snake bites.

Precaution and warning: toxic. Use with caution during pregnancy.

(The picture is only for learning and identification the herb; the specific use of the herb please consult the herbalist or health professionals)

Bile Arisaema (Dannanxing)

Chinese phonetic alphabet/pin yin: dǎn nán xīng

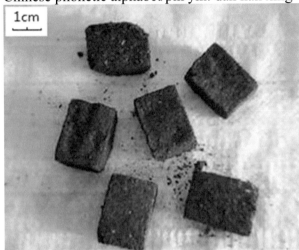

Chinese characters simplified/traditional:胆南星/膽南星

Latin: Arisaema Cum Bile (Common name: Bile Arisaema)

Plant: *Arisaema heterophyllum* Blume. (or *Arisaema erubescens* (Wall.) Schott., *Arisaema amurense* Maxim.) (See Jackinthepulpit Tuber)

TCM prepared in ready-to-use forms (medicinal parts): it's prepared by fermentation of finely powdered Arisaematis Rhizoma with the bile of ox, sheep or pig.

Property and flavor: cold; mild pungent, bitter.

Main and collateral channels: lung, liver and spleen meridians.

Administration and dosage: 3-6 g.

Indication: cough with phlegm, yellow thick sputum, seizure, dizziness.

Precaution and warning: toxic.

(The picture is only for learning and identification the herb; the specific use of the herb please consult the herbalist or health professionals)

Mustard Seed (Jiezi)

Chinese phonetic alphabet/pin yin: jiè zǐ

Chinese characters simplified/traditional:芥子/芥子

Chinese nickname's alphabet (Nickname's Chinese characters): Baijiezi/ Lacaizi/(白芥子/辣菜子)

Latin: Sinapis Semen seu Brassicae Semen (Common name: Mustard Seed or Sinalbin)

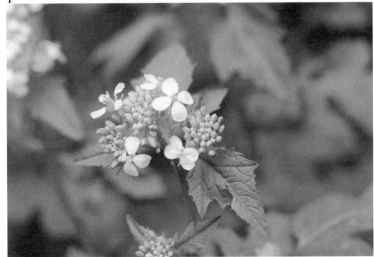

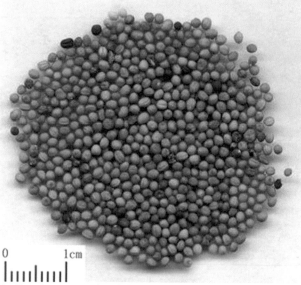

Plant: *Sinapis alba* L. (or *Brassica juncea* (L.) Czern. et Coss.)
TCM prepared in ready-to-use forms (medicinal parts): it's dried mature seed.
Property and flavor: warm; pungent.
Main and collateral channels: lung meridian.
Administration and dosage: 3-9 g. Appropriate amount for topical application.

Indication: cough with phlegm, chest pain, joint numbness, swollen and pain. (The picture is only for learning and identification the herb; the specific use of the herb please consult the herbalist or health professionals)

Platycodon Root (Jiegeng)
Chinese phonetic alphabet/pin yin: jié gěng
Chinese characters simplified/traditional:桔梗/桔梗
Chinese nickname's alphabet (Nickname's Chinese characters): Lingdanghua/ Daolaji/ Baiyao(铃铛花/道拉基/白药)

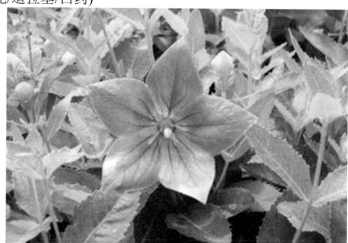

Latin: Platycodonis Radix (Common name: Platycodon Root or Chinese Bellflower Root)
Plant: *Platycodon grandiflorum* (Jacq.) A. DC.

Property and flavor: neutral; bitter, pungent.
Main and collateral channels: lung meridian.
Administration and dosage: 3-10 g.
Indication: cough with phlegm, hoarse voice, sore throat and carbuncle spit pus.
It is taken as food in some part of China.

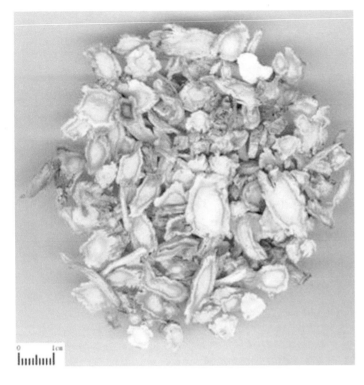

TCM prepared in ready-to-use forms (medicinal parts): it's dried root which harvested in spring or autumn.
(The picture is only for learning and identification the herb; the specific use of the herb please consult the herbalist or health professionals)

Inula Flower (Xuanfuhua)

Chinese phonetic alphabet/pin yin: xuán fù huā
Chinese characters simplified/traditional:旋覆花/旋覆花
Chinese nickname's alphabet (Nickname's Chinese characters): Jinfohua/ Liuyueju(金佛花/六月菊)

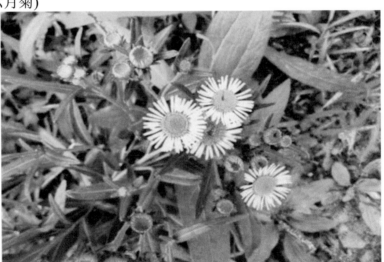

Latin: Inulae Flos (Common name: Inula Flower or Inulic)
Plant: *Inula japonica* Thunb. (or *Inula britannica* L.)
Property and flavor: mild warm; bitter, pungent and salty.

Main and collateral channels: lung, spleen, stomach and large intestine meridians.
Administration and dosage: 3-9 g, wrap-boiling.
Indication: cough caused by chill (*Fenghan*) cold, profuse sputum, chest fullness, asthmatic cough, vomiting, ructation and belching.
It is key herb to treat hiccup and asthma.

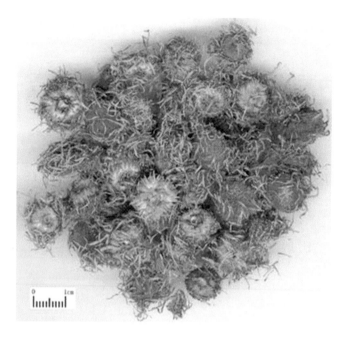

TCM prepared in ready-to-use forms (medicinal parts): it's dried capitulum. (The picture is only for learning and identification the herb; the specific use of the herb please consult the herbalist or health professionals)

Snakegourd Fruit (Gualou)

Chinese phonetic alphabet/pin yin: guā lóu

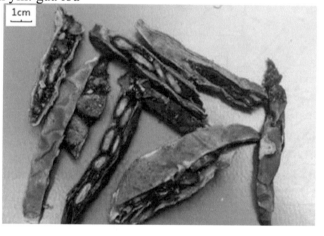

Chinese characters simplified/traditional:瓜蒌/瓜蔞

Chinese nickname's alphabet (Nickname's Chinese characters): Gualou/ Wangbai/ Yaogua(栝楼/王白/药瓜)

Latin: Trichosanthis Fructus (Common name: Snakegourd Fruit)

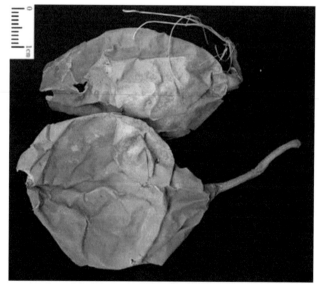

Plant: *Trichosanthes kirilowii* Maxim. (or *Trichosanthes rosthornii* Harms.)

TCM prepared in ready-to-use forms (medicinal parts): it's dried mature fruit.

Property and flavor: cold; sweet, mild bitter.

Main and collateral channels: lung, stomach and large intestine meridians.

Administration and dosage: 9-15 g.

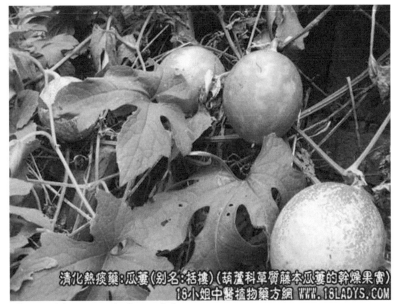

Indication: cough caused by heat, phlegm thick yellow, chest pain, acute mastitis, thoracic tightness, constipation, intestinal carbuncle and swelling.

It is key herb to treat heat-phlegm and chest tightness.

Precaution and warning: Incompatible with Common Monkshood Mother Root, Short-pedicel Aconite Root, Kusnezoff Monkshood Root, Common Monkshood Daughter Root and their prepared one.

(The picture is only for learning and identification the herb; the specific use of the herb please consult the herbalist or health professionals)

Tendrilleaf Fritilary Bulb (Chuanbeimu)

Chinese phonetic alphabet/pin yin: chuān bèi mǔ

Chinese characters simplified/traditional:川贝母/川貝母

Chinese nickname's alphabet (Nickname's Chinese characters): Chuanbei (川贝)

Latin: Fritillariae Cirrhosae Bulbus (Common name: Tendrilleaf Fritilary Bulb)

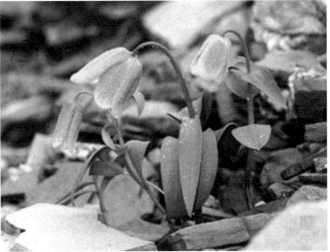

Plant: *Fritillaria przewalskii* Maxim ex Batal. (or *Fritillaria cirrhosa* D. Don., *Fritillaria unibracteata* Hsiao et K. C. Hisa., *Fritillaria delavayi* Franch., *Fritillaria taipaiensis* P. Y. Li., *Fritillaria unibracteata* Hsiao et K. C. Hisa var. *wabuensis* (S. Y. Yang et S. C. Yue) Z. D. Liu, S. Wang et S. C. Chen.)

TCM prepared in ready-to-use forms (medicinal parts): it's dried bulb which harvested between June and October.

Property and flavor: mild cold; bitter, sweet.

Main and collateral channels: lung and heart meridians.

Administration and dosage: 3-10 g. Ground into powder for oral administration (taking it after mixing it with water), 1-2 g per time.

It is key herb to treat chronic cough and excessive phlegm.
Precaution and warning:
Incompatible with Common Monkshood Mother Root, Short-pedicel Aconite Root, Kusnezoff Monkshood Root, Common Monkshood Daughter Root ant their prepared one.

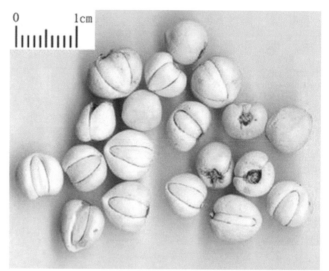

Indication: dry cough, sputum with blood, scrofula and acute mastitis.
(The picture is only for learning and identification the herb; the specific use of the herb please consult the herbalist or health professionals)

Thunberg Fritillary Bulb (Zhebeimu)
Chinese phonetic alphabet/pin yin: zhè bèi mǔ
Chinese characters simplified/traditional:浙贝母/浙贝母

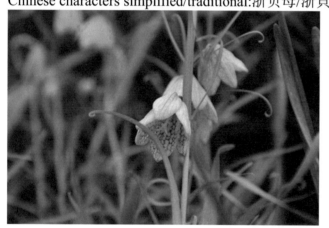

Chinese nickname's alphabet (Nickname's Chinese characters): Tubeimu/ Zhebei/ Xiangbeimu(土贝母/浙贝/象贝母)
Latin: Fritillariae Thunbergii Bulbus
(Common name: Thunberg Fritillary Bulb)
Plant: *Fritillaria thunbergii* Miq.

TCM prepared in ready-to-use forms (medicinal parts): it's dried bulb which harvested in summer.
Property and flavor: cold; bitter.
Main and collateral channels: lung and heart meridians.
Administration and dosage: 5-10 g.
Indication: cough with thick phlegm, mastitis, scrofula, sores and skin infections.
It is key herb to treat heat-phlegm.

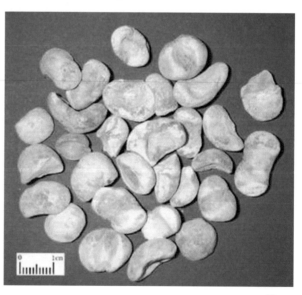

Precaution and warning: Incompatible with Common Monkshood Mother Root, Short-pedicel Aconite Root, Kusnezoff Monkshood Root, Common Monkshood Daughter Root ant their prepared one.
(The picture is only for learning and identification the herb; the specific use of the herb please consult the herbalist or health professionals)

Paniculate Bolbostemma (Tubeimu)
Chinese phonetic alphabet/pin yin: tǔ bèi mǔ
Chinese characters simplified/traditional:土贝母/土貝母
Chinese nickname's alphabet (Nickname's Chinese characters): Jiabeimu/ Dikudan/ Tubei(假贝母/地苦胆/土贝)

Latin:
Bolbostemmatis
Rhizoma
(Common name:
Paniculate
Bolbostemma)
Plant:
Bolbstemma
paniculatum
(Maxim.)
Franquent.

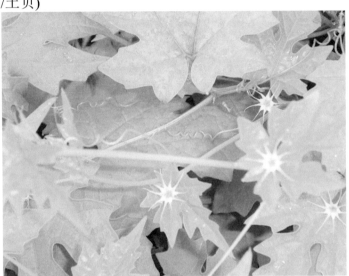

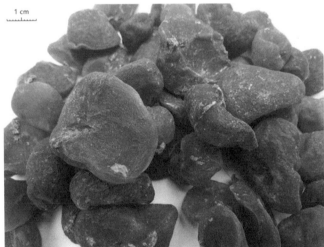

TCM prepared in ready-to-use forms (medicinal parts): it's dried tuber which harvested in autumn.
Property and flavor: mild cold; bitter.
Main and collateral channels: lung and spleen meridians.
Administration and dosage: 5-10 g.
Indication: mastitis, scrofula and phlegm mass.

(The picture is only for learning and identification the herb; the specific use of the herb please consult the herbalist or health professionals)

Hubei Fritillary Bulb (Hubeibeimu)
Chinese phonetic alphabet/pin yin: hú běi bèi mǔ
Chinese characters simplified/traditional:湖北贝母/湖北贝母
Chinese nickname's alphabet (Nickname's Chinese characters): Banbei/ Jiaobei/ Fengjiebeimu(板贝/窖贝/奉节贝母)

Latin: Fritillariae Hupehensis Bulbus (Common name: Hubei Fritillary Bulb)
Plant: *Fritillaria hupehensis* Hsiao et K. C. Hisa.
TCM prepared in ready-to-use forms (medicinal parts): it's dried bulb which harvested in summer.
Property and flavor: cool; mild bitter.
Main and collateral channels: lung and heart meridians.

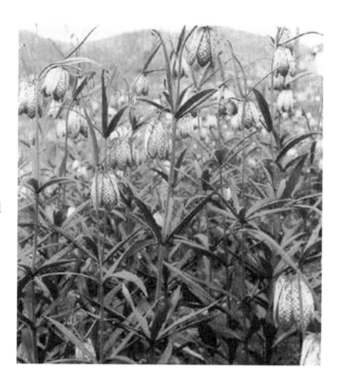

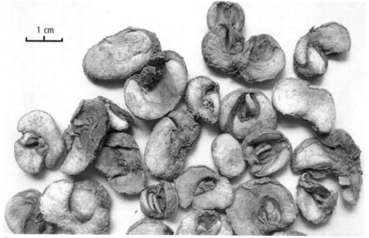

Administration and dosage: 3-9 g, ground into powder for oral administration with water.
Indication: cough, profuse sputum, scrofula, skin infection, swelling and abscess.

Precaution and warning: incompatible with Common Monkshood Mother Root, Short-pedicel Aconite Root, Kusnezoff Monkshood Root, Common Monkshood Daughter Root ant their prepared one.
(The picture is only for learning and identification the herb; the specific use of the herb please consult the herbalist or health professionals)

Sinkiang Fritillary Bulb (Yibeimu)
Chinese phonetic alphabet/pin yin: yī bèi mǔ
Chinese characters simplified/traditional:伊贝母/伊貝母
Chinese nickname's alphabet (Nickname's Chinese characters): Tianshanbeimu/ Xinjiangbeimu(天山贝母/新疆贝母)
Latin: Fritillariae Pallidiflorae Bulbus (Common name: Sinkiang Fritillary Bulb)

Plant: *Fritillaria pallidiflora* Schrenk. (or *Fritillaria walujewii* Regel.) TCM prepared in ready-to-use forms (medicinal parts): it's dried bulb which harvested from May to July.

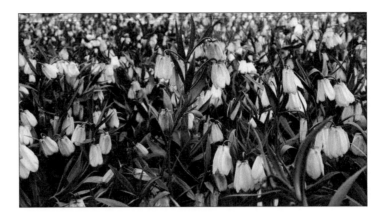

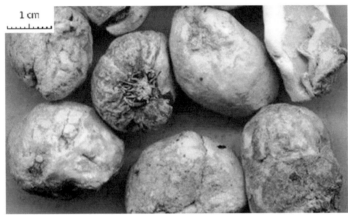

Property and flavor: mild cold; sweet, bitter. Main and collateral channels: lung and heart meridians. Administration and dosage: 3-9 g. Indication: dryness cough, chronic cough and expectoration of phlegm with blood.

Precaution and warning: incompatible with Common Monkshood Mother Root, Short-pedicel Aconite Root, Kusnezoff Monkshood Root, Common Monkshood Daughter Root ant their prepared one.
(The picture is only for learning and identification the herb; the specific use of the herb please consult the herbalist or health professionals)

Ussuri Fritillary Bulb (Pingbeimu)

Chinese phonetic alphabet/pin yin: píng bèi mǔ
Chinese characters simplified/traditional:平贝母/平貝母
Chinese nickname's alphabet (Nickname's Chinese characters): Pingbei(平贝)
Latin: Fritillariae Ussuriensis Bulbus (Common name: Ussuri Fritillary Bulb)
Plant: *Fritillaria ussurienisis* Maxim.
TCM prepared in ready-to-use forms (medicinal parts): it's dried bulb which harvested in spring.

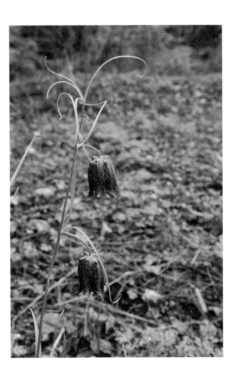

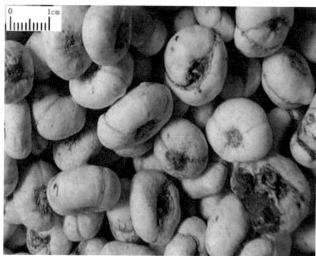

Property and flavor: mild cold; bitter, sweet.
Main and collateral channels: lung and heart meridians.
Administration and dosage: 3-9 g. Ground into powder for oral administration with water, 1-2 g per time.
Indication: dryness cough, cough caused by consumptive disease, expectoration of phlegm with blood.

Precaution and warning: incompatible with Common Monkshood Mother Root, Short-pedicel Aconite Root, Kusnezoff Monkshood Root, Common Monkshood Daughter Root ant their prepared one.
(The picture is only for learning and identification the herb; the specific use of the herb please consult the herbalist or health professionals)

Bamboo Shavings (Zhuru)

Chinese phonetic alphabet/pin yin: zhú rú

Chinese characters simplified/traditional:竹茹/竹茹

Chinese nickname's alphabet (Nickname's Chinese characters): Zhupi/Qingzhuri(竹皮/青竹茹)

Latin: Bambusae Caulis in Taenias (Common name: Bamboo Shavings)

Plant: *Bambusa tuldoides* Munro. (or *Sinocalamus beecheyanus* (Munro.) McClure. var. *pubescens* P. F. Li, *Phyllostachys nigra* (Lodd.) Munro var. *henonis* (Mitf.) Stapf. ex Rendle.)

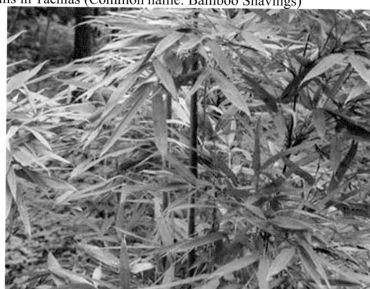

TCM prepared in ready-to-use forms (medicinal parts): it's dried the middle layer/shaving of stem.
Property and flavor: mild cold; sweet.

Main and collateral channels: lung, stomach, heart and gallbladder meridians.
Administration and dosage: 5-10 g.
Indication: cough with heat phlegm, vomiting, insomnia, apoplexy, vomiting of pregnancy and fetal irritability.
(The picture is only for learning and identification the herb; the specific use of the herb please consult the herbalist or health professionals)

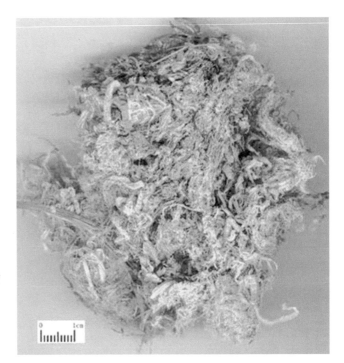

Giant Typhonium Rhizome (Yubaifu)

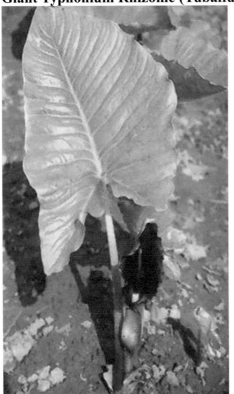

Chinese phonetic alphabet/pin yin: yú bái fù
Chinese characters simplified/traditional: 禹白附/禹白附
Chinese nickname's alphabet (Nickname's Chinese characters): Naibaifu/ Yebanxia/ Baifuzi(奶白附/野半夏/白附子)
Latin: Typhonii Rhizoma (Common name: Giant Typhonium Rhizome)
Plant: *Typhonium giganteum* Engl.
TCM prepared in ready-to-use forms (medicinal parts): it's dried rhizome tuber which harvested in autumn.
Property and flavor: warm; pungent.
Main and collateral channels: stomach and liver meridians.
Procedure: remove the herb's peel, washed until it become white, steam, sun-dry then fumigate it by sulfur.

Administration and dosage: 3-6 g, usually used after being processed. Appropriate amount of unprocessed one is mashed for boiling or being ground into powder and mixed with liquor before applied to the *pars affecta* for topical application.
Indication: apoplexy, phlegm, dysphasia, headache, sore throat, pharyngitis and tetanus; external used for scrofula and snakebite.

Precaution and warning: toxic. Be caution for use by pregnant women. Unprocessed one should be used cautiously for oral administration.
(The picture is only for learning and identification the herb; the specific use of the herb please consult the herbalist or health professionals)

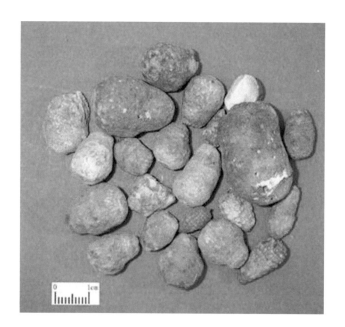

Bamboo Juice (Zhuli)
Chinese phonetic alphabet/pin yin: zhú lì
Chinese characters simplified/traditional:竹沥/竹瀝

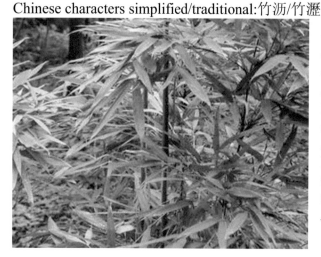

Chinese nickname's alphabet (Nickname's Chinese characters): Zhuzhi/Zhuyou(竹汁/竹油)
Latin: Bambusae Succus (Common name: Bamboo Juice)
Plant: *Phyllostachys nigra* (Lodd.) Munro var. *henonis* (Mitf.) Stapf. ex Rendle (or *Bambusa tuldoides* Munro.)

TCM prepared in ready-to-use forms (medicinal parts): it's the juice get by fire /scorch green bamboo shoot.
Property and flavor: cold; sweet, bitter.
Main and collateral channels: heart, liver and heart meridians.
Administration and dosage: 30-60 g, drink of used in pill or paste.
Indication: phlegm, apoplexy, convulsion, epilepsy and tetanus.

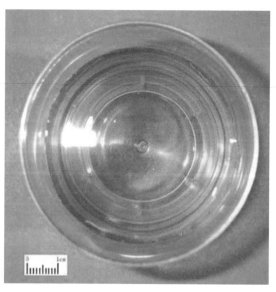

(The picture is only for learning and identification the herb; the specific use of the herb please consult the herbalist or health professionals)

Willowleaf Swallowwort Rhizome (Baiqian)

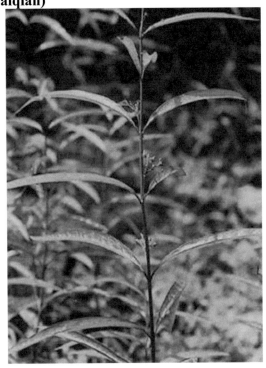

Chinese phonetic alphabet/pin yin: bái qián
Chinese characters simplified/traditional:白前/白前
Chinese nickname's alphabet (Nickname's Chinese characters):
Liuyebaiqian/ Yuanhuayebaiqian (柳叶白前/芫花叶白前)
Latin: Cynanchi Stauntonii Rhizoma et Radix (Common name: Willowleaf Swallowwort Rhizome)
Plant: *Cynanchum glaucescens* (Decne.) Hand.-Mazz. (or *Cynanchum stauntonii* (Decne.) Schltr.)

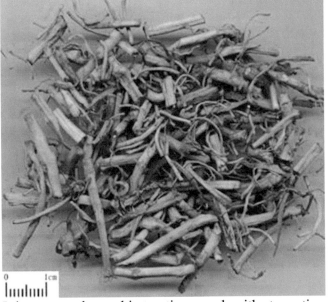

TCM prepared in ready-to-use forms (medicinal parts): it's dried rhizome and root which harvested in autumn.
Property and flavor: mild warm; pungent, bitter.
Main and collateral channels: lung meridian.
Administration and dosage: 3-10 g.
Indication: cough, sputum, chest tightness and dyspnea.

It is commonly used in treating cough with stagnation of sputum.
(The picture is only for learning and identification the herb; the specific use of the herb please consult the herbalist or health professionals)

Hogfennel Root (Qianhu)
Chinese phonetic alphabet/pin yin: qián hú
Chinese characters simplified/traditional:前胡/前胡

Chinese nickname's alphabet (Nickname's Chinese characters): Shanduhuo/ Louguicai/ Yimacai(山独活/罗鬼菜/姨妈菜)
Latin: Peucedani Radix (Common name: Hogfennel Root)
Plant: *Peucedanum praeruptorum* Dunn.

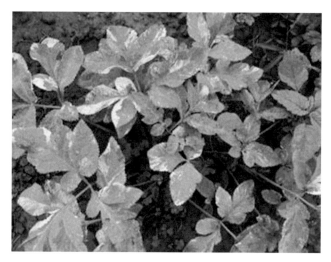

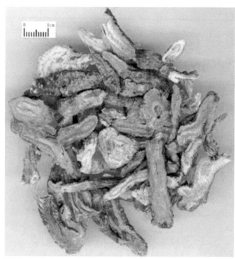

TCM prepared in ready-to-use forms (medicinal parts): it's dried root which harvested in winter or spring.
Property and flavor: mild cold; pungent, bitter.
Main and collateral channels: lung meridian.
Administration and dosage: 3-10 g.
Indication: cough and excessive phlegm, thick yellow sputum.
(The picture is only for learning and identification the herb; the specific use of the herb please consult the herbalist or health professionals)

Kelp (Kunbu)

Chinese phonetic alphabet/pin yin: kūn bù
Chinese characters simplified/traditional: 昆布/昆布
Chinese nickname's alphabet (Nickname's Chinese characters): Haidai/ Ezhangcai(海带/鹅掌菜)
Latin: Laminariae Thallus seu Eckloniae Thallus (Common name: Kelp or Tangle)
Plant: *Ecklonia kurome* Okam. (or *Laminaria japonica* Aresch.)
TCM prepared in ready-to-use forms (medicinal parts): it's dried thalline which harvested in summer or autumn.
Property and flavor: cold; salty.

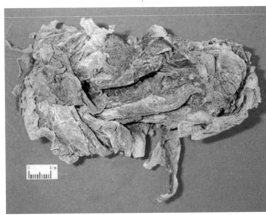

Main and collateral channels: liver, stomach and kidney meridians.
Administration and dosage: 6-12 g.
Indication: goiter, scrofula, testicular swelling and pain, edema and phlegm; promote urination.
It is taken as food in some part of China.

(The picture is only for learning and identification the herb; the specific use of the herb please consult the herbalist or health professionals)

Seaweed (Haizao)

Chinese phonetic alphabet/pin yin: hǎi zǎo
Chinese characters simplified/traditional:
海藻/海藻
Chinese nickname's alphabet
(Nickname's Chinese characters):
Luoshou/ Hailuo/ Wucai(落首/海萝/乌菜)
Latin: Sargassum (Common name: Seaweed)
Plant: *Sargassum fusiforme* (Harv.) Setch. (or *Sargassum pallidum* (Turn.) C. Ag.)
TCM prepared in ready-to-use forms (medicinal parts): it's dried algae which harvested in summer or autumn.
Property and flavor: cold; bitter, salty.
Main and collateral channels: liver, stomach and kidney meridians.
Administration and dosage: 6-12 g.

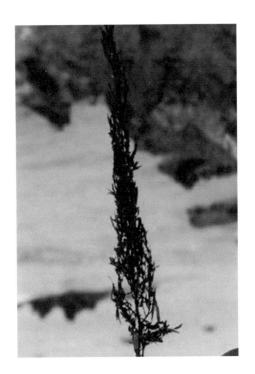

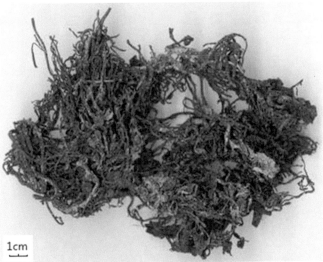

Indication: goiter, scrofula, testicular swelling and pain, edema and phlegm.
Precaution and warning: incompatible with Liquorice Root.
(The picture is only for learning and identification the herb; the specific use of the herb please consult the herbalist or health professionals)

Tabasheer (Tianzhuhuang)

Chinese phonetic alphabet/pin yin: tiān zhú huáng

Chinese characters simplified/traditional:天竺黄/天竺黄

Chinese nickname's alphabet (Nickname's Chinese characters): Zhuhuang/ Zhugao(竹黄/竹膏)

Latin: Bambusae Concretio Silicea (Common name: Tabasheer)

Plant: *Bambusa textilis* McClure. (or *Schizostachyum chinense* Rendle.)

TCM prepared in ready-to-use forms (medicinal parts): it's dried masses secretion/ material in stem which harvested between November and December.

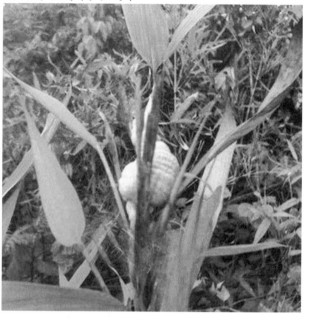

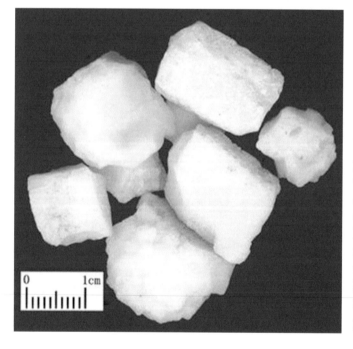

Property and flavor: cold; sweet.

Main and collateral channels: heart and liver meridians.

Administration and dosage: 3-9 g.

Indication: fever, coma, phlegm heat shock carbuncle, convulsions and night crying.

(The picture is only for learning and identification the herb; the specific use of the herb please consult the herbalist or health professionals)

Airpotato Yam Rhizome (Huangyaozi)

Chinese phonetic alphabet/pin yin: huáng yào zǐ

Chinese characters simplified/traditional:黄药子/黄藥子

Chinese nickname's alphabet (Nickname's Chinese characters): Huangyao/ Huangdu(黄药/黄独)

Latin: Dioscoreae Bulbiferae Rhizoma (Common name: Airpotato Yam Rhizome)

Plant: *Dioscorea bulbifera* L.
TCM prepared in ready-to-use forms (medicinal parts): it's dried rhizome which harvested in autumn.
Property and flavor: cool; bitter, pungent.
Main and collateral channels: liver, stomach, heart and lung meridians.

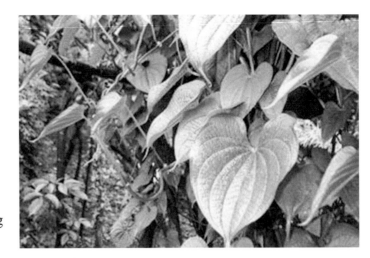

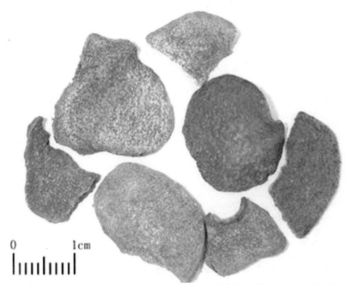

Administration and dosage: 15-25 g. Appropriate amount for topical application.
Indication: goiter, sores, carbuncle, sore throat, hemoptysis, hematemesis, epistaxis, insect and snake bites.
Precaution and warning: toxic.

(The picture is only for learning and identification the herb; the specific use of the herb please consult the herbalist or health professionals)

Arc Shell (Walengzi)
Chinese phonetic alphabet/pin yin: wǎ léng zǐ

Chinese characters simplified/traditional: 瓦楞子/瓦楞子
Chinese nickname's alphabet (Nickname's Chinese characters): Hanzike(蚶子壳)
Latin: Arcae Concha (Common name: Arc Shell)
Animal: *Arca subcrenata* Lischke. (or *Arca granosa* Linnaeus., *Arca inflata* Reeve.)

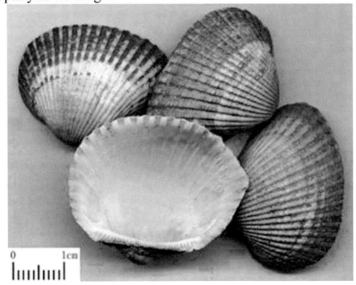

TCM prepared in ready-to-use forms (medicinal parts): it's dried shell which harvested in autumn or winter.
Property and flavor: neutral; salty.
Main and collateral channels: lung and stomach meridians.
Administration and dosage: 9-15 g. It should be decocted first.
Indication: scrofula, goiter, blood stasis, abdominal lump and acid regurgitation.
(The picture is only for learning and identification the herb; the specific use of the herb please consult the herbalist or health professionals)

Clam Shell (Haigeqiao)

Chinese phonetic alphabet/pin yin: hǎi gě qiào
Chinese characters simplified/traditional:海蛤壳/海蛤殼
Chinese nickname's alphabet (Nickname's Chinese characters): Haige/Geke(海蛤/蛤壳)
Latin: Meretricis Concha seu Cyclinae Concha (Common name: Clam Shell)

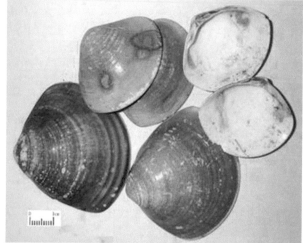

Animal: *Meretrix meretrix* Linnaeus. (or *Cyclina sinensis* (Gmelin.))
TCM prepared in ready-to-use forms (medicinal parts): it's dried shell which harvested in summer or autumn.
Property and flavor: cool; bitter, salty.
Main and collateral channels: lung, kidney and stomach meridians.

Administration and dosage: 6-15 g. It should be decocted first, ground into powder for wrap-boiling. Appropriate amount for topical application, ground it into extreme fine powder for spreading or being mixed it with oil for application.
Indication: excessive phlegm, cough, chest pain, blood stasis, scrofula, goiter and acid regurgitation; external use to treat eczema, scald and burns.
(The picture is only for learning and identification the herb; the specific use of the herb please consult the herbalist or health professionals)

Pumice Stone (Haifushi)

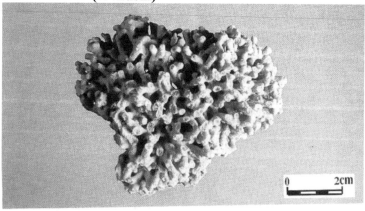

Chinese phonetic alphabet/pin yin: hǎi fú shí
Chinese characters simplified/traditional:海浮石/海浮石

Chinese nickname's alphabet (Nickname's Chinese characters): Shuipaoshi/
Fuhaishi(水泡石/浮海石)
Latin: Pumex (Common name: Pumice Stone, Costazia or Bryozoatum)
Mineral: main component SiO_2.
TCM prepared in ready-to-use forms (medicinal parts): it's *Costazia aculeata* Canu. et
Bassler or other species dried skeleton, or Lava from a volcano formed a porous rock.
Property and flavor: cold; salty.
Main and collateral channels: stomach, kidney, liver and large intestine meridians.
Administration and dosage: 6-10 g. It should be decocted first.
Indication: cough caused by heat, sputum sticky, scrofula and goiter.
(The picture is only for learning and identification the herb; the specific use of the
herb please consult the herbalist or health professionals)

Chlorite Schist (Mengshi)
Chinese phonetic alphabet/pin yin: méng shí
Chinese characters simplified/traditional:礞石/礞石
Chinese nickname's alphabet (Nickname's Chinese characters): Qingmengshi/
Heiyunmu(青礞石/黑云母)
Latin: Chloriti Lapis (Common name: Chlorite Schist, Vermiculite Schist or
Hydrobiotite Schist)

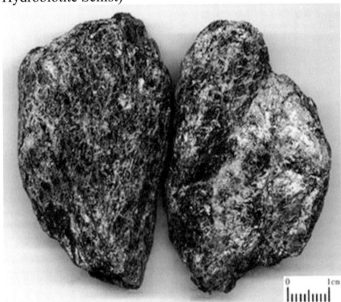

Mineral: main component $K(Mg \cdot Fe)_2(Al \cdot Si_3O_{10})(OH \cdot F)_2$
TCM prepared in ready-to-use forms (medicinal parts): it's cleaned mineral of biotite schist or mainly composed of calcite, dolomite, gold mica, sericite, quartz and the other minerals aggregation.
Property and flavor: neutral; sweet, salty.
Main and collateral channels: lung, heart and liver meridians.
Administration and dosage: usually used in pill or powder, 3-6 g. 10-15 g wrapped for
decoction, it should be decocted first.
Indication: the demonstration of stubborn phlegm, cough with wheezing, mania,
convulsion and epilepsy.
(The picture is only for learning and identification the herb; the specific use of the
herb please consult the herbalist or health professionals)

Mica-schist (Jinmengshi)
Chinese phonetic alphabet/pin yin: jīn méng shí
Chinese characters simplified/traditional:金礞石/金礞石

Chinese nickname's alphabet (Nickname's Chinese characters): Lanshi/ Susushi(烂石/酥酥石)

Latin: Micae Lapis Aureus (Common name: Mica-schist)

Mineral: main component $K(Mg\cdot Fe)_2(Al\cdot Si_5O_{10})(OH\cdot F)_2$ with a little hornblende $((Ca,Na)_{2-3}(Mg^{2+},Fe^{2+},Fe^{3+},Al^{3+})_5[(Al,Si)_4O_{11}](OH)_2)$ and SiO_2. It is usually a rock schist of metamorphic group. TCM prepared in ready-to-use forms (medicinal parts): it's cleaned mineral.

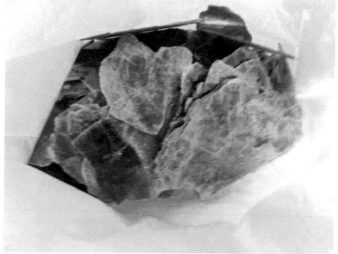

Property and flavor: neutral; sweet and salty.

Main and collateral channels: lung, heart and liver meridians.

Administration and dosage: usually used in pill or powder, 3-6 g. 10-15 g for decoction, decocted wrap-in cloth first.

Indication: the stubborn phlegm bind, cough, wheezing, epilepsy, manic psychosis, vexation, oppression in the chest and convulsion.

(The picture is only for learning and identification the herb; the specific use of the herb please consult the herbalist or health professionals)

Bitter Apricot (Kuxingren)

Chinese phonetic alphabet/pin yin: kǔ xìng rén

Chinese characters simplified/traditional:苦杏仁/苦杏仁

Chinese nickname's alphabet (Nickname's Chinese characters): Xingren(杏仁)

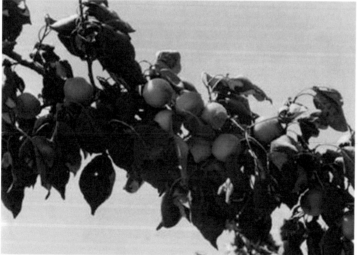

Latin: Armeniacae Semen Amarum (Common name: Bitter Apricot or Bitter Almond)
Plant: *Prunus armeniaca* L. (or *Prunus armeniaca* L. var. *ansu* Maxim., *Prunus mandshurica* (Maxim.) Koechne., *Prunus sibirica* L.)

TCM prepared in ready-to-use forms (medicinal parts): it's ripe seed.

Property and flavor: mild warm; bitter.

Main and collateral channels: lung and large intestine meridians.
Administration and dosage: 5-10 g, unprocessed for decoction, added when the decoction is nearly done.
Indication: cough and wheezing, excessive phlegm, blood deficiency, constipation.

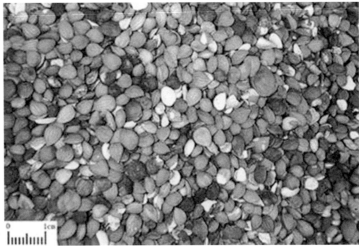

It is key herb to treat cough and dyspnea.
The sweet one is taken as food in some part of China.
Precaution and warning: toxic, be care of over-dosage for oral administration to avoid poisoning.
(The picture is only for learning and identification the herb; the specific use of the herb please consult the herbalist or health professionals)

Stemona Root (Baibu)
Chinese phonetic alphabet/pin yin: bǎi bù
Chinese characters simplified/traditional: 百部/百部

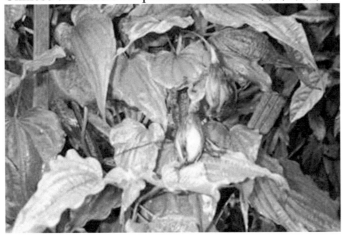

Chinese nickname's alphabet (Nickname's Chinese characters): Baitiaogen(百条根)
Latin: Stemonae Radix (Common name: Stemona Root)
Plant: *Stemona japonica* Bl. (or *Stemona sessilifolia* (Miq.) Miq., *Stemona tuberosa* Lour.)

TCM prepared in ready-to-use forms (medicinal parts): it's dried root tuber which harvested in spring or autumn.
Property and flavor: mild warm; sweet, bitter.
Main and collateral channels: lung meridian.

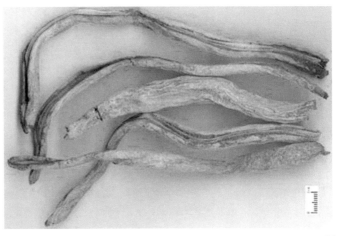

67

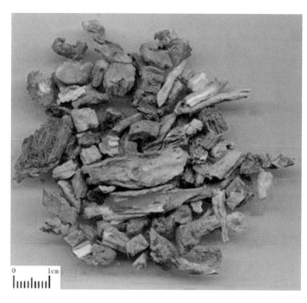

Administration and dosage: 3-9 g. Appropriate amount for topical application, decocted in water or soaked in wine or liquor.
Indication: chronic cough, pulmonary tuberculosis, pertussis; external use for parasite and lice.
It is key herb to treat chronic cough.
(The picture is only for learning and identification the herb; the specific use of the herb please consult the herbalist or health professionals)

Perilla Fruit (Zisuzi)

Chinese phonetic alphabet/pin yin: zǐ sū zǐ

Chinese characters simplified/traditional:紫苏子/紫蘇子

Chinese nickname's alphabet (Nickname's Chinese characters): Suzi/ Heisuzi(苏子/黑苏子)

Latin: Perillae Fructus (Common name: Perilla Fruit)

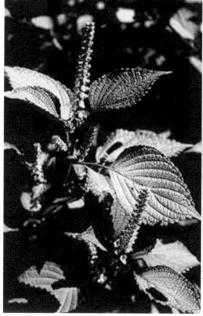

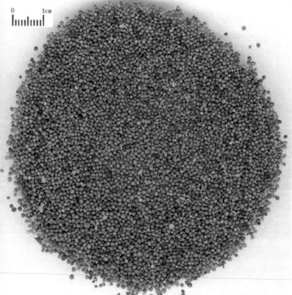

Plant: *Perilla frutescens* (L.) Britt.   TCM prepared in ready-to-use forms (medicinal parts): it's mature seed.

Property and flavor: warm; pungent.

Main and collateral channels: lung meridian.

Administration and dosage: 3-10 g.

Indication: phlegm stagnation, cough, asthma, constipation.

It is taken as food in some part of China.

(The picture is only for learning and identification the herb; the specific use of the herb please consult the herbalist or health professionals)

White Mulberry Root-bark (Sangbaipi)
Chinese phonetic alphabet/pin yin: sāng bái pí
Chinese characters simplified/traditional:桑白皮/桑白皮

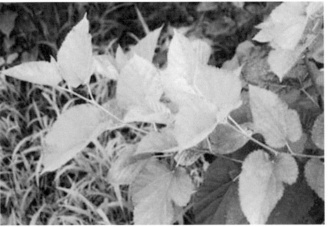

Chinese nickname's alphabet (Nickname's Chinese characters): Sanggenpi/ Sangpi/ Baisangpi(桑根皮/桑皮/白桑皮)
Latin: Mori Cortex
(Common name: White Mulberry Root-bark)
Plant: *Morus alba* L.

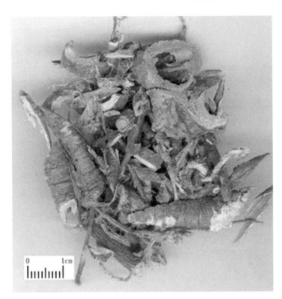

TCM prepared in ready-to-use forms (medicinal parts): it's dried root bark which harvested in winter.
Property and flavor: cold; sweet.
Main and collateral channels: lung meridian.
Administration and dosage: 6-12 g.
Indication: cough, edema, oliguria and swelling.
(The picture is only for learning and identification the herb; the specific use of the herb please consult the herbalist or health professionals)

Pepperweed Seed (Tinglizi)

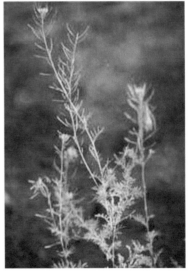

Chinese phonetic alphabet/pin yin: tíng lì zì
Chinese characters simplified/traditional:葶苈子/葶藶子
Chinese nickname's alphabet (Nickname's Chinese characters): Dashi/ Dingli(大室/丁历)
Latin: Descurainiae Semen seu Lepidii Semen
(Common name: Pepperweed Seed, Tansymustard Seed or Draba Nemorosa Seed)
Plant: *Descurainia Sophia* (L.) Webb ex Prantl.
(or *Lepidium apetalum* Willd., *Lepidium virginicum* L., *Draba nemorosa* L.)
TCM prepared in ready-to-use forms (medicinal parts): it's dried mature seed.

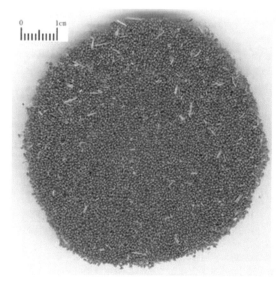

Property and flavor: highly cold; pungent, bitter.

Main and collateral channels: lung and bladder meridians.

Administration and dosage: 3-10 g, wrap-boiling.

Indication: profuss sputum, cough, asthma, chest tightness, abdominal edema and dysuria.

(The picture is only for learning and identification the herb; the specific use of the herb please consult the herbalist or health professionals)

Tatarian Aster Root (Ziyuan)

Chinese phonetic alphabet/pin yin: zǐ yuān

Chinese characters simplified/traditional: 紫苑/紫苑

Chinese nickname's alphabet(Nickname's Chinese characters): Ziwan/ Qingyuan(紫菀/青菀)

Latin: Asteris Radix et Rhizoma (Common name: Tatarian Aster Root)

Plant: *Aster tataricus* L. f.

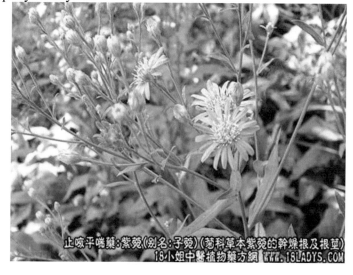

止咳平喘藥：紫菀(別名：子菀)(菊科草本紫菀的幹燥根及根莖)
18小姐中醫植物藥方網 WWW.18LADYS.COM

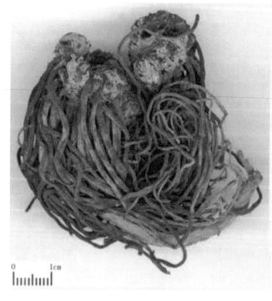

TCM prepared in ready-to-use forms (medicinal parts): it's dried root and rhizome which harvested in spring or autumn.

Property and flavor: warm; pungent, bitter.

Main and collateral channels: lung meridian.

Administration and dosage: 5-10 g.

Indication: excessive phlegm, acute and chronic cough, wheezing, hemoptysis and dysuria.

(The picture is only for learning and identification the herb; the specific use of the herb please consult the herbalist or health professionals)

Common Coltsfoot Flower (Kuandonghua)

Chinese phonetic alphabet/pin yin: kuǎn dōng huā

Chinese characters simplified/traditional:款冬花/款冬花

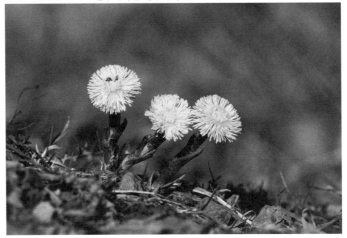

Chinese nickname's alphabet (Nickname's Chinese characters): Kandenghua/Aidonghua(看灯花/艾冬花)
Latin: Farfarae Flos (Common name: Common Coltsfoot Flower)
Plant: *Tussilago farfara* L.

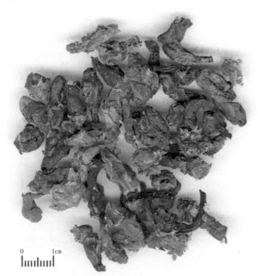

TCM prepared in ready-to-use forms (medicinal parts): it's dried flower bud.
Property and flavor: warm; mild bitter, pungent.
Main and collateral channels: lung meridian.
Administration and dosage: 5-10 g.
Indication: cough, asthmatic, hemoptysis, excessive phlegm.
(The picture is only for learning and identification the herb; the specific use of the herb please consult the herbalist or health professionals)

Loquat Leaf (Pipaye)

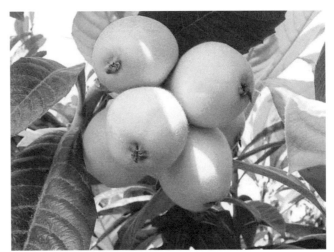

Chinese phonetic alphabet/pin yin: pí pā yè
Chinese characters simplified/traditional:枇杷叶/枇杷葉
Chinese nickname's alphabet (Nickname's Chinese characters): Baye(巴叶)
Latin: Eriobotryae Folium (Common name: Loquat Leaf)

Plant: *Eriobotrya japonica* (Thunb.) Lindl.

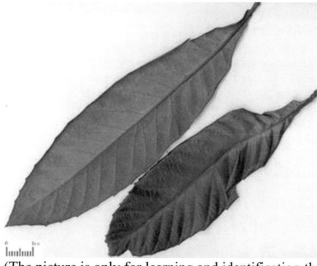

TCM prepared in ready-to-use forms (medicinal parts): it's dried leaf which harvested all year round.
Property and flavor: mild cold; bitter.
Main and collateral channels: lung and stomach meridians.
Administration and dosage: 5-10 g.
Indication: cough, dyspnea, ructation, vomiting and vexation.

(The picture is only for learning and identification the herb; the specific use of the herb please consult the herbalist or health professionals)

Dutohmanspipe Fruit (Madouling)

Chinese phonetic alphabet/pin yin: mǎ dōu líng
Chinese characters simplified/traditional:马兜铃/馬兜鈴

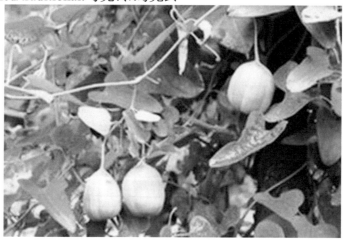

Chinese nickname's alphabet (Nickname's Chinese characters): Shuimaxiangguo/ Sheshenguo(水马香果/蛇参果)
Latin: Aristolochiae Fructus (Common name: Dutohmanspipe Fruit)

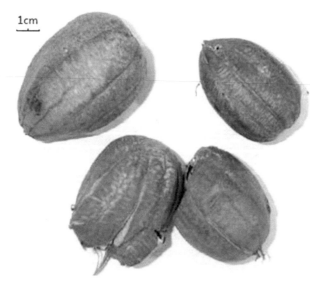

1cm

Plant: *Aristolochia debilis* Sieb. et Zucc. (or *Aristolochia contorta* Bge.)
TCM prepared in ready-to-use forms (medicinal parts): it's dried mature fruit.
Property and flavor: mild cold; bitter.
Main and collateral channels: lung and large intestine meridians.
Administration and dosage: 3-9 g.

Indication: cough and wheezing, phlegm with blood, hemorrhoids, swelling and pain.
Precaution and warning: the herb contain aristolochic acid which may induce kidney damage, it should be used cautiously for child and aged. Contraindicated for pregnant woman, infant and the patients suffering from renal insufficiency.
(The picture is only for learning and identification the herb; the specific use of the herb please consult the herbalist or health professionals)

Ginkgo Seed (Baiguo)
Chinese phonetic alphabet/pin yin: bái guǒ

Chinese characters simplified/traditional:白果/白果
Chinese nickname's alphabet (Nickname's Chinese characters): Yinxingzi/ Fozhijia(银杏子/佛指甲)
Latin: Ginkgo Semen (Common name: Ginkgo Seed or Maidenhair Tree Seed)
Plant: *Ginkgo biloba* L.

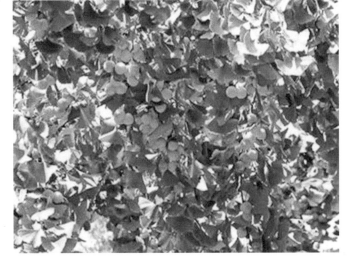

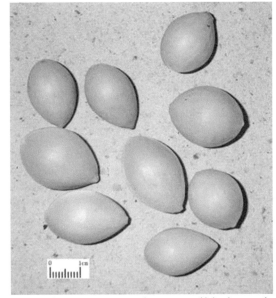

TCM prepared in ready-to-use forms (medicinal parts): it's dried mature seed.
Property and flavor: neutral; sweet, bitter and astringent.
Main and collateral channels: heart and lung meridians.
Administration and dosage: 5-10 g.
Indication: profuse sputum, wheezing and cough, leucorrhea cloudiness, enuresis.
Precaution and warning: slightly toxic, especially unprocessed one is poisonous.
It is taken as food in some part of China.

Attention: to protect the rare wild plant, please don't use the herb from wild plant.
(The picture is only for learning and identification the herb; the specific use of the herb please consult the herbalist or health professionals)

Boat-fruited Sterculia Seed (Pangdahai)
Chinese phonetic alphabet/pin yin: pàng dà hǎi
Chinese characters simplified/traditional:胖大海/胖大海
Chinese nickname's alphabet (Nickname's Chinese characters): Dahazi/ Dadongguo(大海子/大洞果)

Latin: Sterculiae Lychnophorae Semen (Common name: Boat-fruited Sterculia Seed)
Plant: *Sterculia lychnophora* Hance.
TCM prepared in ready-to-use forms (medicinal parts): it's dried ripe seed.
Property and flavor: cold; sweet.

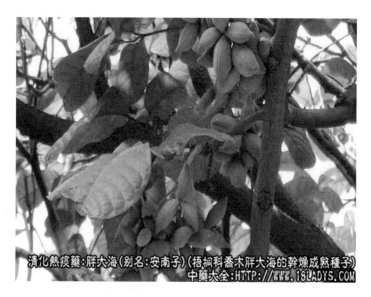

清化熱痰藥:胖大海(別名:安南子)(梧桐科喬木胖大海的乾燥成熟種子)
中藥大全:HTTP://WWW.18LADYS.COM

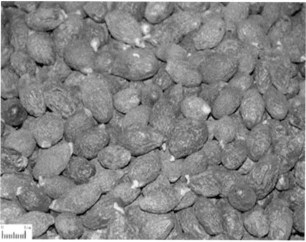

Main and collateral channels: lung and large intestine meridians.
Administration and dosage: 2-3 pieces soaked in boiling water or decocted for oral administration.
Indication: hoarseness, dry cough, sore throat, constipations, headache and red eyes.
It is taken as tea in some part of China.

(The picture is only for learning and identification the herb; the specific use of the herb please consult the herbalist or health professionals)

Datura Flower (Yangjinhua)
Chinese phonetic alphabet/pin yin: yáng jīn huā

Chinese characters simplified/traditional: 洋金花/洋金花
Chinese nickname's alphabet (Nickname's Chinese characters): Shanqiehua/Mantuoluohuan(山茄花/曼陀罗花)
Latin: Daturae Flos (Common name: Datura Flower)
Plant: *Datura metel* L.

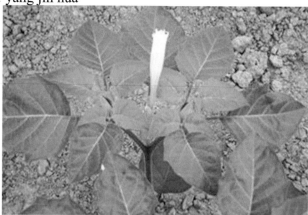

TCM prepared in ready-to-use forms (medicinal parts): it's dried flower.
Property and flavor: warm; pungent.
Main and collateral channels: liver and lung meridians.

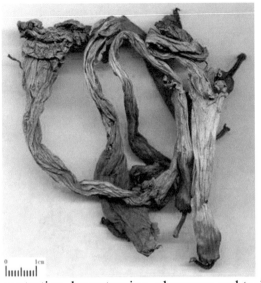

Administration and dosage: 0.3-0.6 g, usually used in pills or powder; or smoke it for several times (no more than 1.5 g per day). Appropriate amount for topical application.

Indication: treat asthma, cough, epigastrium and abdominal pain caused by cold/chill (*Hanliang*), painful *bi* disorder, chronic infantile convulsion; external use for surgical anesthesia.

It is key herb to treat dry cough.

Precaution and warning: toxic, contraindicated for pregnant women and patients suffering from exterior contration, hypertension, glaucoma and tachycardia.

(The picture is only for learning and identification the herb; the specific use of the herb please consult the herbalist or health professionals)

Roselle Calyx (Meiguiqie)

Chinese phonetic alphabet/pin yin: méi guì qié

Chinese characters simplified/traditional: 玫瑰茄/玫瑰茄

Chinese nickname's alphabet (Nickname's Chinese characters): Hongjinmei/Hongmeiguo(红金梅/红梅果)

Latin: Hibisci Calyx (Common name: Roselle Calyx)

Plant: *Hibicus sabdariffa* L.

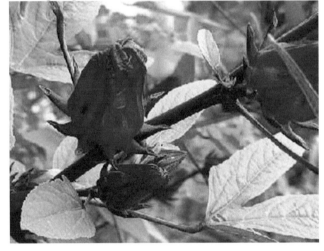

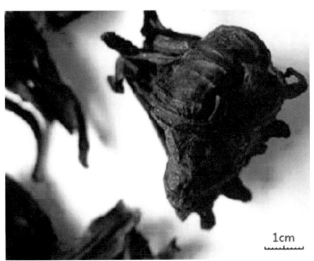

TCM prepared in ready-to-use forms (medicinal parts): it's dried calyx with flower.

Property and flavor: cool; acidity.

Main and collateral channels: kidney meridian.

Administration and dosage: 9-15 g, soaked in boiling water or decocted for oral administration.

Indication: hypertension, cough and heat-shock; alleviate a hangover.

(The picture is only for learning and identification the herb; the specific use of the herb please consult the herbalist or health professionals)

Japanese Ardisia Herb (Aidicha)

Chinese phonetic alphabet/pin yin: ǎi dì chá
Chinese characters simplified/traditional:矮地茶/矮地茶

Chinese nickname's alphabet (Nickname's Chinese characters): Pingdimu/ Buchulin/ Zijinniu(平地木/不出林/紫金牛)
Latin: Ardisiae Japonicae Herba (Common name: Japanese Ardisa Herb)
Plant: *Ardisa japonica* (Thunb.) Blume.

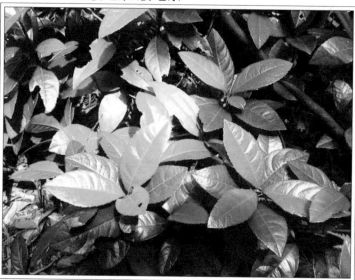

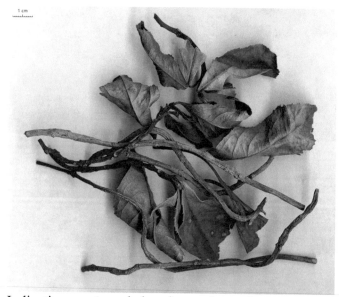

TCM prepared in ready-to-use forms (medicinal parts): it's dried whole herb which harvested in summer or autumn.
Property and flavor: neutral; pungent, mild bitter.
Main and collateral channels: lung and liver meridians.
Administration and dosage: 15-30 g.

Indication: acute and chronic cough, profuse sputum, phlegm with blood, jaundice, amenorrhea and traumatic injuries.
(The picture is only for learning and identification the herb; the specific use of the herb please consult the herbalist or health professionals)

Greater Celandine Herb (Baiqucai)

Chinese phonetic alphabet/pin yin: bái qū cài
Chinese characters simplified/traditional:白屈菜/白屈菜
Chinese nickname's alphabet (Nickname's Chinese characters): Dihuanglian/ Shanhuanglian/ Duanchangcao(地黄连/山黄连/断肠草)
Latin: Chelidonii Herba (Common name: Greater Celandine Herb)

Plant: *Chelidonium majus* L.
TCM prepared in ready-to-use forms (medicinal parts): it's dried whole herb which harvested in summer or autumn.
Property and flavor: cool; bitter.
Main and collateral channels: lung and stomach meridians.
Administration and dosage: 9-18 g.

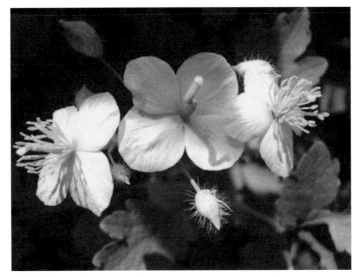

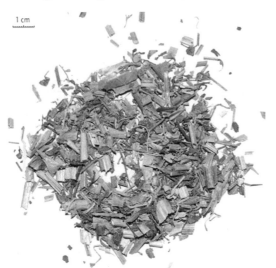

Indication: painful in epigastria and abdominal, cough, panting and pertussis; external use for insect or snake bites.
Precaution and warning: slightly toxic.
(The picture is only for learning and identification the herb; the specific use of the herb please consult the herbalist or health professionals)

Lindley Eupatorium Herb (Yemazhui)

Chinese phonetic alphabet/pin yin: yě mǎ zhuī
Chinese characters simplified/traditional:野马追/野馬追

Chinese nickname's alphabet (Nickname's Chinese characters): Baiguding/ Lunyezelan(白鼓钉/ 轮叶泽兰)
Latin: Eupatorii Lindleyani Herba (Common name: Lindley Eupatorium Herb)
Plant: *Eupatorium lindleyanum* DC.

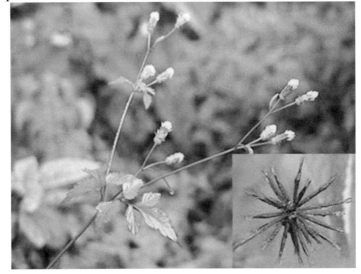

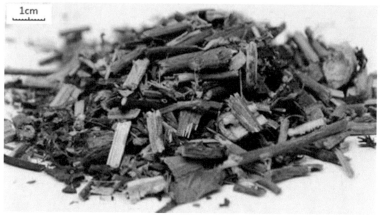

TCM prepared in ready-to-use forms (medicinal parts): it's dried aerial part which harvested in autumn.
Property and flavor: neutral; bitter.

Main and collateral channels: lung meridian.
Administration and dosage: 30-60 g.
Indication: excessive phlegm, cough and wheezing.
(The picture is only for learning and identification the herb; the specific use of the herb please consult the herbalist or health professionals)

Chinese Honeylocust Abnormal Fruit (Zhuyazao)
Chinese phonetic alphabet/pin yin: zhū yá zào
Chinese characters simplified/traditional:猪牙皂/豬牙皂

Chinese nickname's alphabet (Nickname's Chinese characters): Jixizi/ Yazao(鸡栖子/牙皂)
Latin: Gleditsiae Fructus Abnormalis (Common name: Chinese Honeylocust Abnormal Fruit)
Plant: *Gleditsia sinensis* Lam.

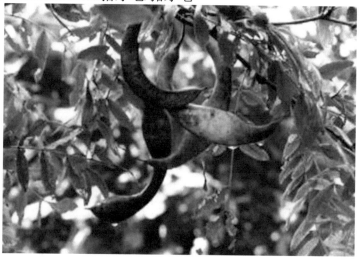

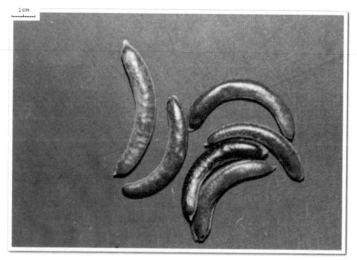

TCM prepared in ready-to-use forms (medicinal parts): it's dried sterile fruit.
Property and flavor: warm; pungent, salty.
Main and collateral channels: lung and large intestine meridians.

Administration and dosage: 1-1.5 g, usually used in pills or powder. Topical application in appropriate amount. Ground it into powder for blowing into nose to sneeze or for applying to the *pars affecta.*

Indication: coma, epilepsy, dyspnea and cough with phlegm, dry stool; external use for swelling abscess.

Precaution and warning: slightly toxic. Contraindicated during pregnancy or patients with hemoptysis or hematemesis.

(The picture is only for learning and identification the herb; the specific use of the herb please consult the herbalist or health professionals)

Big Gleditsia (Dazaojiao)

Chinese phonetic alphabet/pin yin: dà zào jiǎo

Chinese characters simplified/traditional:大皂角/大皂角

Chinese nickname's alphabet (Nickname's Chinese characters): Zaojiao/ Zaojia(皂角/皂荚)

Latin: Gleditsiae Sinensis Fructus (Common name: Big Gleditsia)

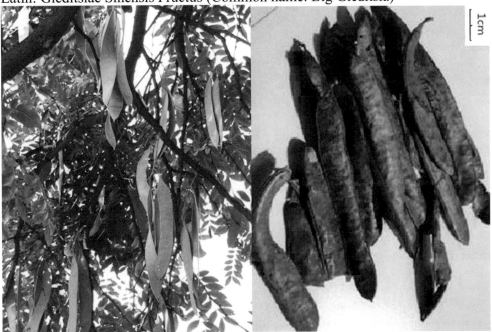

Plant: *Gleditsia sinensis* Lam.   TCM prepared in ready-to-use forms (medicinal parts): it's dried ripe fruit.

Property and flavor: warm; pungent.

Main and collateral channels: lung and large intestine meridians.

Administration and dosage:1-1.5 g, usually used in pills or powder. Topical application in appropriate amount. Ground it into powder for blowing into nose to sneeze or for applying to the *pars affecta.*

Indication: syncope, epilepsy, abundant expectoration, dyspnea and cough with phlegm.

Precaution and warning: slightly toxic. Contraindicated during pregnancy or patients with hemoptysis or hematemesis.

(The picture is only for learning and identification the herb; the specific use of the herb please consult the herbalist or health professionals)

Tenacious Condorvine Stem (Tongguanteng)

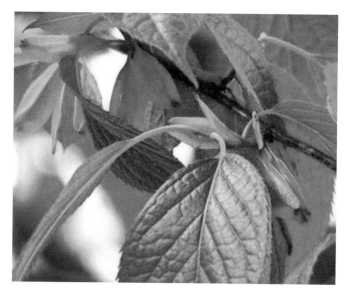

Chinese phonetic alphabet/pin yin: tōng guān téng
Chinese characters simplified/traditional:通关藤/通關藤
Latin: Marsdeniae Tenacissimae Caulis
(Common name: Tenacious Condorvine Stem)
Plant: *Marsdenia tenacissima* (Roxb.) Wight et Arn.

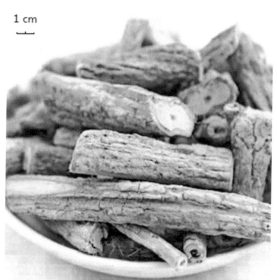

1 cm

TCM prepared in ready-to-use forms (medicinal parts): it's dried lianoid stem which harvested in summer or autumn.
Property and flavor: mild cold; bitter.
Main and collateral channels: lung meridian.
Administration and dosage: 20-30 g. Topical application in appropriate amount.
Indication: cough, wheezing, excessive phlegm, postpartum agalactia, painful swelling, sore, abscess and oligogalactia.

(The picture is only for learning and identification the herb; the specific use of the herb please consult the herbalist or health professionals)

Muskmelon Seed (Tianguazi)
Chinese phonetic alphabet/pin yin: tián guā zǐ

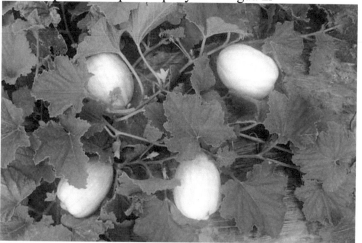

Chinese characters simplified/traditional :甜瓜子/甜瓜子
Chinese nickname's alphabet (Nickname's Chinese characters): Xiangguazi(香瓜子)
Latin: Melo Semen (Common name: Muskmelon Seed)

Plant: *Cucumis melo* L.
TCM prepared in ready-to-use forms (medicinal parts): it's dried ripe seed.
Property and flavor: cold; sweet.
Main and collateral channels: lung, stomach and large intestine meridians.
Administration and dosage: 9-30 g.
Indication: dryness cough, constipation, abscess, traumatic injury, blood stasis, sinew injury and fracture.

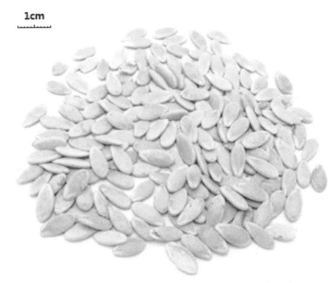

(The picture is only for learning and identification the herb; the specific use of the herb please consult the herbalist or health professionals)

Decurrent Hogfennel Root (Zihuaqianhu)

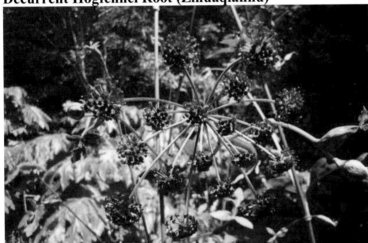

Chinese phonetic alphabet/pin yin: zǐ huā qián hú
Chinese characters simplified/traditional: 紫花前胡/紫花前胡
Chinese nickname's alphabet (Nickname's Chinese characters): Tudanggui/ Yajiaoqi(土当归/鸭脚七)

Latin: Peucedani Decursivi Radix (Common name: Decurrent Hogfennel Root)

Plant: *Peucedanum decursivum* (Miq.) Maxim. (or *Abelmoschus manihot* (L.) Medic.)
TCM prepared in ready-to-use forms (medicinal parts): it's dried root and rhizome which harvested in autumn or winter.
Property and flavor: mild cold; pungent, bitter.
Main and collateral channels: lung meridian.

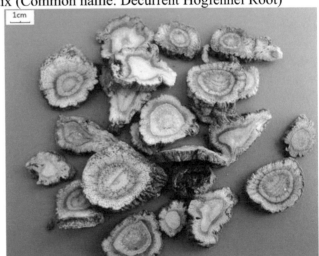

Administration and dosage: 3-9 g, decocted or used in pills and powder.

Indication: yellow thick phlegm, cough and excessive phlegm.
(The picture is only for learning and identification the herb; the specific use of the herb please consult the herbalist or health professionals)

Funneled Physochlaina Root (Huashanshen)

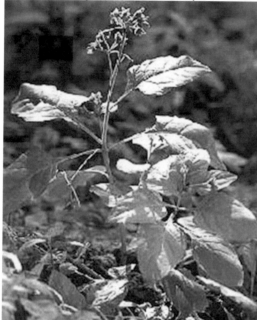

Chinese phonetic alphabet/pin yin: huá shān shēn
Chinese characters simplified/traditional:华山参/華山参
Chinese nickname's alphabet (Nickname's Chinese characters): Qinshen/ Baimaoshen(秦参/白毛参)
Latin: Physochlainae Radix (Common name: Funneled Physochlaina Root)
Plant: *Physochlaina infundibularis* Kuang.
TCM prepared in ready-to-use forms (medicinal parts): it's dried root which harvested in spring.

Property and flavor: warm; sweet, mild bitter.
Main and collateral channels: lung and heart meridians.
Administration and dosage: 0.1-0.2 g.
Indication: wheezing with cough, profuse sputum, fright palpitations and insomnia.

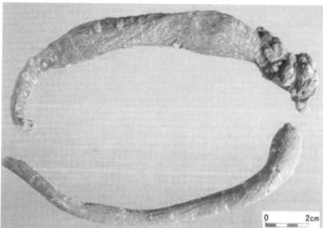

Precaution and warning: poisonous. Contraindicated for patient with glaucoma. Used with caution during pregnancy and in patient with serious prostatic swelling.
(The picture is only for learning and identification the herb; the specific use of the herb please consult the herbalist or health professionals)

Dahurian Rhododendron Leaf (Manshanhong)

Chinese phonetic alphabet/pin yin: mǎn shān hóng
Chinese characters simplified/traditional:满山红/滿山紅
Chinese nickname's alphabet (Nickname's Chinese characters): Yingshanhong/ Dujuanhua(映山红/杜鹃花)
Latin: Rhododendri Daurici Folium (Common name: Dahurian Rhododendron Leaf)

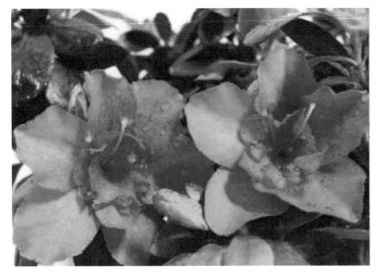

Plant: *Rhododendron dauricum* L.
TCM prepared in ready-to-use forms (medicinal parts): it's dried leaf which harvested in summer or autumn.
Property and flavor: cold; bitter, pungent.
Main and collateral channels: lung and spleen meridians.

Administration and dosage: 25-50 g. 6-12 g, soaked in 40% alcohol.
Indication: cough, wheezing and excessive phlegm.
(The picture is only for learning and identification the herb; the specific use of the herb please consult the herbalist or health professionals)

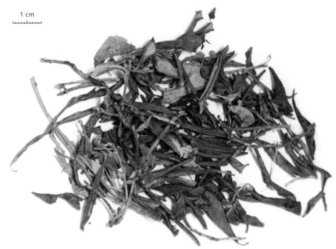

1 cm

Dragon's Tongue Leaf (Longliye)

Chinese phonetic alphabet/pin yin: lóng lì yè
Chinese characters simplified/traditional:龙脷叶/龍脷葉
Chinese nickname's alphabet (Nickname's Chinese characters): Longsheye/Niu'erye(龙舌叶/牛耳叶)
Latin: Sauropi Folium (Common name: Dragon's Tongue Leaf)

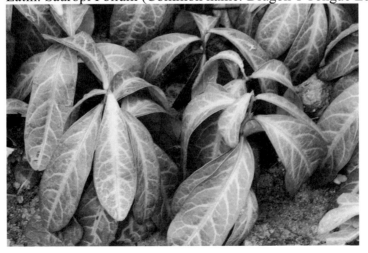

Plant: *Sauropus spatulifolius* Beille.
TCM prepared in ready-to-use forms (medicinal parts): it's dried leaf which harvested in summer or autumn.
Property and flavor: neutral; sweet, bland.
Main and collateral channels: lung and stomach meridians.

Administration and dosage: 9-15 g.
Indication: cough, sore throat, hoarse and constipation.
(The picture is only for learning and identification the herb; the specific use of the herb please consult the herbalist or health professionals)

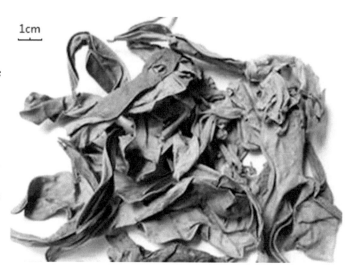

Stalactite (Zhongrushi)
Chinese phonetic alphabet/pin yin: zhōng rǔ shí

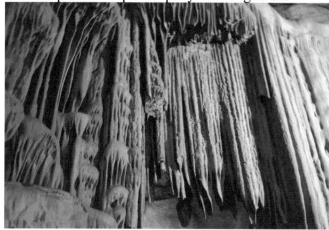

Chinese characters simplified/traditional: 钟乳石/鐘乳石
Chinese nickname's alphabet (Nickname's Chinese characters): Shizhongru(石钟乳)
Latin: Stalactitum
(Common name: Stalactite)
Mineral: main component: $CaCO_3$

TCM prepared in ready-to-use forms (medicinal parts): it's cleaned mineral.
Property and flavor: warm; sweet.
Main and collateral channels: lung, kidney and stomach meridians.
Administration and dosage: 3-9 g. It should be decocted first.

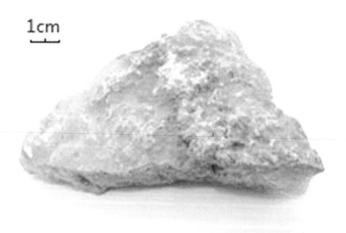

Indication: panting and cough with phlegm, stomachache with acid regurgitation and agalactia.
(The picture is only for learning and identification the herb; the specific use of the herb please consult the herbalist or health professionals)

Manchurian Lilac Bark (Baomazipi)
Chinese phonetic alphabet/pin yin: bào mǎ zǐ pí
Chinese characters simplified/traditional:暴马子皮/暴馬子皮

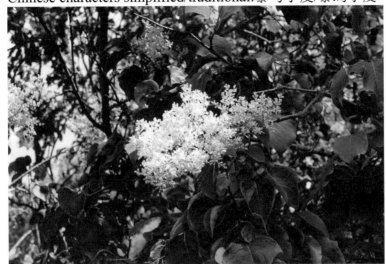

Chinese nickname's alphabet (Nickname's Chinese characters): Dingxiangpi(丁香皮)
Latin: Syringae Cortex (Common name: Manchurian Lilac Bark)

Plant: *Syringa reticulata* (Bl.) Hara. var. *mandshutica* (Maxim.) Hara.
TCM prepared in ready-to-use forms (medicinal parts): it's dried stem bark or branch bark which harvested in spring or autumn.
Property and flavor: mild cold; bitter.

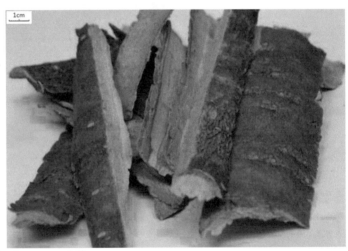

Main and collateral channels: lung meridian.
Administration and dosage: 30-45 g.
Indication: wheezing and cough with excessive phlegm.
(The picture is only for learning and identification the herb; the specific use of the herb please consult the herbalist or health professionals)

Hempleaf Negundo Chastetree Leaf (Mujingye)
Chinese phonetic alphabet/pin yin: mǔ jīng yè
Chinese characters simplified/traditional:牡荆叶/牡荊葉
Chinese nickname's alphabet (Nickname's Chinese characters): Huangjingtiao/ Wuzhigan(黄荆条/五指柑)
Latin: Viticis Negundo Folium (Common name: Hempleaf Negundo Chastetree Leaf)

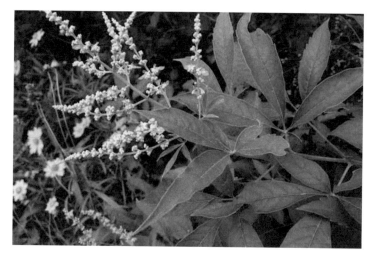

Plant: *Vitex negundo* L. var. *cannabifolia* (Sieb. et Zucc.) Hand.-Mazz.
TCM prepared in ready-to-use forms (medicinal parts): it's dried leaf which harvested in summer or autumn.
Property and flavor: neutral; mild bitter, pungent.

Main and collateral channels: lung meridian.
Administration and dosage: 9-15 g. Topical application in appropriate amount, mashed into mud. It can be used as fume-wash therapy.
Indication: cough and profuse sputum.

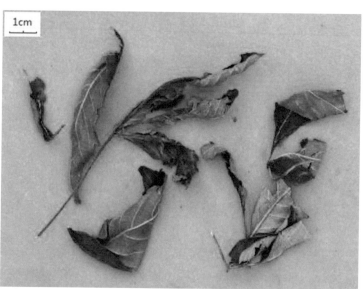

(The picture is only for learning and identification the herb; the specific use of the herb please consult the herbalist or health professionals)

An Shen Yao(安神药)-herbs to tranquilize

An Shen Yao is a kind of herbs which's the major functions are to tranquilize, and treat epilepsy, convulsion.

Cinnabar (Zhusha)
Chinese phonetic alphabet/pin yin: zhū shā

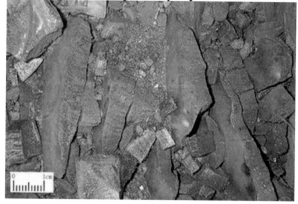

Chinese characters simplified/traditional:朱砂/朱砂
Chinese nickname's alphabet (Nickname's Chinese characters): Dansha/Chensha(丹砂/辰砂)
Latin: Cinnabaris (Common name: Cinnabar)
Mineral: main component HgS

TCM prepared in ready-to-use forms (medicinal parts): it's cleaned mineral.
Property and flavor: mild cold; sweet.
Main and collateral channels: heart meridian.
Administration and dosage: 0.1-0.5 g, it is usually used in pills or powder; used in decoction is inadvisable. Appropriate amount for topical application.
Indication: palpitations, insomnia, irritable, epilepsy, convulsion, blurred vision, stomatitis, pharyngitis, sore swollen and skin infection.
It is key herb to treat insomnia and uneasy.
Precaution and warning: toxic, large dosage or long-term administration is inadvisable. Contraindicated for pregnant woman and patients with hepatic or renal insufficiency.
(The picture is only for learning and identification the herb; the specific use of the herb please consult the herbalist or health professionals)

Magnetite (Cishi)
Chinese phonetic alphabet/pin yin: cí shí
Chinese characters simplified/traditional:磁石/磁石
Chinese nickname's alphabet (Nickname's Chinese characters): Xuanshi/ Xitieshi(玄石/吸铁石)

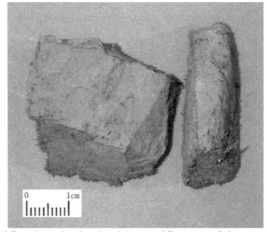

Latin: Magnetitum (Common name: Magnetite)
Mineral: main component Fe_3O_4
TCM prepared in ready-to-use forms (medicinal parts): it's cleaned mineral.
Property and flavor: cold; salty.
Main and collateral channels: liver, heart and kidney meridians.
Administration and dosage: 9-30 g. It should be decocted first.
Indication: palpitations, dizziness, blurred vision, tinnitus, insomnia, asthma.
(The picture is only for learning and identification the herb; the specific use of the herb please consult the herbalist or health professionals)

Skeleton Fossil (Longgu)

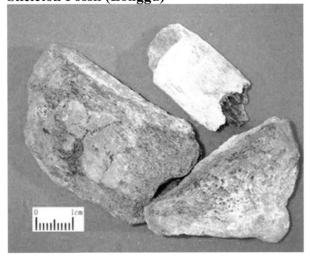

Chinese phonetic alphabet/pin yin: lóng gǔ
Chinese characters simplified/traditional:龙骨/龍骨
Chinese nickname's alphabet (Nickname's Chinese characters): Luhuyisheng/ Najiagu(陆虎遗生/那伽骨)
Latin: Draconis Os (Common name: Skeleton Fossil)
Mineral: skeleton fossil (main component: apatite and calcite)

TCM prepared in ready-to-use forms (medicinal parts): it's cleaned mineral.
Property and flavor: neutral; astringent, sweet.
Main and collateral channels: heart, liver, kidney and large intestine meridians.
Administration and dosage: 15-30 g. It should be decocted first.
Indication: epilepsy, palpitation, insomnia, delirium, dizziness, blurred vision and seminal emission.
Attention: It is illegal for some kinds of skeleton fossil's trade and destroying, use it abide by the law.
(The picture is only for learning and identification the herb; the specific use of the herb please consult the herbalist or health professionals)

Amber (Hupo)
Chinese phonetic alphabet/pin yin: hǔ pò
Chinese characters simplified/traditional:琥珀/琥珀

Chinese nickname's alphabet (Nickname's Chinese characters): Shoupo/ Jiangzhu(兽魄/江珠)
Latin: Ambrum seu Succinum (Common name: Amber or Lamber)
Mineral: fossiled resin, main component $C_{10}H_{16}O$

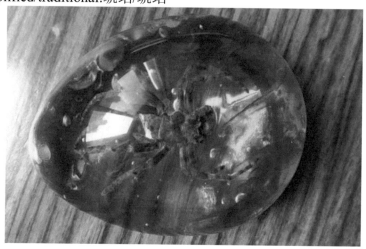

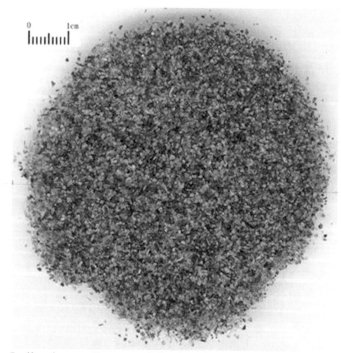

TCM prepared in ready-to-use forms (medicinal parts): it's the brownish fossil resin is taken from a pine tree which has been buried underground for a long time.
Property and flavor: neutral; sweet.
Main and collateral channels: heart, liver and bladder meridians.
Administration and dosage: 1.5-3 g. It is usually used in pill or powder.

Indication: epilepsy, palpitation, insomnia, delirium, convulsion, blood stasis, bloody strangury, dysmenorrhea and amenorrhea.

(The picture is only for learning and identification the herb; the specific use of the herb please consult the herbalist or health professionals)

Pearl (Zhenzhu)
Chinese phonetic alphabet/pin yin: zhēn zhū
Chinese characters simplified/traditional:珍珠/珍珠

Chinese nickname's alphabet (Nickname's Chinese characters): Bangzhu/ Zhuzi(蚌珠/珠子)
Latin: Margarita seu Pernulo (Common name: Pearl)
Mineral: It is formed in bivalve irritated by foreign substance.

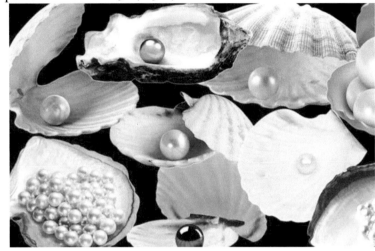

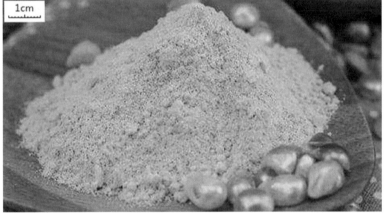

Property and flavor: cold; sweet, salty. Main and collateral channels: heart and liver meridians.

TCM prepared in ready-to-use forms (medicinal parts): pearl (or its power), it is a hard object produced within the soft tissue (specifically the mantle) of a living shelled mollusk or another animal, such as aconulariid.
Administration and dosage: 0.1-0.3 g, it is usually used in pills or powder. Topical application in appropriate amount.
Indication: insomnia, epileptic, convulsion, cataract, palpitation, sore and ulcer.
(The picture is only for learning and identification the herb; the specific use of the herb please consult the herbalist or health professionals)

Spine Date Seed (Suanzaoren)
Chinese phonetic alphabet/pin yin: suān zǎo rén
Chinese characters simplified/traditional:酸枣仁/酸棗仁
Chinese nickname's alphabet (Nickname's Chinese characters): Zaoren/ Suanzaohe(枣仁/酸枣核)
Latin: Ziziphi Spinosae Semen (Common name: Spine Date Seed or Wild Jujube Seed)

Plant: *Ziziphus jujuba* Mill. var. *spinosa* (Bge.) Hu ex H. F. Chou.
TCM prepared in ready-to-use forms (medicinal parts): it's mature seed.

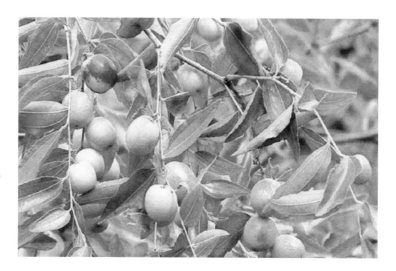

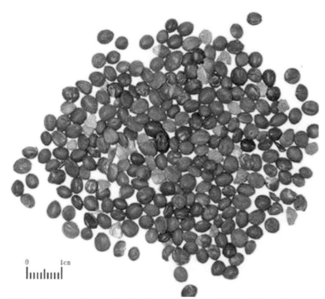

Property and flavor: neutral; sweet, acidity.
Main and collateral channels: liver, gallbladder and heart meridians.
Administration and dosage: 10-15 g.
Indication: insomnia, palpitation, hyperhidrosis, diabetes and vexation.
It is key herb to tranquilize by nourishing the heart.
It is taken as food in some part of China.

(The picture is only for learning and identification the herb; the specific use of the herb please consult the herbalist or health professionals)

Thinleaf Milkwort Root (Yuanzhi)

Chinese phonetic alphabet/pin yin: yuǎn zhì
Chinese characters simplified/traditional:远志/遠志
Chinese nickname's alphabet (Nickname's Chinese characters): Yaorao/ Jiyuan(yuan) (蓘绕/ 棘蒬(蒬))

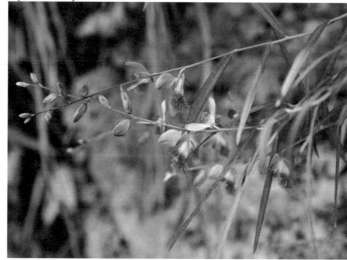

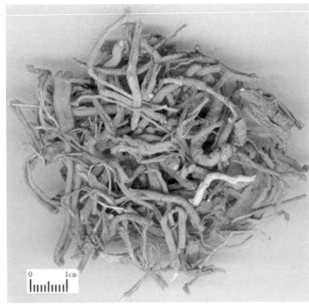

Latin: Polygalae Radix (Common name: Thinleaf Milkwort Root)
Plant: *Polygala tenuifolia* Willd. (or *Polygala sibirica* L.)
TCM prepared in ready-to-use forms (medicinal parts): it's dried root which harvested in spring or autumn.
Property and flavor: warm; bitter, pungent.
Main and collateral channels: heart, kidney and lung meridians.

Administration and dosage: 3-10 g.
Indication: insomnia, amnesia, palpitation, trance, forgetfulness, sore and ulcer, breast swelling and pain.
(The picture is only for learning and identification the herb; the specific use of the herb please consult the herbalist or health professionals)

Chinese Arbovitae Kernel (Baiziren)
Chinese phonetic alphabet/pin yin: bǎi zǐ rén
Chinese characters simplified/traditional:柏子仁/柏子仁
Chinese nickname's alphabet (Nickname's Chinese characters): Baishi/ Cebaizi(柏实/ 侧柏子)
Latin: Platycladi Semen (Common name: Chinese Arbovitae Kernel)

Plant: *Platycladus orientalis* (L.) Franco.
TCM prepared in ready-to-use forms (medicinal parts): it's dried ripe kernel.
Property and flavor: neutral; sweet.

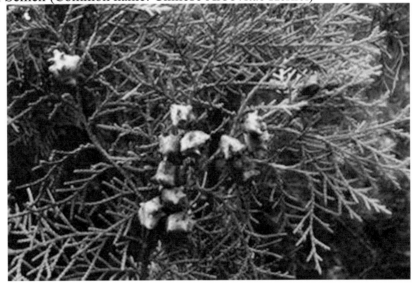

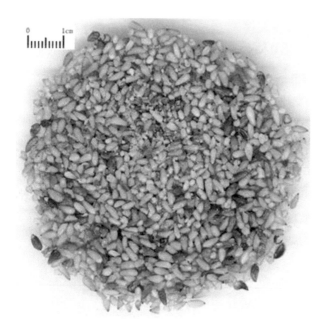

Main and collateral channels: heart, kidney and large intestine meridians.
Administration and dosage: 3-10 g.
Indication: vexation, insomnia, palpitations, night sweating, constipation.
(The picture is only for learning and identification the herb; the specific use of the herb please consult the herbalist or health professionals)

Tuber Fleeceflower Stem (Yejiaoteng)
Chinese phonetic alphabet/pin yin: yè jiāo téng
Chinese characters simplified/traditional:夜交藤/夜交藤

Chinese nickname's alphabet (Nickname's Chinese characters): Qiteng/ Shouwuteng(棋藤/首乌藤)
Latin: Polygoni Multiflori Caulis (Common name: Tuber Fleeceflower Stem)

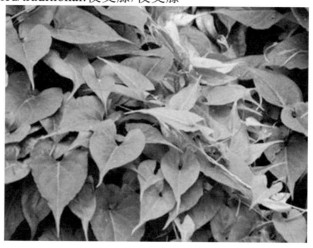

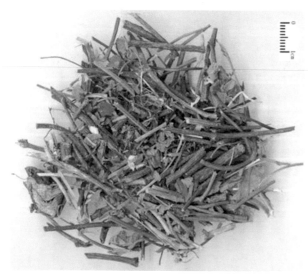

Plant: *Polygonum multiflorum* Thunb. (or *Fallopia multiflora* (Thunb.) Harald.)
TCM prepared in ready-to-use forms (medicinal parts): it's dried lianoid cane with leaf which harvested between October and December.
Property and flavor: neutral; sweet.

Main and collateral channels: heart and liver meridians.
Administration and dosage: 9-15 g. Topical application in appropriate amount, decocted for bathing.
Indication: insomnia, blood deficiency, painful *bi* disorder; external use for pruritus, rubella.
(The picture is only for learning and identification the herb; the specific use of the herb please consult the herbalist or health professionals)

Silktree Albizia Bark (Hehuanpi)
Chinese phonetic alphabet/pin yin: hé huān pí
Chinese characters simplified/traditional:合欢皮/合歡皮

Chinese nickname's
alphabet
(Nickname's Chinese
characters): Hehunpi/
Hehuanmu Pi (合昏
皮/合欢木皮)
Latin: Albiziae
Cortex (Common
name: Silktree
Albizia Bark)
Plant: *Albizia
julibrissin* Durazz.

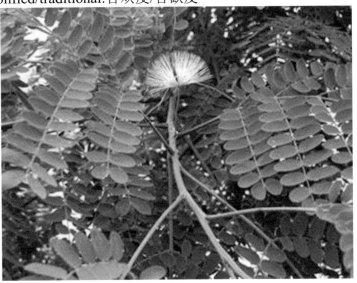

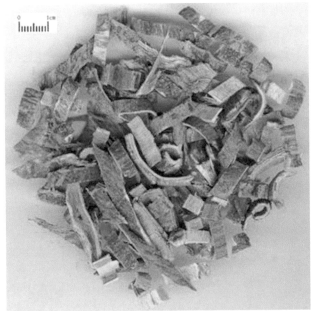

TCM prepared in
ready-to-use forms
(medicinal parts): it's dried
stem bark which harvested
in summer or autumn.
Property and flavor:
neutral; sweet.
Main and collateral
channels: heart, liver and
lung meridians.
Administration and
dosage: 6-12 g. Topical
application in appropriate
amount, ground into
powder.

Indication: insomnia, swelling and sore, depression and traumatic injury.
(The picture is only for learning and identification the herb; the specific use of the
herb please consult the herbalist or health professionals)

Coral (Shanhu)

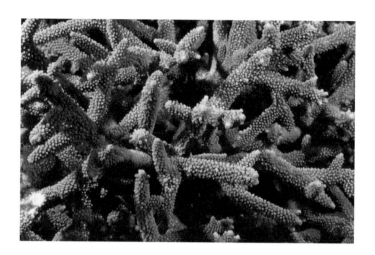

Chinese phonetic
alphabet/pin yin:
shān hú
Chinese characters
simplified/tradition
al:珊瑚/珊瑚
Latin: Coral
(Common name:
Coral)

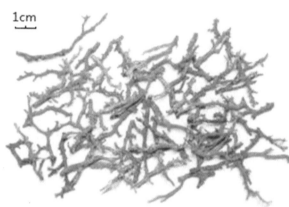

1cm

Animal: *Corallium rubrum*
(Linnaeus.) (or *Corallium
japonicum* Kishinouye. Or
other species of *Corallium.*)
TCM prepared in
ready-to-use forms
(medicinal parts): just coral,
it's calcareous skeleton
remains of marine
invertebrates in the class
Anthozoa
of phylum Cnidaria.

Property and flavor: neutral; sweet.
Administration and dosage: 0.3-0.6 g. Topical application in appropriate amount,
ground into powder and apply to *pars affecta*.
Indication: cataract, epilepsy and vomit.
Attention: to protect the environment, please don't use the herb from wild. It is illegal
for some kinds of coral's trade and destroying, use it abide by the law.
(The picture is only for learning and identification the herb; the specific use of the
herb please consult the herbalist or health professionals)

Vermiculite (Jinjingshi)

Chinese phonetic
alphabet/pin yin: jīn jīng
shí
Chinese characters
simplified/traditional:金精
石/金精石
Chinese nickname's
alphabet (Nickname's
Chinese characters):
Zhishi/ Maojin(蛭石/猫金)
Latin: Vermiculitum
(Common name:
Vermiculite)

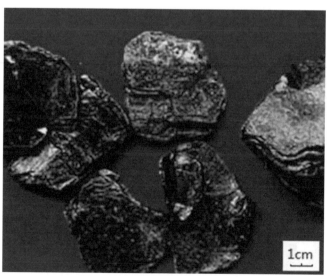

1cm

Mineral: main component $(Mg,Fe)_3[(Si,Al)_4O_{10}](OH)_2 \cdot 4H_2O$

TCM prepared in ready-to-use forms (medicinal parts): it's cleaned mineral.

Property and flavor: cold; salty.

Main and collateral channels: heart, liver and kidney meridians.

Administration and dosage: 3-6 g. It should be decocted first or used in pill or powder.

Indication: cataract, palpitation, insomnia and vexation.

Precaution and warning: slightly toxic.

(The picture is only for learning and identification the herb; the specific use of the herb please consult the herbalist or health professionals)

Fluorite (Zishiying)

Chinese phonetic alphabet/pin yin: zǐ shí yīng

Chinese characters simplified/traditional:紫石英/紫石英

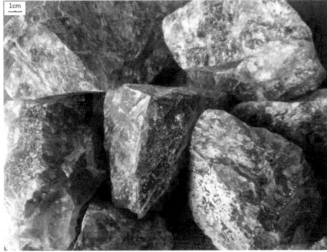

Chinese nickname's alphabet (Nickname's Chinese characters): Yingshi/ Fushi(萤石/氟石)

Latin: Fluoritum (Common name: Fluorite)

Mineral: main component CaF_2

TCM prepared in ready-to-use forms (medicinal parts): it's cleaned mineral.

Property and flavor: warm; sweet.

Main and collateral channels: kidney, heart and lung meridians.

Administration and dosage: 9-15 g. It should be decocted first.

Indication: palpitations, insomnia and vexation; relieve uneasiness of mind and body tranquilization; relieve the wheezing and cough.

(The picture is only for learning and identification the herb; the specific use of the herb please consult the herbalist or health professionals)

Lotus Plumule (Lianzixin)

Chinese phonetic alphabet/pin yin: lián zǐ xīn

Chinese characters simplified/traditional:
莲子心/蓮子心

Chinese nickname's alphabet (Nickname's Chinese characters):
Kuyi/ Lianxin(苦薏/莲心)

Latin: Nelumbinis Plumula (Common name: Lotus Plumule)

Plant: *Nelumbo nucifera* Gaertn.

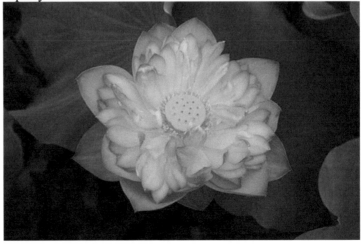

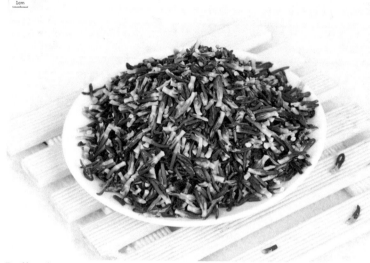

TCM prepared in ready-to-use forms (medicinal parts): it's dried young cotyledon and radicle of the ripe seed.
Property and flavor: cold; bitter.
Main and collateral channels: heart and kidney meridians.
Administration and dosage: 2-5 g.

Indication: coma, insomnia, seminal emission and hematemesis.
(The picture is only for learning and identification the herb; the specific use of the herb please consult the herbalist or health professionals)

Ping Gan Xi Feng Yao(平肝熄风药)-herbs for liver wind

Ping Gan Xi Feng Yao is a kind of herbs which's the major functions are to treat convulsion, epilepsy, dizziness, headache, dim vision.

Abalone Shell (Shijueming)

Chinese phonetic alphabet/pin yin: shí jué míng
Chinese characters simplified/traditional:石决明/石决明

Chinese nickname's alphabet (Nickname's Chinese characters): Jiukongluo/ Qianliguang/ Zhenzhumu(九孔螺 /千里光/真珠母)
Latin: Haliotidis Concha (Common name: Abalone Shell)

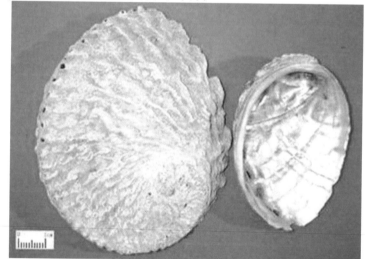

Animal: *Haliotis diversicolor* Reeve. (or *Haliotis discus hannai* Ino., *Haliotis ovina* Gmelin., *Haliotis ruber* (Leach.), *Haliotis asinina* L., *Haliotis laevigata* (Donovan.), *Haliotis gigantea discns* Reeve.)
TCM prepared in ready-to-use forms (medicinal parts): it's shell which harvested in summer or autumn.
Property and flavor: cold; salty.
Main and collateral channels: liver meridian.
Administration and dosage: 6-20 g. It should be decocted first.
Indication: headache, dizziness, red eyes, blurred vision and nyctalopia.

It is key herb to treat dizziness, red eyes and pain.
(The picture is only for learning and identification the herb; the specific use of the herb please consult the herbalist or health professionals)

Oysters Shell (Muli)
Chinese phonetic alphabet/pin yin: mǔ lì
Chinese characters simplified/traditional:牡蛎/牡蠣

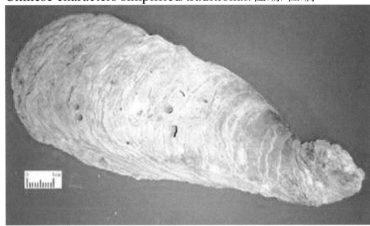

Chinese nickname's alphabet (Nickname's Chinese characters): Hao/Hailizi(蚝/海蛎子)
Latin: Ostreae Concha (Common name: Oysters Shell)

Animal: *Ostrea gigas* Thunberg. (or *Ostrea talienwhanensis* Crosse., *Ostrea rivularis* Gould.)
TCM prepared in ready-to-use forms (medicinal parts): it's shell which harvested all year round.
Property and flavor: mild cold; salty.
Main and collateral channels: liver, gallbladder and kidney meridians.
Administration and dosage: 9-30 g. It should be decocted first.
Indication: palpitation, insomnia, dizziness, tinnitus, phlegm, blood stasis, scrofula, abdominal lump; processed one can treat night sweating, seminal emission, profuse and yellow vaginal discharge, stomachache with acid regurgitation.
(The picture is only for learning and identification the herb; the specific use of the herb please consult the herbalist or health professionals)

Hematite (Zheshi)
Chinese phonetic alphabet/pin yin: zhě shí
Chinese characters simplified/traditional:赭石/赭石

Chinese nickname's alphabet (Nickname's Chinese characters): Daizheshi(代赭石)
Latin: Haematitum (Common name: Hematite)
Mineral: main component Fe_2O_3
TCM prepared in ready-to-use forms (medicinal parts): it's cleaned mineral.
Property and flavor: cold; bitter.
Main and collateral channels: liver, heart, lung and stomach meridians.

Administration and dosage: 9-30 g. It should be decocted first.

Indication: dizziness and tinnitus, vomiting, hiccup, ructation, panting, hematemesis, epistaxis and metrorrhagia with spotting.

Precaution and warning: use with caution during pregnancy.

(The picture is only for learning and identification the herb; the specific use of the herb please consult the herbalist or health professionals)

Nacre (Zhenzhumu)

Chinese phonetic alphabet/pin yin: zhēn zhū mǔ

Chinese characters simplified/traditional:珍珠母/珍珠母

Chinese nickname's alphabet (Nickname's Chinese characters): Bangke/ Mingzhumu/ Zhumu(蚌壳/明珠母/珠母)

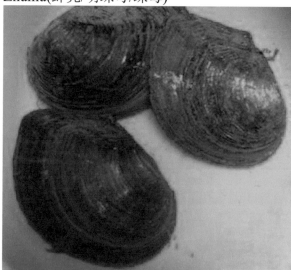

Latin: Margaritifera Concha (Common name: Nacre or Mother of Pearl)
Animal: *Hyriopsis cumingii* (Lea). (or *Cristaria plicata* (Leach.), *Pteria martensii* (Dunker.))
TCM prepared in ready-to-use forms (medicinal parts): it's shell.
Property and flavor: cold; salty.
Main and collateral channels: liver and heart meridians.
Administration and dosage: 10-25 g. It should be decocted first.

Indication: headache, dizziness, irritability, insomnia, red eyes, eye congest, and palpitations.

(The picture is only for learning and identification the herb; the specific use of the herb please consult the herbalist or health professionals)

Puncturevine Caltrop Fruit (Jili)

Chinese phonetic alphabet/pin yin: jí lí

Chinese characters simplified/traditional:蒺藜/蒺藜

Chinese nickname's alphabet (Nickname's Chinese characters): Cijili/ Jilizi/ Baijili (刺蒺藜/蒺藜子/白蒺藜)

Latin: Tribuli Fructus (Common name: Puncturevine Caltrop Fruit)

TCM prepared in ready-to-use forms (medicinal parts): it's dried ripe fruit.

Plant: *Tribulus terrestris* L.

Property and flavor: mild warm; pungent.

Main and collateral channels: liver meridian.

Administration and dosage: 6-10 g.

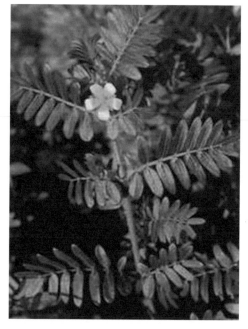

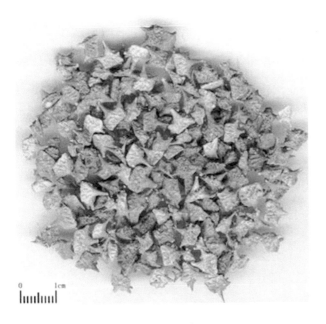

Indication: headache, dizziness, chest pain, acute mastitis, red eye, cataract, rubella, itching. It is key herb to improve eyesight.
Precaution and warning: slightly toxic. (The picture is only for learning and identification the herb; the specific use of the herb please consult the herbalist or health professionals)

Dogbane Leaf (Luobumaye)

Chinese phonetic alphabet/pin yin: luó bù má yè

Chinese characters simplified/traditional:罗布麻叶/羅布麻葉

Chinese nickname's alphabet (Nickname's Chinese characters): Chayehua/ Zeqima/ Yechaye(茶叶花/泽漆麻/野茶叶)

Latin: Apocyni Veneti Folium (Common name: Dogbane Leaf)

Plant: *Apocynum venetum* L.

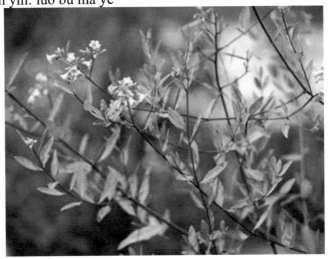

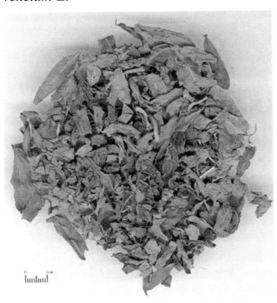

TCM prepared in ready-to-use forms (medicinal parts): it's dried leaf which harvested in summer.
Property and flavor: cool; sweet, bitter.
Main and collateral channels: liver meridian.
Administration and dosage: 6-12 g.
Indication: dizziness, palpitations, insomnia, edema, oliguria and hypertension.
(The picture is only for learning and identification the herb; the specific use of the herb please consult the herbalist or health professionals)

Antelope Horn (Lingyangjiao)

Chinese phonetic alphabet/pin yin: líng yáng jiǎo

Chinese characters simplified/traditional:羚羊角/羚羊角

Chinese nickname's alphabet (Nickname's Chinese characters): Lingjiao(羚角) Latin: Saigae Tataricae Cornu (Common name: Antelope Horn) Animal: *Saiga tatarica* Linnaeus. TCM prepared in ready-to-use forms (medicinal parts): it's horn.

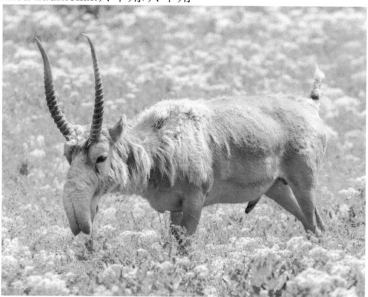

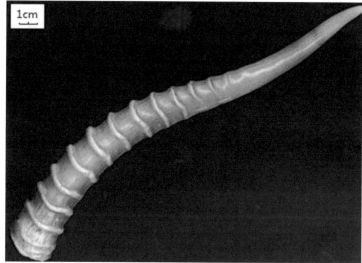

Property and flavor: cold; sally.
Main and collateral channels: liver and heart meridians.
Administration and dosage: 1-3 g, decocted alone for more than 2 hours. Ground into powder or with water: 0.3-0.6 g per time.

Indication: fever, epilepsy, syncope, eclamptic, convulsions, headache, dizziness, red eyes, scales, dim vision, carbuncle, manic psychosis, sore and skin infection.
It is key herb to treat fever and epilepsy.

Attention: to protect the rare wild animals, don't use it from wild animal.
(The picture is only for learning and identification the herb; the specific use of the herb please consult the herbalist or health professionals)

Gambir Plant (Gouteng)

Chinese phonetic alphabet/pin yin: gōu téng

Chinese characters simplified/traditional:钩藤/鉤藤

Chinese nickname's alphabet (Nickname's Chinese characters): Diaogouteng/ Yingzhuafeng(钓钩藤/鹰爪风)

Latin: Uncariae Ramulus cum Uncis (Common name: Gambir Plant)

Plant: *Uncaria rhynchophylla* (Miq.) Jacks. (or *Uncaria macrophylla* Wall., *Uncaria hirsuta* Havil., *Uncaria sinesis* (Oliv.) Havil., *Uncaria sessilifructus* Roxb.) TCM prepared in ready-to-use forms (medicinal parts): it's dried stalk with hook which harvested in autumn or winter.

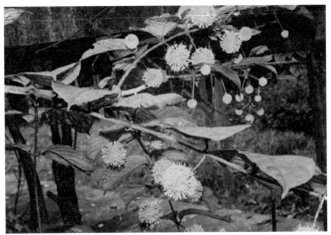

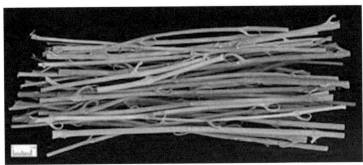

Property and flavor: cool; sweet.
Main and collateral channels: liver and pericardium meridians.
Administration and dosage: 3-12 g, added when the decoction is nearly done.

Indication: headache, epilepsy, dizziness, fever, spasm, convulsions, eclampsia and hypertension.
It is key herb to relieve convulsion with fever.
(The picture is only for learning and identification the herb; the specific use of the herb please consult the herbalist or health professionals)

Tall Gastrodia Tuber (Tianma)
Chinese phonetic alphabet/pin yin: tiān má
Chinese characters simplified/traditional:天麻/天麻
Chinese nickname's alphabet (Nickname's Chinese characters): Chijian/ Guiduyou/Mingtianma(赤箭/鬼督邮/明天麻)
Latin: Gastrodiae Rhizoma (Common name: Tall Gastrodia Tuber)
Plant: *Gastrodia elata* Bl.
TCM prepared in ready-to-use forms (medicinal parts): it's dried tuber which harvested in winter or spring.
Property and flavor: neutral; sweet.
Main and collateral channels: liver meridian.
Administration and dosage: 3-10 g.

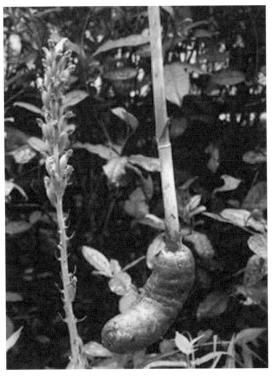

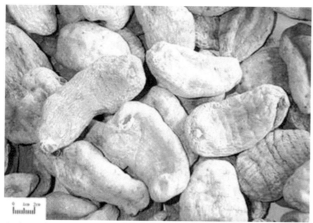

Indication: headache, dizziness, limb numbness, infantile convulsion, epilepsy, tetanus and arthralgia.
It is key herb to treat vertigo.
Attention:
to protect the rare wild plant, please don't use the herb from wild plant.

(The picture is only for learning and identification the herb; the specific use of the herb please consult the herbalist or health professionals)

Scorpion (Quanxie)

Chinese phonetic alphabet/pin yin: quán xiē

Chinese characters simplified/traditional:全蝎/全蝎

Chinese nickname's alphabet (Nickname's Chinese characters): Xiezi(蝎子)

Latin: Scorpio (Common name: Scorpion)

Animal: *Buthus martensii* Karsch.

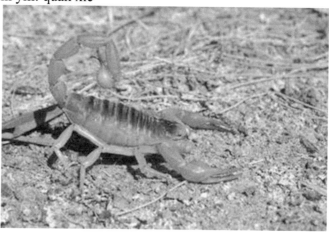

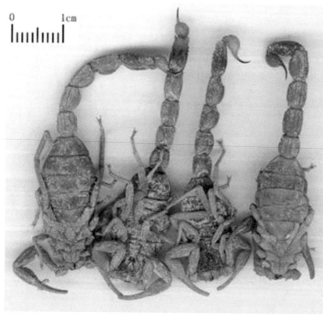

TCM prepared in ready-to-use forms (medicinal parts): it's dried whole insect.
Property and flavor: neutral; pungent.
Main and collateral channels: liver meridian.
Administration and dosage: 3-6 g.
Indication: spasm, apoplexy, hemiplegia, tetanus, rheumatoid, arthritis, headache, sore, scrofula, convulsion, hemiplegia, tetanus, sore and ulcer.

It is key herb to treat spasms or twitching.
Precaution and warning: toxic. Contraindicated during pregnancy.

Attention: to protect the rare wild animals, please don't use it from wild animal. (The picture is only for learning and identification the herb; the specific use of the herb please consult the herbalist or health professionals)

Centipede (Wugong)

Chinese phonetic alphabet/pin yin: wú gōng
Chinese characters simplified/traditional:蜈蚣/蜈蚣
Chinese nickname's alphabet (Nickname's Chinese characters): Tianlong/ Baijiao(天龙/ 百脚)

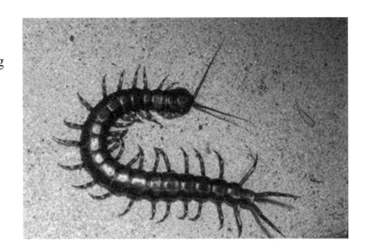

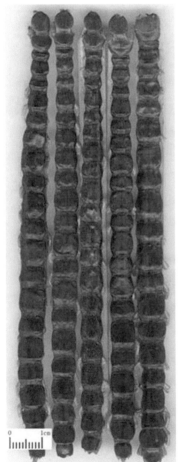

Latin: Scolopendra (Common name: Centipede)
Animal: *Scolopendra subspinipes mutilans* L. Koch.
TCM prepared in ready-to-use forms (medicinal parts): it's dried whole insect.
Property and flavor: warm; pungent.
Main and collateral channels: liver meridian.
Administration and dosage: 3-5 g.
Indication: convulsion, spasm, apoplexy, hemiplegia, tetanus, rheumatoid, arthritis, headache, sore, scrofula, insect and snake bites.
It is key herb to treat spasms or twitching.
Precaution and warning: toxic.
Contraindicated during pregnancy.
Attention: to protect the rare wild animals, please don't use it from wild animal.
(The picture is only for learning and identification the herb; the specific use of the herb please consult the herbalist or health professionals)

Earthworm (Dilong)
Chinese phonetic alphabet/pin yin: dì lóng
Chinese characters simplified/traditional:地龙/地龍

Chinese nickname's alphabet (Nickname's Chinese characters): Qiuyin(蚯蚓)
Latin: Pheretima (Common name: Earthworm)
Animal: *Pheretima aspergillum* (E. Perrier.)
(or *Pheretima vulgaris* Chen., *Pheretima guillelmi* (Michaelsen.), *Pheretima pectinifera* Michaelsen.)

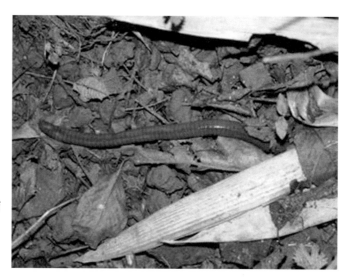

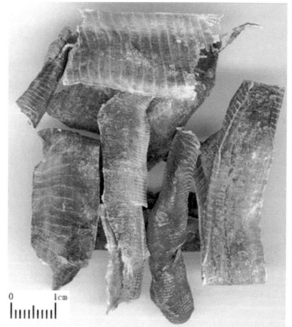

TCM prepared in ready-to-use forms (medicinal parts): it's dried body.
Property and flavor: cold; salty.
Main and collateral channels: liver, spleen and bladder meridians.
Administration and dosage: 5-10 g.
Indication: fever, convulsion, epilepsy, coma, joint pain, numbness, hemiplegia, cough, oliguria, edema and hypertension.
(The picture is only for learning and identification the herb; the specific use of the herb please consult the herbalist or health professionals)

Stiff Silkworm (Jiangcan)
Chinese phonetic alphabet/pin yin: jiāng cán

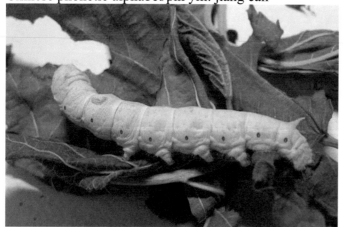

Chinese characters simplified/traditional: 僵蚕/僵蠶
Chinese nickname's alphabet (Nickname's Chinese characters): Baijiangcan/ Tianchong/ Jiangchong(白僵蚕/ 天虫/僵虫)

Latin: Bombyx Batryticatus (Common name: Stiff Silkworm or Silkworm infected by fungus (*Beauveria bassiana* (Bals.) Vuillant))

Herb: larva *Bombyx mori* Linnaeus. died of infection of *Beauveria bassiana* (Bals.) Vuillant.

TCM prepared in ready-to-use forms (medicinal parts): it's dried fatal infected whole body.

Property and flavor: neutral; salty, pungent.

Main and collateral channels: liver, lung and stomach meridians.

Administration and dosage: 5-10 g.

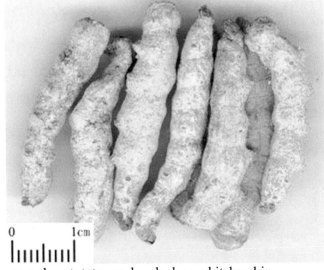

Indication: epilepsy, convulsion, sore throat, tetanus, headache and itchy skin.

(The picture is only for learning and identification the herb; the specific use of the herb please consult the herbalist or health professionals)

Erosaria Shell (Zibeichi)

Chinese phonetic alphabet/pin yin: zǐ bèi chǐ

Chinese characters simplified/traditional:紫贝齿/紫貝齒

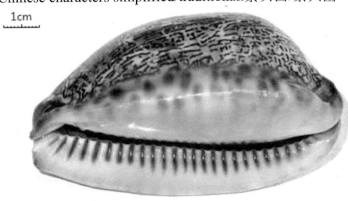

Chinese nickname's alphabet (Nickname's Chinese characters): Zibei/ Wenbei/ Zibeizi(紫贝/文贝/紫贝子)

Latin: Cypraeae Violacae Concha (Common name: Erosaria Shell or Cowrie Shell)

Animal: *Cypraea lymx* (Linnaeus.) (or *Cypraea tigris* Linnaeus., *Mauritia arabica* (Linnaeus.))

TCM prepared in ready-to-use forms (medicinal parts): it's shell.

Property and flavor: neutral; salty.

Main and collateral channels: liver meridian.

Administration and dosage: 10-15 g. It should be decocted first or used in pill or powder.

Indication: insomnia, dizziness, red eyes, scales.

(The picture is only for learning and identification the herb; the specific use of the herb please consult the herbalist or health professionals)

Henbane Seed (Tianxianzi)

Chinese phonetic alphabet/pin yin: tiān xiān zǐ

Chinese characters simplified/traditional:天仙子/天仙子

Chinese nickname's alphabet (Nickname's Chinese characters): Liangdangzi/ Miguanzi/ Xunyazi(莨菪子/米罐子/熏牙子)

Latin: Hyoscyami Semen (Common name: Henbane Seed)
Plant: *Hyoscyamus niger* L.
TCM prepared in ready-to-use forms (medicinal parts): it's dried mature seed.
Property and flavor: warm; bitter, pungent.
Main and collateral channels: heart, stomach and liver meridians.

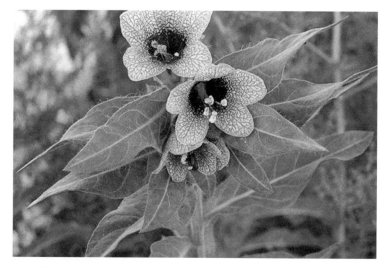

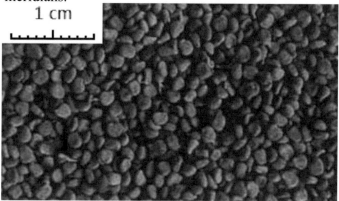

1 cm

Administration and dosage: 0.06-0.6 g.
Indication: painful spasm in abdominal, wheezing cough, depressive psychosis and manic psychosis.
Attention:
to protect the rare wild pla nt, please don't use the herb from wild plant.

Precaution and warning: highly toxic. Contraindicated in patients suffering from heart disease, tachypragia, glaucoma or pregnant woman.
(The picture is only for learning and identification the herb; the specific use of the herb please consult the herbalist or health professionals)

Common St. John's Wort Herb (Guanyejinsitao)
Chinese phonetic alphabet/pin yin: guàn yè jīn sī táo
Chinese characters simplified/traditional:贯叶金丝桃/貫葉金絲桃

Chinese nickname's alphabet (Nickname's Chinese characters): Guanyelianqiao/ Qiancenglou/ Ganshanbian(贯叶连翘/千层楼/赶山鞭)
Latin: Hyperici Perforati Herba (Common name: Common St. John's Wort Herb)

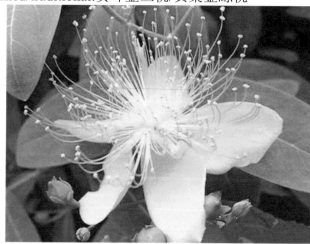

Plant: *Hypericum perforatum* L.
TCM prepared in ready-to-use forms (medicinal parts): it's dried up-ground-part

which harvested in summer or autumn at flowering.

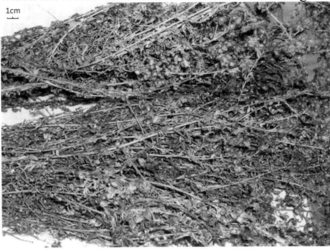

Property and flavor: cold; pungent.
Main and collateral channels: liver meridian.
Administration and dosage: 2-3 g.
Indication: moodiness, joint pain and swelling and acute mastitis; lactagogue.
(The picture is only for learning and identification the herb; the specific use of the herb please consult the herbalist or health professionals)

Hedge Prinsepia Nut (Ruiren)

Chinese phonetic alphabet/pin yin: ruǐ rén
Chinese characters simplified/traditional:蕤仁/蕤仁
Chinese nickname's alphabet (Nickname's Chinese characters): Ruihe/ Bairuiren/ Yuren(蕤核/白桵仁/棫仁)

Latin: Prinsepiae Nux (Common name: Hedge Prinsepia Nut)
Plant: *Prinsepia uniflora* Batal. (or *Prinsepia uniflora* Batal. var. *serrata* Rehd.)
TCM prepared in ready-to-use forms (medicinal parts): it's dried ripe kernel which harvested in autumn.

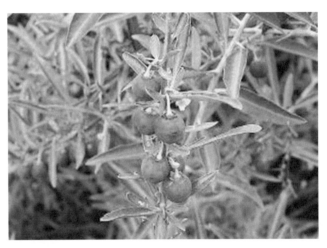

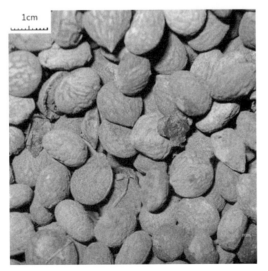

Property and flavor: mild cold; sweet.
Main and collateral channels: liver meridian.
Administration and dosage: 5-9 g.
Indication: red painful eyes, blepharitis, dim or blurring vision and photophobia.
(The picture is only for learning and identification the herb; the specific use of the herb please consult the herbalist or health professionals)

Fruit of Silybum Marianum (Shuifeiji)

Chinese phonetic alphabet/pin yin: shuǐ fēi jì

Chinese characters simplified/traditional:水飞蓟/水飛薊

Chinese nickname's alphabet (Nickname's Chinese characters): Naiji/ Laoshujin(奶蓟/老鼠筋)

Latin: Silybi Fructus (Common name: Fruit of Silybum Marianum)

Plant: *Silybum marianum* (L.) Gaertn.

TCM prepared in ready-to-use forms (medicinal parts): it's dried ripe fruit.

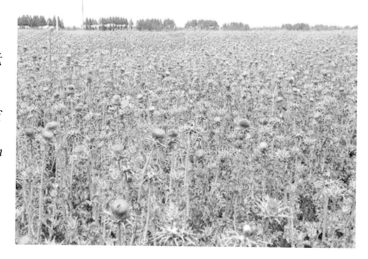

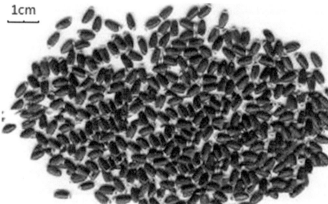

Property and flavor: cool; bitter.

Main and collateral channels: liver and gallbladder meridians.

Administration and dosage: used for preparation of Chinese patent medicine.

Indication: hypochondriac pain, jaundice and hepatitis.

(The picture is only for learning and identification the herb; the specific use of the herb please consult the herbalist or health professionals)

Mile Swertia Herb (Qingyedan)

Chinese phonetic alphabet/pin yin: qīng yè dǎn

Chinese characters simplified/traditional:青叶胆/青葉膽

Chinese nickname's alphabet (Nickname's Chinese characters): Ganyancao/ Qingyudan/Qidanyao(肝炎草/青鱼胆/七疸药)

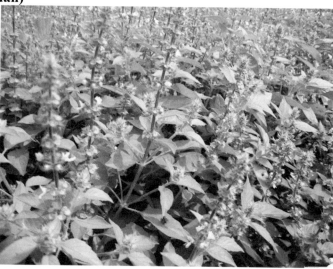

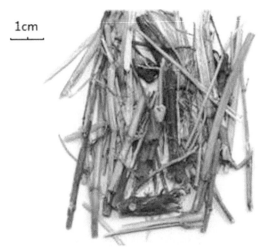

1cm

Latin: Swertiae Mileensis Herba (Common name: Mile Swertia Herb)
Plant: *Swertia mileensis* T. N. Ho et W. L. Shih.
TCM prepared in ready-to-use forms (medicinal parts): it's dried herb which harvested in autumn.
Property and flavor: cold; bitter, sweet.
Main and collateral channels: liver, gallbladder and bladder meridians.

Administration and dosage: 10-15 g.
Indication: jaundice, gallbladder distention, hypochondriac pain and pyretic stranguria with pain.
Precaution and warning: used with cautiously in people with deficiency and cold.
(The picture is only for learning and identification the herb; the specific use of the herb please consult the herbalist or health professionals)

Kai Qiao Yao(开窍药)-herbs for inducing resuscitation
Kai Qiao Yao is a kind of herbs which's the major functions are to treat coma, epilepsy, hemiplegia, apoplexy.

Musk (Shexiang)
Chinese phonetic alphabet/pin yin: shè xiāng

Chinese characters simplified/traditional:麝香/麝香
Chinese nickname's alphabet (Nickname's Chinese characters): Dangmenzi/ Xiangqizi(当门子/香脐子)
Latin: Moschus
(Common name: Musk)

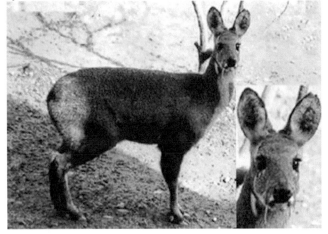

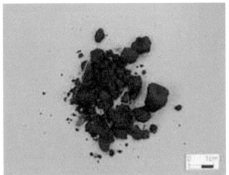

Animal: *Moschus berezovskii* Flerov. (or *Moschus moschiferus* L., *Moschus sifanicus* Przewalki.)
TCM prepared in ready-to-use forms (medicinal parts): it's dried adult male animal's secretion or secretory gland.
Property and flavor: warm; pungent.

← secretion

Main and collateral channels: heart and spleen meridians. Administration and dosage: 0.03-0.1 g, usually used in pills or powder. Appropriate amount for topical application. Indication: coma, apoplexy, syncope, amenorrhea, abdominal pain, dystocia, heartache, carbuncle, scrofula, sore throat, pain or flutter, arthralgia, numbness and traumatic injuries.

secretory gland ⟶

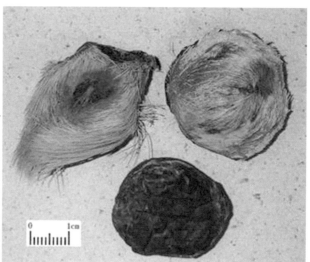

It is key herb to induce resuscitation.

Precaution and warning: contraindicate with pregnant woman.

Attention: to protect the rare wild animals, don't use it from wild animal.

(The picture is only for learning and identification the herb; the specific use of the herb please consult the herbalist or health professionals)

Borneol (Bingpian)
Chinese phonetic alphabet/pin yin: bīng piàn

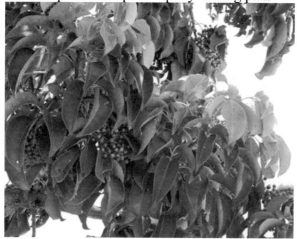

Chinese characters simplified/traditional:冰片/冰片
Chinese nickname's alphabet (Nickname's Chinese characters): Longnao(龙脑)
Latin: Borneolum (Common name: Borneol)
Plant: *Cinnamomum camphora* (L.) Presl. (or *Dryobalanop sarornatica* Gaerta. f., *Blumea balsamifera* DC.)

TCM prepared in ready-to-use forms (medicinal parts): it's refined crystal get form branches and leaves, main component: $C_{10}H_{18}O$.
Property and flavor: cool; pungent, bitter.
Main and collateral channels: heart, spleen and lung meridians.

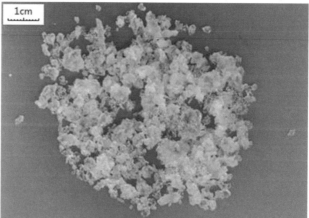

Administration and dosage: 0.3-0.9 g, usually used in pills or powder. Appropriate

amount for topical application, ground into powder and apply to *pars affecta*.
Indication: fever, coma, convulsion due to phlegm syncope, apoplexy, red eyes, aphtha, sore throat, heart pain and ear pus.
Precaution and warning: use with caution during pregnancy.
Attachment: Synthetic Borneol is the production of turpentine which is made by a series of chemical methods, its $C_{10}H_{18}O$ content should not less 55%.
(The picture is only for learning and identification the herb; the specific use of the herb please consult the herbalist or health professionals)

Grassleaf Sweetflag Rhizome (Shichangpu)

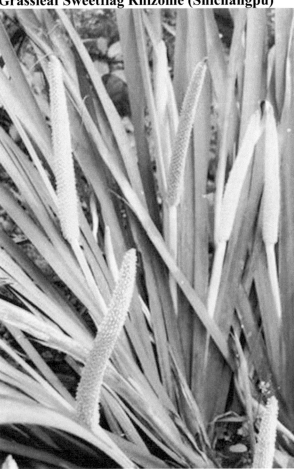

Chinese phonetic alphabet/pin yin: shí chāng pú
Chinese characters simplified/traditional:石菖蒲/石菖蒲
Chinese nickname's alphabet (Nickname's Chinese characters): Jiujiechangpu/ Shuijianchangpu/ Shanchangpu(九节菖蒲/水剑菖蒲/山菖蒲)
Latin: Acori Tatarinowii Rhizoma (Common name: Grassleaf Sweetflag Rhizome)
Plant: *Acorus tatarinowii* Schott.
TCM prepared in ready-to-use forms (medicinal parts): it's dried rhizome which harvested in autumn or winter.
Property and flavor: warm; pungent, bitter.
Main and collateral channels: heart and stomach meridians.

Administration and dosage: 3-10 g.
Indication: diarrhea, coma, epilepsy, insomnia, tinnitus, forgetfulness, traumatic injury and carbuncles; appetizer.

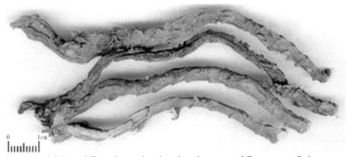

(The picture is only for learning and identification the herb; the specific use of the herb please consult the herbalist or health professionals)

Storax (Suhexiang)

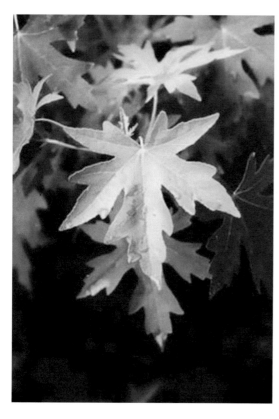

Chinese phonetic alphabet/pin yin: sū hé xiāng

Chinese characters simplified/traditional:苏合香/蘇合香

Chinese nickname's alphabet (Nickname's Chinese characters): Suheyou(苏合油)

Latin: Styrax (Common name: Storax)

Plant: *Liquidambar orientalis* Mill.

TCM prepared in ready-to-use forms (medicinal parts): it's purified balsam obtained from the truck.

Property and flavor: warm; pungent.

Main and collateral channels: heart and spleen meridians.

Administration and dosage: 0.3-1 g, used in pills or powder.

Indication: sputum, faint, heart pain, epilepsy; aromatic resuscitation.
It is key herb to treat coma with body and limbs cold.
(The picture is only for learning and identification the herb; the specific use of the herb please consult the herbalist or health professionals)

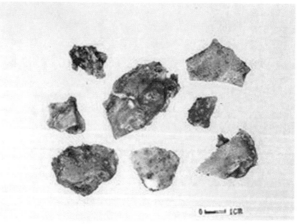

Benzoin (Anxixiang)

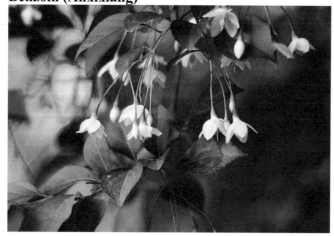

Chinese phonetic alphabet/pin yin: ān xī xiāng

Chinese characters simplified/traditional: 安息香/安息香

Chinese nickname's alphabet (Nickname's Chinese characters): Zhuobeiluoxiang(拙贝罗香)

Latin: Benzoinum (Common name: Benzoin)

Plant: *Styrax tonkinensis* (Pierre.) Craib. ex Hart.

TCM prepared in ready-to-use forms (medicinal parts): it's dried resin collected from the truck.

Property and flavor: neutral; pungent, bitter.

Main and collateral channels: heart and spleen meridians.

Administration and dosage: 0.6-1.5 g, generally used in pills or powder.

Indication: syncope, coma, apoplexy, heart pain and infantile convulsion.

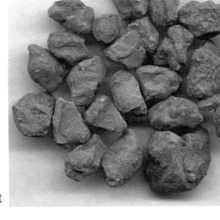

(The picture is only for learning and identification the herb; the specific use of the herb please consult the herbalist or health professionals)

Sandalwood (Tanxiang)

Chinese phonetic alphabet/pin yin: tán xiāng

Chinese characters simplified/traditional:檀香/檀香

Chinese nickname's alphabet (Nickname's Chinese characters): Baitan/ Yuxiang(白檀/浴香)

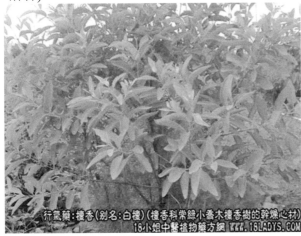

Latin: Santali Albi Lignum (Common name: Sandalwood)

Plant: *Santalum album* L.

TCM prepared in ready-to-use forms (medicinal parts): it's dried heart wood with oil obtained from the truck.

Property and flavor: warm; pungent.

Main and collateral channels: spleen, stomach, heart and lung meridians.

Administration and dosage: 2-5 g. It can be used for fumigating therapy.

Indication: heart pain, pain in the epigastrium and abdomen, dysphagia and vomiting.

Attention: to protect the rare wild plant, please don't use the herb from wild plant.

(The picture is only for learning and identification the herb; the specific use of the herb please consult the herbalist or health professionals)

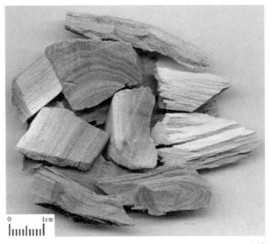

Bu Yi Yao(补益药)- tonic

Bu Yi Yao is a kind of herbs which's the major functions are tonic, build up a good physique and improve one's health (**caution**: not all tonic is good for everyone).

Ginseng (Renshen)

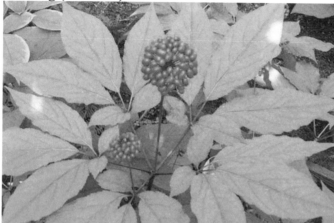

Chinese phonetic alphabet/pin yin: rén shēn
Chinese characters simplified/traditional:人参/人參
Chinese nickname's alphabet (Nickname's Chinese characters): Tujing/ Shencao/ Huangshen/ Dijing(土精/神草/黄参/地精)

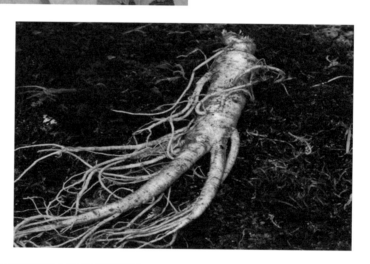

Latin: Ginseng Radix et Rhizoma (Common name: Ginseng)
Plant: *Panax ginseng* C. A. Mey
TCM prepared in ready-to-use forms (medicinal parts): it's dried root which harvested in September or October.

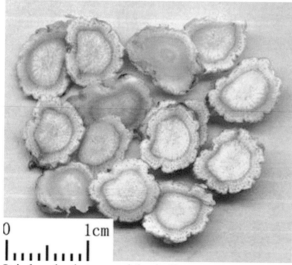

0   1cm

Property and flavor: mild warm; sweet, mild bitter.
Main and collateral channels: spleen, lung, heart and kidney meridians.
Administration and dosage: 3-9 g. Decocted separately and added it into decoction; or ground it into powder for oral administration: 2 g per time, twice a day.
Indication: collapse caused by weak, cold limbs, cough, diabetes, chronic insomnia, cardiogenic shock and palpitation; appetizer.

It is key herb to nourish vitality.
It is taken as food in some part of China.
Precaution and warning: incompatible with Black False Hellebore and Flying

Squirrel's Faeces.

Attachment: Red Ginseng is the steamed and dried root of cultivar *Panax ginseng* C. A. Mey.

(The picture is only for learning and identification the herb; the specific use of the herb please consult the herbalist or health professionals)

Tangshen (Dangshen)
Chinese phonetic alphabet/pin yin: dǎng shēn
Chinese characters simplified/traditional:党参/黨参

Chinese nickname's alphabet (Nickname's Chinese characters): Shangdangrenshen/ Shitoushen/ Zhonglingcao(上党人参/狮头参/中灵草)
Latin: Codonopsis Radix (Common name: Tangshen)

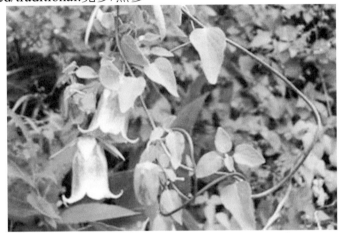

Plant: *Codonopsis pilosula* (Franch.) Nannf. (or *Codonopsis pilosula* Nannf. var. *modesta* (Nannf.) L. T. Shen., *Codonopsis tangshen* Oliv.)

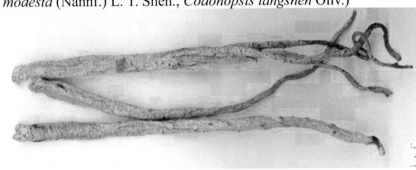

TCM prepared in ready-to-use forms (medicinal parts): it's dried root which harvested in autumn.

Property and flavor: neutral; sweet.
Main and collateral channels: lung and spleen meridians.
Administration and dosage: 9-30 g.
Indication: palpitations, shortness of breath, asthma and cough, less food intake, diabetes, weakness and fatigue.
Precaution and warning: incompatible with Black False Hellebore.

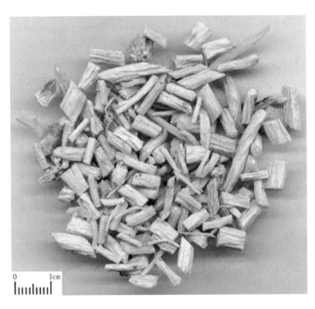

(The picture is only for learning and identification the herb; the specific use of the herb please consult the herbalist or health professionals)

Medicinal Changium Root (Mingdangshen)

Chinese phonetic alphabet/pin yin: míng dǎng shēn
Chinese characters simplified/traditional:明党参/明黨參

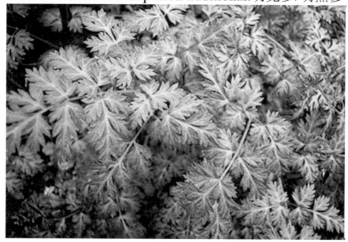

Chinese nickname's alphabet (Nickname's Chinese characters): Shanluobo/ Fenshashen(山萝卜/粉沙参)
Latin: Changii Radix (Common name: Medicinal Changium Root)
Plant: *Changium smyrnioides* Wolff.

TCM prepared in ready-to-use forms (medicinal parts): it's dried root which harvested in April and May.
Property and flavor: mild cold; sweet, mild bitter.
Main and collateral channels: lung, spleen and liver meridians.
Administration and dosage: 6-12 g.
Indication: cough, vomiting, indigestion, dizziness, sore and ulcer.
(The picture is only for learning and identification the herb; the specific use of the herb please consult the herbalist or health professionals)

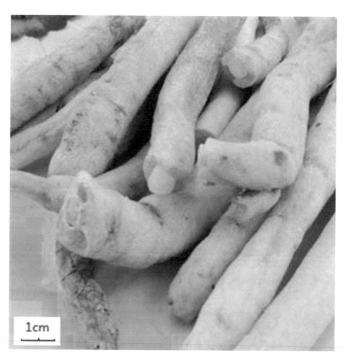

Milkvetch Root (Huangqi)

Chinese phonetic alphabet/pin yin: huáng qí
Chinese characters simplified/traditional:黄芪/黃芪
Chinese nickname's alphabet (Nickname's Chinese characters): Shuzhi/ Baiben/ Baiyaomian(蜀脂/百本/百药棉)
Latin: Astragali Radix (Common name: Milkvetch Root)

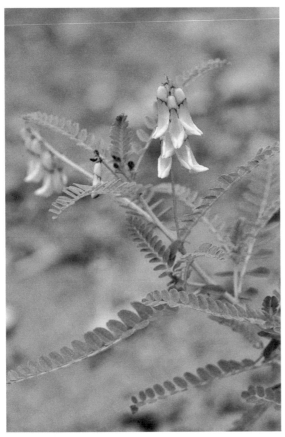

Plant: *Astragalus membranaceus* (Fisch.) Bunge. (or *Astragalus membranaceus* (Fisch.) Bunge. var. *mongholicus* (Bge.) Hsiao.)
TCM prepared in ready-to-use forms (medicinal parts): it's dried root which harvested in spring or autumn.
Property and flavor: mild warm; sweet.
Main and collateral channels: lung and spleen meridians.
Administration and dosage: 9-30 g.
Indication: night sweating, chronic diarrhea, hemiplegia, arthralgia, numbness, edema, weakness, carbuncle and cough.
Attachment: Processing of Prepared Milkvetch Root: stir bake the slice of Milkvetch Root with honey until no more sticky to fingers.

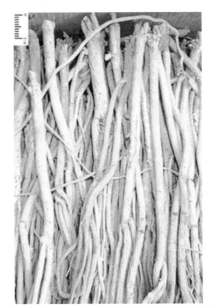
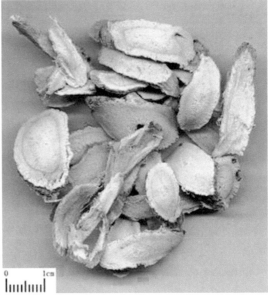

(The picture is only for learning and identification the herb; the specific use of the herb please consult the herbalist or health professionals)

Largehead Atractylodes Rhizome (Baizhu)
Chinese phonetic alphabet/pin yin: bái zhù
Chinese characters simplified/traditional:白术/白朮
Chinese nickname's alphabet (Nickname's Chinese characters): Zhu/ Dongbaizhu(术/冬白术)

Latin: Atractylodis Macrocephalae Rhizoma (Common name: Largehead Atractylodes Rhizome)
Plant: *Atractylodes macrocephala* Koidz.
TCM prepared in ready-to-use forms (medicinal parts): it's dried rhizome which harvested in November or December.

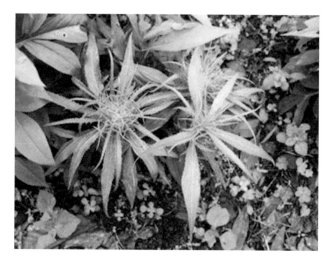

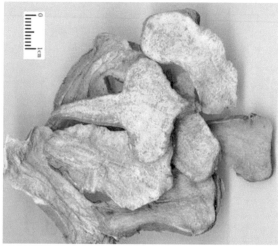

Main and collateral channels: spleen and stomach meridians.
Administration and dosage: 6-12 g.
Indication: diarrhea, excessive phlegm, dizziness, edema, night sweating, fetal irritability; appetizer.
(The picture is only for learning and identification the herb; the specific use of the herb please consult the herbalist or health professionals)

Common Yam Rhizome (Shanyao)
Chinese phonetic alphabet/pin yin: shān yào

Chinese characters simplified/traditional:山药/山藥
Chinese nickname's alphabet (Nickname's Chinese characters): Shuyu/ Shanyu/ Huai(Huai)shanyao(薯蓣/山芋/淮(怀)山药)
Latin: Dioscoreae Rhizoma (Common name: Common Yam Rhizome or Chinese Yam Rhizome)
Plant: *Dioscorea opposita* Thunb.

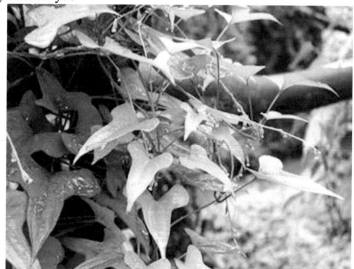

TCM prepared in ready-to-use forms (medicinal parts): it's dried rhizome which harvested in winter.
Property and flavor: neutral; sweet.
Main and collateral channels: spleen, lung and kidney meridians.

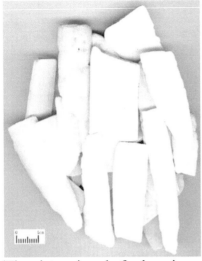

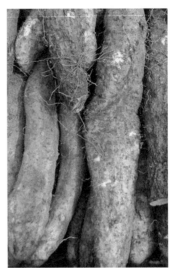

Administration and dosage: 15-30 g.
Indication: diarrhea, spermatorrhea, leucorrhea, thirst, impotence, cough and dyspnea; appetizer.
It is taken as food in some part of China.

(The picture is only for learning and identification the herb; the specific use of the herb please consult the herbalist or health professionals)

Panthaica Yam Rhizome (Huangshanyao)
Chinese phonetic alphabet/pin yin: huáng shān yào
Chinese characters simplified/traditional:黄山药/黄山藥

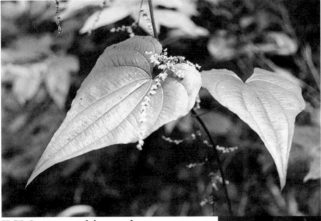

Chinese nickname's alphabet (Nickname's Chinese characters): Huangjiang/Jianghuangcao(黄姜/姜黄草)
Latin: Dioscorea Panthaicae Rhizoma (Common name: Panthaica Yam Rhizome)
Plant: *Dioscorea panthaica* Prain et Burk.

TCM prepared in ready-to-use forms (medicinal parts): it's dried rhizome which harvested in autumn.
Property and flavor: neutral; bitter, mild pungent.
Main and collateral channels: stomach and heart meridians.
Administration and dosage: 15-30 g. Topical application in appropriate amount, mashed and applied to *pars affecta*.

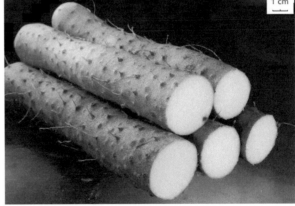

Indication: stomachache, vomiting and diarrhea with abdominal pain, traumatic injuries; external use for abscess, swelling and toxin, scrofula, phlegm nodule.
(The picture is only for learning and identification the herb; the specific use of the herb please consult the herbalist or health professionals)

Liquorice Root (Gancao)
Chinese phonetic alphabet/pin yin: gān cǎo

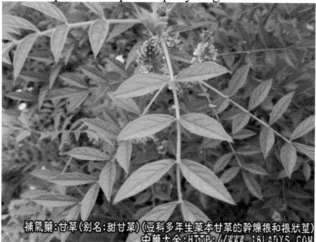

Chinese characters simplified/traditional:甘草/甘草
Chinese nickname's alphabet (Nickname's Chinese characters): Guolao/ Tiancao/ Tiangenzi(国老/甜草/甜根子)
Latin: Glycyrrhizae Radix et Rhizoma (Common name: Liquorice Root or Licorice Root)
Plant: *Glycyrrhiza uralensis* Fisch. (or *Glycyrrhiza inflata* Bat., *Glycyrrhiza glabra* L.)

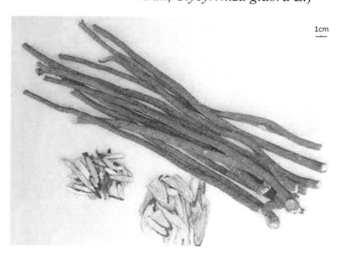

TCM prepared in ready-to-use forms (medicinal parts): it's dried rhizome and root which harvested in spring or autumn.
Property and flavor: neutral; sweet.
Main and collateral channels: heart, lung, spleen and stomach meridians.
Administration and dosage: 2-10 g.

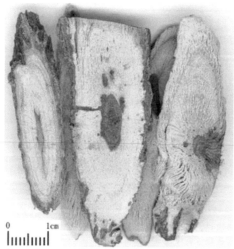

Indication: cough, fatigue, cough, skin infection, excessive phlegm, abdominal pain, palpitation and shortness of breath; ease of drug toxicity; improve strength; clear away heat and toxic material.
It is commonly used in coordinating the drug actions of a prescription.
It is taken as food in some part of China.
Precaution and warning: incompatible with Seaweed, Peking Euphorbia Root, Knoxia Root, Gansui Root and Lilac Daphne Flower Bud.

Attachment: Processing of Prepared Liquorice Root: stir-bake the slice of Liquorice Root with honey until it becomes deep yellow and not sticky to the fingers, take out and cool in the air.
(The picture is only for learning and identification the herb; the specific use of the herb please consult the herbalist or health professionals)

Heterophylly Falsestarwort Root (Taizishen)

Chinese phonetic alphabet/pin yin: tài zǐ shēn
Chinese characters simplified/traditional:太子参/太子參

Chinese nickname's alphabet (Nickname's Chinese characters): Hai'ershen/Tongshen(孩儿参/童参)
Latin: Pseudostellariae Radix (Common name: Heterophylly Falsestarwort Root)
Plant: *Pseudostellaria heterophylla* (Miq.) Pax ex Pax et Hoffm

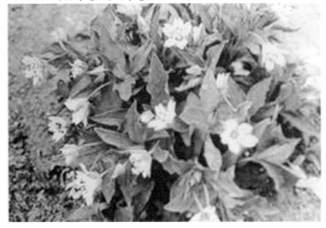

.

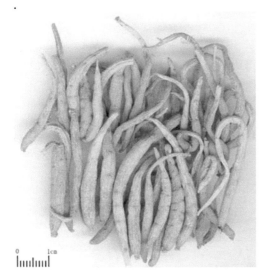

TCM prepared in ready-to-use forms (medicinal parts): it's dried root tuber which harvested in summer.
Property and flavor: neutral; sweet, mild bitter.
Main and collateral channels: spleen and lung meridians.
Administration and dosage: 9-30 g.
Indication: poor appetite, weakness after illness, night sweating, thirst and dry cough.
(The picture is only for learning and identification the herb; the specific use of the herb please consult the herbalist or health professionals)

American Ginseng (Xiyangshen)

Chinese phonetic alphabet/pin yin: xī yáng shēn
Chinese characters simplified/traditional:西洋参/西洋參
Chinese nickname's alphabet (Nickname's Chinese characters): Huaqishen(花旗参)
Latin: Panacis Quinquefolii Radix (Common name: American Ginseng)
Plant: *Panax quinquefolius* L.
TCM prepared in ready-to-use forms (medicinal parts): it's dried root which harvested in autumn.

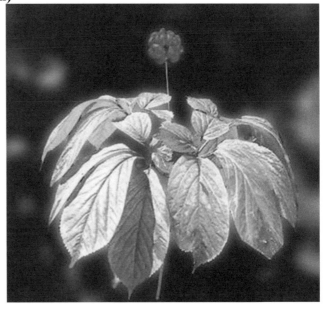

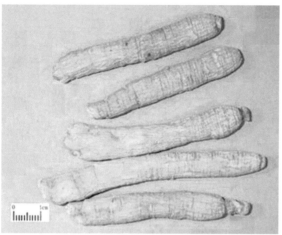

Property and flavor: cool; sweet, mild bitter.
Main and collateral channels: heart, lung and kidney meridians.
Administration and dosage: 3-6 g, decocted alone and mixed with another decoction before taking.
Indication: cough, phlegm with blood, thirst, vexation and fatigue.
Precaution and warning: incompatible with Black False Hellebore.

Attention: to protect the rare wild plant, please don't use the herb from wild plant. (The picture is only for learning and identification the herb; the specific use of the herb please consult the herbalist or health professionals)

Manyprickle Acanthopanax (Ciwujia)

Chinese phonetic alphabet/pin yin: cì wǔ jiā
Chinese characters simplified/traditional:刺五加/刺五加
Chinese nickname's alphabet (Nickname's Chinese characters): Kanguaibangzi/
Laohuliao(坎拐棒子/老虎潦)

Latin:
Acanthopanacis
Senticosi Radix et
Rhizoma seu
Caulis (Common
name:
Manyprickle
Acanthopanax)
Plant:
*Acanthopanax
senticosus* (Rupr.
et Maxim.) Harms.

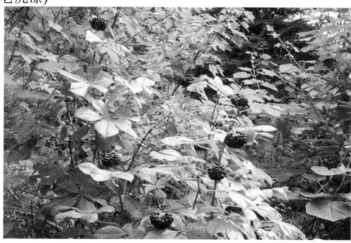

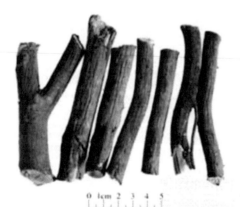

TCM prepared in ready-to-use forms (medicinal parts): it's dried root and rhizome or stem which harvested in autumn.
Property and flavor: warm; pungent and mild bitter.
Main and collateral channels: spleen, kidney and heart meridians.

◄─── root

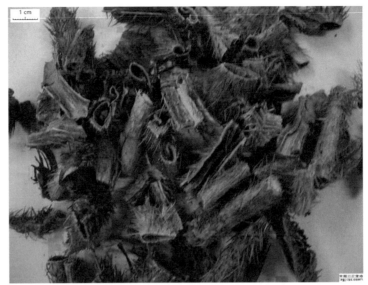

Administration and dosage: 9-27 g.
Indication: soreness and weakness of waist and knees, poor appetite, chronic cough, insomnia, bruises and fracture; robust.

stem (bark) ⟶

(The picture is only for learning and identification the herb; the specific use of the herb please consult the herbalist or health professionals)

Chinese Date (Dazao)
Chinese phonetic alphabet/pin yin: dà zǎo
Chinese characters simplified/traditional:大枣/大棗

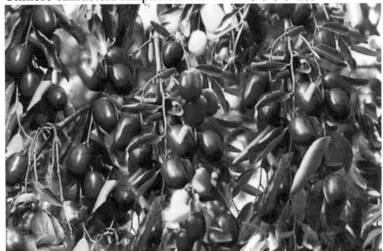

Chinese nickname's alphabet (Nickname's Chinese characters): Hongzao(红枣)
Latin: Jujubae Fructus (Common name: Chinese Date)
Plant: *Ziziphus jujuba* Mill.

TCM prepared in ready-to-use forms (medicinal parts): it's dried mature fruit.
Property and flavor: warm; sweet.
Main and collateral channels: spleen, stomach and heart meridians.
Administration and dosage: 6-15 g.
Indication: diarrhea, colpitis; appetizer.
It is taken as food in some part of China.
(The picture is only for learning and identification the herb; the specific use of the herb please consult the herbalist or health professionals)

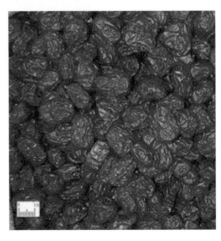

Axillary Choerospondias Fruit (Guangzao)
Chinese phonetic alphabet/pin yin: guǎng zǎo
Chinese characters simplified/traditional:广枣/廣棗

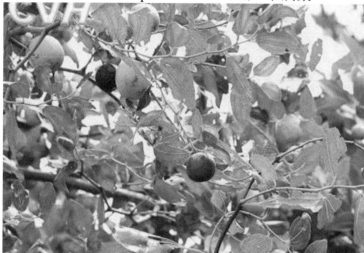

Latin: Choerospondiatis Fructus (Common name: Axillary Choerospondias Fruit)
Plant: *Choerospondias axillaris* (Roxb.) Burtt et Hill.
TCM prepared in ready-to-use forms (medicinal parts): it's dried ripe fruit.

Property and flavor: neutral; sweet, acidity.
Administration and dosage: 1.5-2.5 g.
Indication: blood stasis, heart pain, palpitations, shortness of breath, vexation.
(The picture is only for learning and identification the herb; the specific use of the herb please consult the herbalist or health professionals)

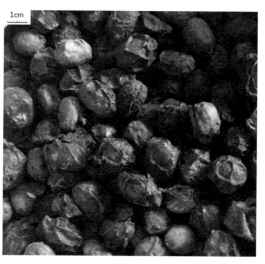

White Hyacinth Bean (Baibiandou)
Chinese phonetic alphabet/pin yin: bái biǎn dòu

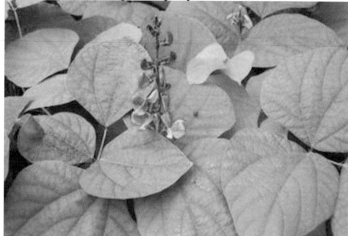

Chinese characters simplified/ traditional:白扁豆/ 白扁豆
Chinese nickname's alphabet (Nickname's Chinese characters): (Bian)Biandou/ Nanbiandou((扁)藊 豆/南扁豆)

Latin: Lablab Semen Album (Common name: White Hyacinth Bean or White Lentils)
Plant: *Dolicho Lablab* L.
TCM prepared in ready-to-use forms (medicinal parts): it's dried mature seed.
Property and flavor: mild warm; sweet.
Main and collateral channels: spleen and stomach meridians.
Administration and dosage: 9-15 g.
Indication: diarrhea, leucorrhea excessive, vomiting, abdominal and chest distension and tightness; appetizer.
It is taken as food in some part of China.
(The picture is only for learning and identification the herb; the specific use of the herb please consult the herbalist or health professionals)

Honey (Fengmi)
Chinese phonetic alphabet/pin yin: fēng mì

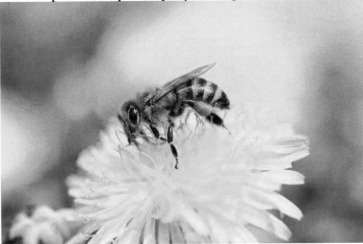

Chinese characters simplified/ traditional:蜂蜜/蜂蜜
Chinese nickname's alphabet (Nickname's Chinese characters): Mi/ Fengtang(蜜/蜂糖)
Latin: Mel (Common name: Honey)

Animal: *Apis cerana* Linnaeus. (or *Apis mellifera* Linnaeus.)
TCM prepared in ready-to-use forms (medicinal parts): it's a saccharine fluid deposited by the animal (bee).
Property and flavor: neutral; sweet.
Main and collateral channels: lung, spleen and large intestine meridians.
Administration and dosage: 15-30 g.
Indication: constipation, epigastrium and abdomen pain; relieve dry cough; detoxic; topical application: unhealing sore and ulcer, scald and burn.
It is taken as food in some part of China.
Precaution and warning: used with cautiously for diabetics.
(The picture is only for learning and identification the herb; the specific use of the herb please consult the herbalist or health professionals)

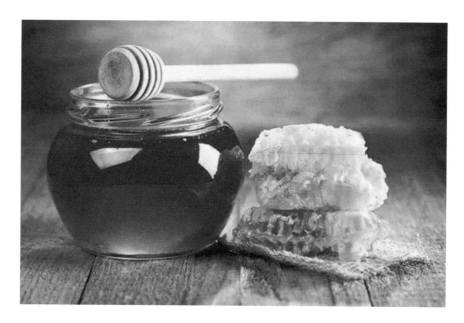

Maltose (Yitang)
Chinese phonetic alphabet/pin yin: yí táng
Chinese characters simplified/traditional:饴糖/飴糖

Chinese nickname's
alphabet (Nickname's
Chinese characters):
Xing/ Jiaoyi/
Tangyi(饧/胶饴/糖饴)
Latin:
Saccharum Granorum
(Common name:
Maltose or Malt Sugar)
Plant: *Hordeurn
vulgare* L.

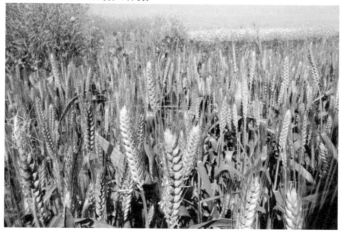

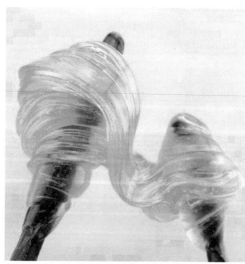

TCM prepared in ready-to-use forms
(medicinal parts): it's the sugar produced
by fermentation and saccharification of
grain. Its main component is
$C_{12}H_{22}O_{11} \cdot H_2O$.
Property and flavor: warm; sweet.
Main and collateral channels: spleen,
stomach and lung meridians.
Administration and dosage: 15-20 g,
dissolved in decoction or used in pill or
paste.
Indication: abdominal pain, dry cough,
vomiting, sore throat and constipation.
Precaution and warning: used with
cautiously for diabetics.
(The picture is only for learning and identification the herb; the specific use of the
herb please consult the herbalist or health professionals)

Bigflower Rhodiola Root (Hongjingtian)

Chinese phonetic alphabet/pin yin: hóng jǐng tiān

Chinese characters simplified/traditional:红景天/紅景天

Chinese nickname's alphabet (Nickname's Chinese characters): Saoluoma'erbu(扫罗玛布尔)

Latin: Rhodiolae Crenulatae Radix et Rhizoma (Common name: Bigflower Rhodiola Root)

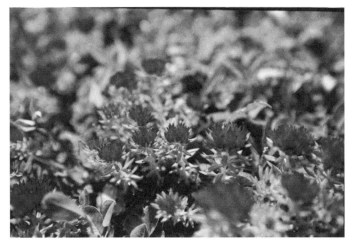

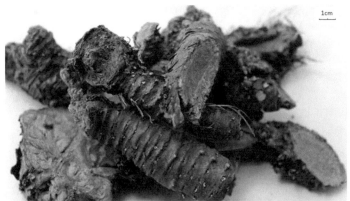

Plant: *Rhodiola crenulata* (Hook. f. et Thomas.) H. Ohba. *(or Rhodiola rosea* L.)

TCM prepared in ready-to-use forms (medicinal parts): it's dried root and rhizome which harvested in autumn.

Property and flavor: neutral; bitter, sweet.

Main and collateral channels: lung and heart meridians.

Administration and dosage: 3-6 g.

Indication: cough, blood stasis, heart pain, hemiplegia, fatigue, hemoptysis and traumatic injury.

(The picture is only for learning and identification the herb; the specific use of the herb please consult the herbalist or health professionals)

Gynostemma Herb (Jiaogulan)

Chinese phonetic alphabet/pin yin: jiǎo gǔ lán

Chinese characters simplified/traditional:绞股蓝/絞股藍

Chinese nickname's alphabet (Nickname's Chinese characters): Qiyedan/ Xiaokuyao(七叶胆/小苦药)

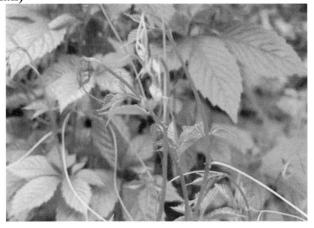

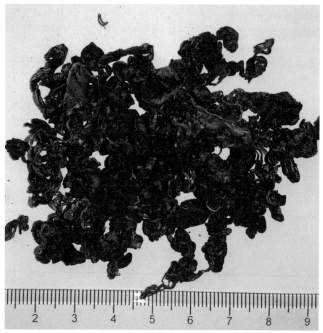

Latin: Gynostemmae Herba (Common name: Gynostemma Herb)
Plant: *Gynostemma pentaphyllum* (Thunb.) Makino.
TCM prepared in ready-to-use forms (medicinal parts): it's dried whole herb which harvested in November or December.
Property and flavor: cool; bitter, mild sweet.
Main and collateral channels: lung, spleen and kidney meridians.

Administration and dosage: 15-30 g, or brew as tea.
Indication: cough, hypertension and expectorant; anti-inflammatory and detoxifying, build up a good physique and improve one's health.
(The picture is only for learning and identification the herb; the specific use of the herb please consult the herbalist or health professionals)

Pilose Antler (Lurong)
Chinese phonetic alphabet/pin yin: lù róng
Chinese characters simplified/traditional:鹿茸/鹿茸
Chinese nickname's alphabet (Nickname's Chinese characters): Banlongzhu(斑龙珠)

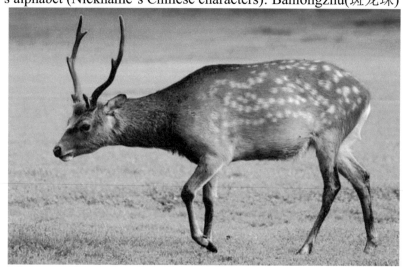

Latin: Cervi Cornu Pantotrichum (Common name: Pilose Antler)
Animal: *Cervus nippon* Temminck (or *Cervus elaphus* L.)

TCM prepared in ready-to-use forms (medicinal parts): it's dried unossified young antler with hair.
Property and flavor: warm; sweet, salty.
Main and collateral channels: kidney and liver meridians.
Administration and dosage: 1-2 g. Ground into powder for oral administration with water.

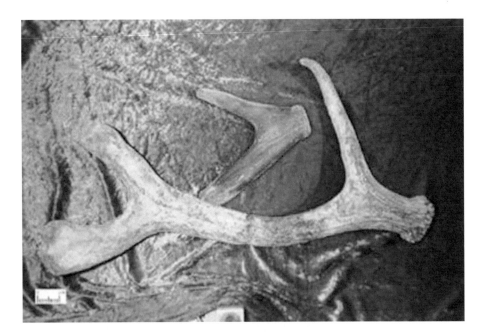

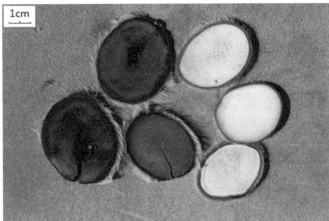

Indication: impotence, spermatorrhea, infertility, emaciation, lassitude, fatigue, chills, dizziness, tinnitus and metrorrhagia; strength the bones and muscles.

It is key herb to treat impotence and premature ejaculation.

Attention: to protect the rare wild animals, don't use it from wild animal.
(The picture is only for learning and identification the herb; the specific use of the herb please consult the herbalist or health professionals)

Deerhorn Glue (Lujiaojiao)

Chinese phonetic alphabet/pin yin: lù jiǎo jiǎo
Chinese characters simplified/traditional:鹿角胶/鹿角膠
Latin: Cervi Cornus Colla (Common name: Deerhorn Glue)
Animal: *Cervus nippon* Temminck (or *Cervus elaphus* L.) (See Pilose Antler)
TCM prepared in ready-to-use forms (medicinal parts): it's solid glue prepared from deerhorn by decoction and concentration.

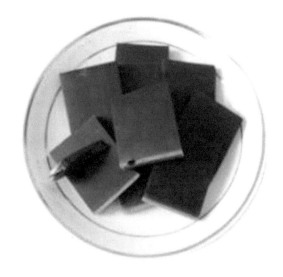

Property and flavor: warm; sweet, salty.
Main and collateral channels: kidney and liver meridians.
Administration and dosage: 3-6 g, taken after dissolving it in boiling decoction.
Indication: soreness and weakness in the waist and knees, menstrual flooding and spotting, impotence and seminal emission, bloody stool, hematuria, swelling and pain.
Attention: to protect the rare wild animals, don't use it from wild animal.
(The picture is only for learning and identification the herb; the specific use of the herb please consult the herbalist or health professionals)

Degelatined Deer-horn (Lujiaoshuang)
Chinese phonetic alphabet/pin yin: lù jiǎo shuāng

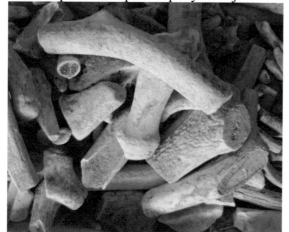

Chinese characters simplified/traditional:鹿角霜/鹿角霜
Chinese nickname's alphabet (Nickname's Chinese characters): Lujiaobaishuang(鹿角白霜)
Latin: Cervi Cornu Degelatinatum (Common name: Degelatined Deer-horn)
Animal: *Cervus nippon* Temminck (or *Cervus elaphus* L.) (See Pilose Antler)

TCM prepared in ready-to-use forms (medicinal parts): it's piece or power of antler removed from gelatin.
Property and flavor: warm; salty, astringent.
Main and collateral channels: liver and kidney meridians.
Administration and dosage: 9-15 g. It should be decocted first.
Indication: profuse white vaginal discharge, metrorrhagia and spotting, enuresis, unhealing sore and ulcer.

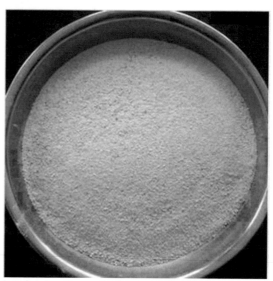

Attention: to protect the rare wild animals, don't use it from wild animal.
(The picture is only for learning and identification the herb; the specific use of the herb please consult the herbalist or health professionals)

Desertliving Cistanche Herb (Roucongrong)
Chinese phonetic alphabet/pin yin: ròu cōng róng
Chinese characters simplified/traditional:肉苁蓉/肉蓯蓉
Chinese nickname's alphabet (Nickname's Chinese characters): Dayun/ Cunyun/ Zongrong/ Dijing(大芸/寸芸/纵蓉/地精)
Latin: Cistanches Herba (Common name: Desertliving Cistanche Herb)

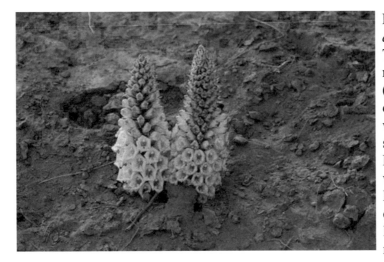

Plant: *Cistanche deserticola* Ma.
TCM prepared in ready-to-use forms (medicinal parts): it's dried succulent stem which harvested in spring.
Property and flavor: warm; sweet, salty.
Main and collateral channels: kidney and large intestine meridians.

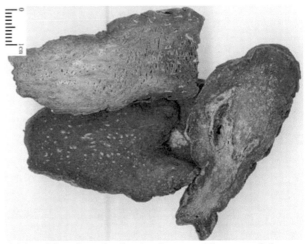

Administration and dosage: 6-10 g.
Indication: impotence, infertility, soreness and weakness of waist and knees, muscles weakness, constipation.
Attention:
to protect the rare wild plant, don't use the herb from wild plant.

(The picture is only for learning and identification the herb; the specific use of the herb please consult the herbalist or health professionals)

Epimedium leaf (Yinyanghuo)

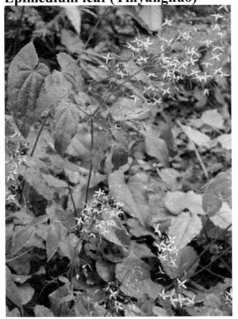

Chinese phonetic alphabet/pin yin: yín yáng huò
Chinese characters simplified/traditional: 淫羊藿/淫羊藿
Chinese nickname's alphabet (Nickname's Chinese characters): Xianlingpi(仙灵脾)
Latin: Epimedii Folium (Common name: Epimedium leaf)
Plant: *Epimedium brevicornum* Maxim. (or *Epimedium sagittatum* (Sieb. Et Zucc) Maxim., *Epimedium pubescens* Maxim., *Epimedium koreanum* Nakai.)
TCM prepared in ready-to-use forms (medicinal parts): it's dried leaf which harvested in summer or autumn.

Property and flavor: warm; sweet, pungent.
Main and collateral channels: liver and kidney meridians.
Administration and dosage: 6-10 g.
Indication: impotence, seminal emission, spermatorrhea, painful *bi* disorder and numbness spasm; strength the bones and muscles.
(The picture is only for learning and identification the herb; the specific use of the herb please consult the herbalist or health professionals)

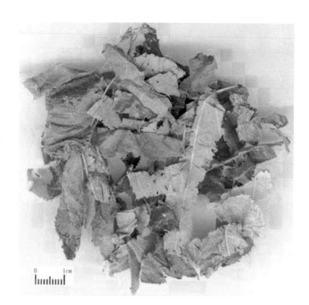

Epimedium Wushanense Leaf (Wushan Yinyanghuo)

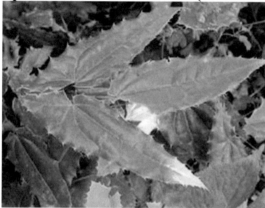

Chinese phonetic alphabet/pin yin: wū shān yín yáng huò
Chinese characters simplified/traditional:巫山淫羊藿/巫山淫羊藿
Latin: Epimedii Wushanensis Folium (Common name: Epimedium Wushanense Leaf)
Plant: *Epimedium wushanense* T. S. Ying.
TCM prepared in ready-to-use forms (medicinal parts): it's dried leaf which harvested in summer or autumn.

Property and flavor: warm; sweet, pungent.
Main and collateral channels: liver and kidney meridians.
Administration and dosage: 3-9 g.
Indication: debilitation, impotence and seminal emission, limp wilting sinew and bone, painful *bi* disorder, joint pain, dizziness, numbness and spasm.

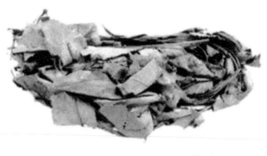

(The picture is only for learning and identification the herb; the specific use of the herb please consult the herbalist or health professionals)

Eucommia Bark (Duzhong)
Chinese phonetic alphabet/pin yin: dù zhòng
Chinese characters simplified/traditional:杜仲/杜仲
Chinese nickname's alphabet (Nickname's Chinese characters): Sixian/ Mumian/ Simianpi(思仙/木绵/丝绵皮)

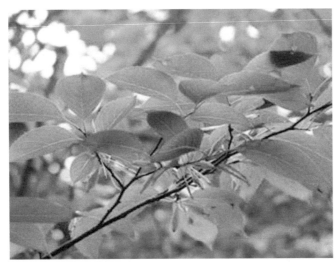

Latin: Eucommiae Cortex
(Common name:
Eucommia Bark)
Plant: *Eucommia ulmoides*
Oliver.
TCM prepared in
ready-to-use forms
(medicinal parts): it's dried
stem bark which harvested
between April and June.
Property and flavor: warm;
sweet.

Main and collateral
channels: liver and
kidney meridians.
Administration and
dosage: 6-10 g.
Indication: pain in
the loins and knee,
muscles weakness,
pregnancy blood
leakage, fetal
irritability and
hypertension.

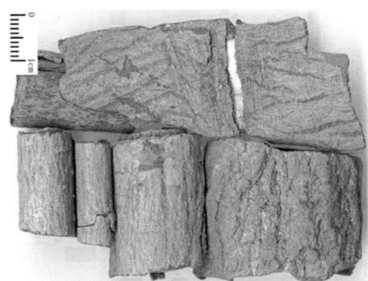

It is key herb to treat soreness and weakness of waist and knees with weakness of the
muscles and bones.

Attention: to protect the rare wild plant, please don't use the herb from wild plant
(The picture is only for learning and identification the herb; the specific use of the
herb please consult the herbalist or health professionals)

Himalayan Teasel Root (Xuduan)

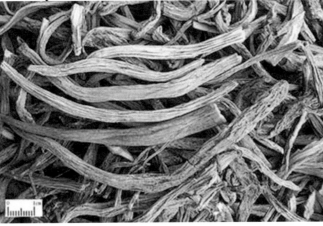

Chinese phonetic
alphabet/pin yin: xù duàn
Chinese characters
simplified/traditional:续断/
續斷
Chinese nickname's
alphabet (Nickname's
Chinese characters): Jiegu/
Chuanduan(接骨/川断)
Latin: Dipsaci Radix
(Common name: Himalayan
Teasel Root)

Plant: *Dipsacus asper* Wall. ex Henry.

TCM prepared in ready-to-use forms (medicinal parts): it's dried root which harvested in autumn.

Property and flavor: mild warm; bitter, pungent.

Main and collateral channels: liver and kidney meridians.

Administration and dosage: 9-15 g. It processed with wine usually used for painful impediment or injuries; processed with salt usually used for soreness and weakness of waist and knees.

Indication: soreness and weakness of waist and knees, painful *bi* disorder, uterine bleeding, menstrual flooding and spotting and traumatic injuries.

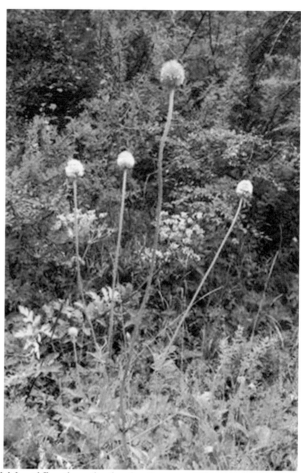

(The picture is only for learning and identification the herb; the specific use of the herb please consult the herbalist or health professionals)

Malaytea Scurfpea Fruit (Buguzhi)

Chinese phonetic alphabet/pin yin: bǔ gǔ zhī

Chinese characters simplified/traditional:补骨脂/補骨脂

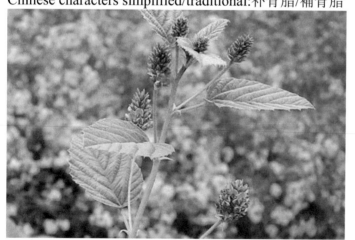

Chinese nickname's alphabet (Nickname's Chinese characters): Poguzhi(破故纸)

Latin: Psoraleae Fructus (Common name: Malaytea Scurfpea Fruit)

Plant: *Psoralea corylifolia* Linn.

TCM prepared in ready-to-use forms (medicinal parts): it's dried mature fruit.

Property and flavor: warm; bitter, pungent.

Main and collateral channels: kidney and spleen meridians.

Administration and dosage: 6-10 g. Topical application: 20%-30% tincture.

Indication: impotence, seminal emission, frequent micturition, pain in the loins and knee and diarrhea; external use for vitiligo and alopecia.
(The picture is only for learning and identification the herb; the specific use of the herb please consult the herbalist or health professionals)

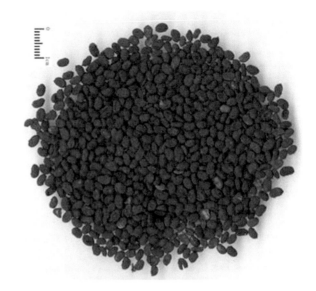

Sharpleaf Glangal Fruit (Yizhiren)
Chinese phonetic alphabet/pin yin: yì zhì rén
Chinese characters simplified/traditional:益智仁/益智仁

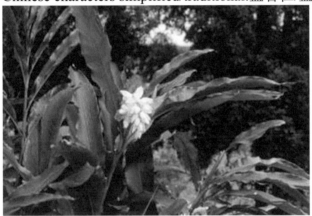

Chinese nickname's alphabet (Nickname's Chinese characters): Yizhi/ Yizhizi(益智/益智子)
Latin: Alpiniae Oxyphyllae Fructus (Common name: Sharpleaf Glangal Fruit)
Plant: *Alpinia oxyphylla* Miq.
TCM prepared in ready-to-use forms (medicinal parts): it's dried mature fruit.

Property and flavor: warm; pungent.
Main and collateral channels: spleen and kidney meridians.
Administration and dosage: 3-10 g.
Indication: diarrhea, seminal emission, abdomen pain caused by cold/chill (*Hanliang*), frequent urination and gonorrhea.
It is taken as food in some part of China.
(The picture is only for learning and identification the herb; the specific use of the herb please consult the herbalist or health professionals)

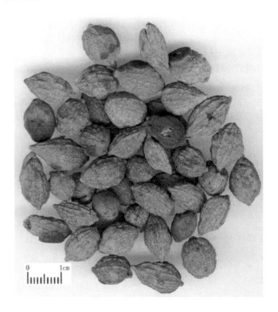

Tokay Gecko (Gejie)

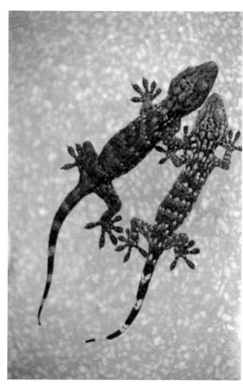

Chinese phonetic alphabet/pin yin: gé jiè
Chinese characters simplified/traditional:蛤蚧/蛤蚧
Chinese nickname's alphabet (Nickname's Chinese characters): Gexie/ Xianchan/ Dabihu(蛤蟹/仙蟾/大壁虎)
Latin: Gecko (Common name: Tokay Gecko or House Lizard)
Animal: *Gekko gecko* L.
TCM prepared in ready-to-use forms (medicinal parts): it's dried body removed internal organs.
Property and flavor: neutral; salty.
Main and collateral channels: lung and kidney meridians.
Administration and dosage: 3-6 g, usually used in pills or powder, or in wine or liquor preparation.
Indication: asthenia, shortness of breath, cough, hemoptysis, impotence, seminal emission and spermatorrhea.

Attention:
to protect the rare wild animals, please don't use it from wild animal.

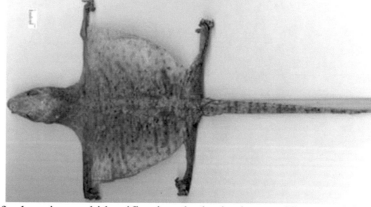

(The picture is only for learning and identification the herb; the specific use of the herb please consult the herbalist or health professionals)

Dodder Seed (Tusizi)

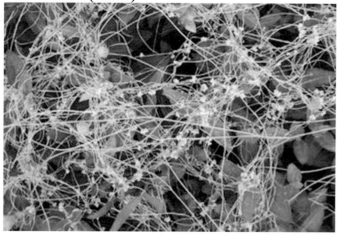

Chinese phonetic alphabet/pin yin: tù sī zǐ
Chinese characters simplified/traditional:菟丝子/菟絲子
Chinese nickname's alphabet (Nickname's Chinese characters): Doujisheng/ Huangsiteng/ Douxuzi(豆寄生/黄丝藤/豆须子)

Latin: Cuscutae Semen (Common name: Dodder Seed or The Seed of Chinese Dodder)
Plant: *Cuscuta chinensis* Lam. (or *Cuscuta australis* R. Br.)
TCM prepared in ready-to-use forms (medicinal parts): it's dried mature seed.
Property and flavor: neutral; pungent, sweet.
Main and collateral channels: liver, kidney and spleen meridians.
Administration and dosage: 6-12 g. Appropriate amount for topical application.

Indication: impotence, seminal emission, blurred vision, frequent micturition, soreness and weakness of waist and knees, dizziness, tinnitus and fetal irritability; external use for vitiligo.
(The picture is only for learning and identification the herb; the specific use of the herb please consult the herbalist or health professionals)

Morinda Root (Bajitian)

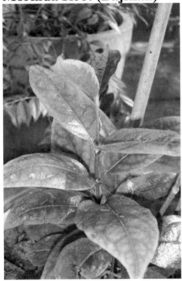

Chinese phonetic alphabet/pin yin: bā jǐ tiān
Chinese characters simplified/traditional:巴戟天/巴戟天
Chinese nickname's alphabet (Nickname's Chinese characters): Jichangfeng/ Tuzichang(鸡肠风/兔子肠)
Latin: Morindae Officinalis Radix (Common name: Morinda Root)
Plant: *Morinda officinalis* How.
TCM prepared in ready-to-use forms (medicinal parts): it's dried root (usually fry by salt) which harvested all year round.
Property and flavor: mild warm; sweet, pungent.

Main and collateral channels: kidney and liver meridians.
Administration and dosage: 3-10 g.
Indication: impotence, seminal emission, infertility, irregular menstruation, abdomen pain caused by cold/chill (*Hanliang*), painful *bi* disorder; strength the bones and muscles.
(The picture is only for learning and identification the herb; the specific use of the herb please consult the herbalist or health professionals)

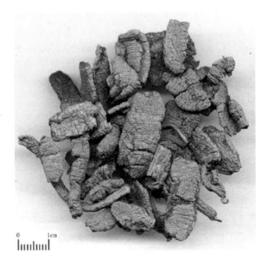

Songaria Cynomorium Herb (Suoyang)

Chinese phonetic alphabet/pin yin: suǒ yáng

Chinese characters simplified/traditional:锁阳/鎖陽

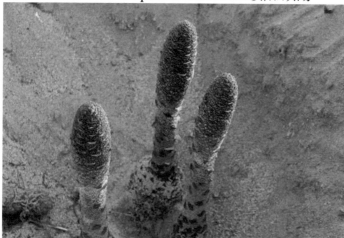

Chinese nickname's alphabet (Nickname's Chinese characters): Bulaoyao/ Dimaoqiu/ Huanggulang/ Xiutiebang/ Suoyanzi(不老药/地毛球/黄骨狼/锈铁棒/锁严子)
Latin: Cynomorii Herba (Common name: Songaria Cynomorium Herb)

Plant: *Cynomorium songaricum* Rupr. TCM prepared in ready-to-use forms (medicinal parts): it's dried succulent/fresh stem which harvested in spring.

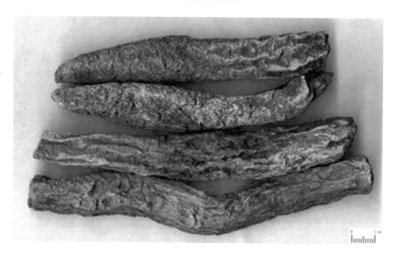

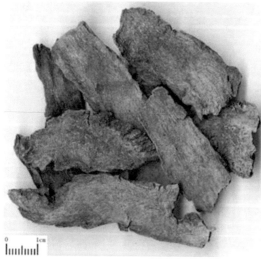

Property and flavor: warm; sweet.
Main and collateral channels: liver, kidney and large intestine meridians.
Administration and dosage: 5-10 g.
Indication: impotence, spermatorrhea, constipation, soreness and weakness of waist and knees.
(The picture is only for learning and identification the herb; the specific use of the herb please consult the herbalist or health professionals)

Fortune's Drynaria Rhizome (Gusuibu)

Chinese phonetic alphabet/pin yin: gǔ suì bǔ

Chinese characters simplified/traditional:骨碎补/骨碎補
Chinese nickname's alphabet (Nickname's Chinese characters): Houjiang/ Maojiang (猴姜/毛姜)
Latin: Drynariae Rhizoma (Common name: Fortune's Drynaria Rhizome)

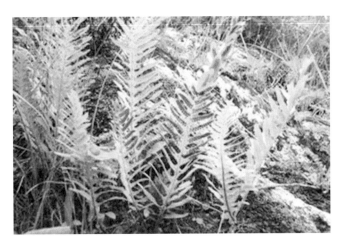

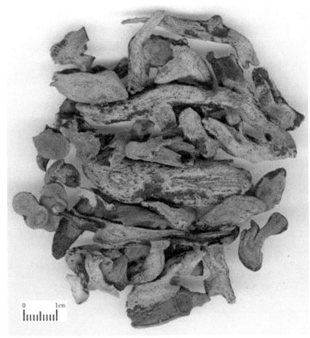

Plant: *Drymaria fortunei* (Kunze.) J. Sm. (or *Davallia mariesii* Moore ex Bak.)
TCM prepared in ready-to-use forms (medicinal parts): it's dried rhizome which harvested all year round.
Property and flavor: warm; bitter.
Main and collateral channels: liver and kidney meridians.
Administration and dosage: 3-9 g, appropriate amount fresh one for topical application.
Indication: tinnitus, traumatic injury, fracture of muscle and bones; external use for alopecia and vitiligo.

It is key herb to treat fracture.
(The picture is only for learning and identification the herb; the specific use of the herb please consult the herbalist or health professionals)

Chinese Caterpillar Fungus (Dongchongxiacao)
Chinese phonetic alphabet/pin yin: dōng chóng xià cǎo
Chinese characters simplified/traditional:冬虫夏草/冬蟲夏草
Chinese nickname's alphabet (Nickname's Chinese characters): Chongcao/ Dongchongcao(虫草/冬虫草)
Latin: Cordyceps (Common name: Chinese Caterpillar Fungus or *Hepialus armoricanus* Larvae infected by Fungus (*Cordyceps Sinensis* (Berk.) Sacc.))
Plant: *Hepialus armoricanus* (larvae) infected by fungus (*Cordyceps sinensis* (Berk.) Sacc.)
TCM prepared in ready-to-use forms (medicinal parts): it's dried the stroma of fungus and dead larval body.

Property and flavor: neutral; sweet

Main and collateral channels: lung and kidney meridians.

Administration and dosage: 3-9 g.

Indication: cough, hemoptysis, impotence, seminal emission, spermatorrhea, waist and knee pain.

Attention:

to protect the rare wild plant, please don't use the herb from wild plant.

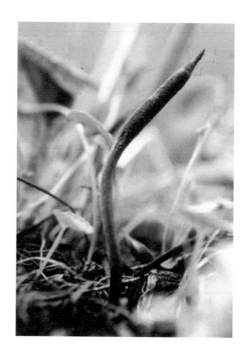

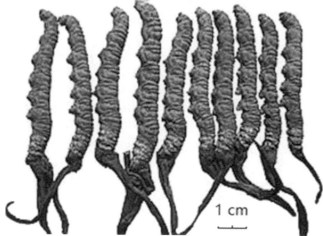

(The picture is only for learning and identification the herb; the specific use of the herb please consult the herbalist or health professionals)

Walnut Seed (Hetaoren)

Chinese phonetic alphabet/pin yin: hé táo rén

Chinese characters simplified/traditional:核桃仁/核桃仁

Chinese nickname's alphabet (Nickname's Chinese characters): Hutaoren/ Hutaorou(胡桃仁/胡桃肉)

Latin: Juglandis Semen (Common name: Walnut Seed or Walnut Kernel)

Plant: *Juglans regia* L.

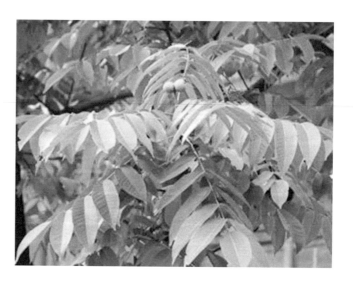

TCM prepared in ready-to-use forms (medicinal parts): it's dried mature kernel.

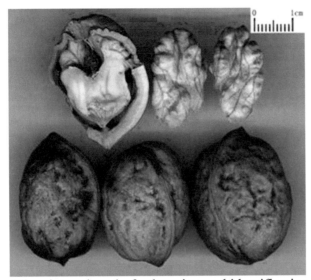

Property and flavor: warm; sweet.
Main and collateral channels: kidney, lung and large intestine meridians.
Administration and dosage: 6-9 g.
Indication: soreness and weakness of waist and knees, impotence, seminal emission, cold cough, constipation.
It is taken as food in some part of China.

(The picture is only for learning and identification the herb; the specific use of the herb please consult the herbalist or health professionals)

Dried Human Placenta (Ziheche)
Chinese phonetic alphabet/pin yin: zǐ hé chē
Chinese characters simplified/traditional:紫河车/紫河車
Chinese nickname's alphabet (Nickname's Chinese characters): Rentaipan/ Taiyi(人胎盘/胎衣)
Latin: Placenta Hominis (Common name: Dried Human Placenta)
Tissue: placenta. It is an organ that connects the developing fetus to the uterine wall to exchange nutriation and waste via the mother's blood supply, block infection, and to produce hormones which support pregnancy.

TCM prepared in ready-to-use forms (medicinal parts): it's boiled than dried human placenta.
Property and flavor: warm; salty, sweet.
Main and collateral channels: lung, heart and kidney meridians.
Administration and dosage: 3.5-5 g.

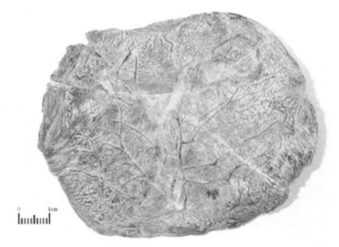

Indication: malnutrition, night sweating, cough, asthma, shortness of breath, impotence, infertility.
(The picture is only for learning and identification the herb; the specific use of the herb please consult the herbalist or health professionals)

Flatstem Milkvetch Seed (Shayuanzi)
Chinese phonetic alphabet/pin yin: shā yuàn zǐ

Chinese characters simplified/traditional:沙苑子/沙苑子

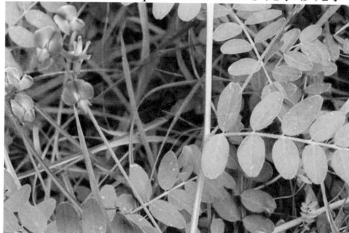

Chinese nickname's alphabet (Nickname's Chinese characters): Bianjinghuangqizi/ Shajili(扁茎黄耆子/ 沙蒺藜)
Latin: Astragali Complanati Semen (Common name: Flatstem Milkvetch Seed)

Plant: *Astragalus complanatus* R. Br.
TCM prepared in ready-to-use forms (medicinal parts): it's dried mature seed.
Property and flavor: warm; sweet.
Main and collateral channels: liver and kidney meridians.
Administration and dosage: 9-15 g.
Indication: spermatorrhea, seminal emission, premature ejaculation, leucorrhea turbidity, dizziness, dim vision, enuresis and frequent urination.

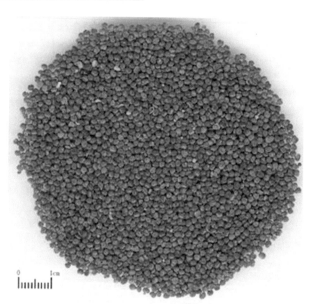

(The picture is only for learning and identification the herb; the specific use of the herb please consult the herbalist or health professionals)

Common Curculigo Rhizome (Xianmao)

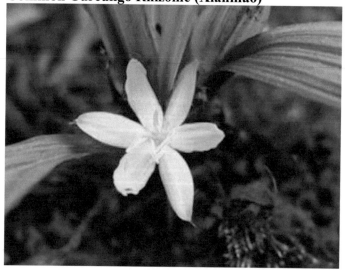

Chinese phonetic alphabet/pin yin: xiān máo
Chinese characters simplified/traditional:仙 茅/仙茅
Chinese nickname's alphabet (Nickname's Chinese characters): Dizong/ Dumaogen(地 棕/独茅根)

Latin: Curculiginis Rhizoma (Common name: Common Curculigo Rhizome)
Plant: *Curculigo orchioides* Gaertn.
TCM prepared in ready-to-use forms (medicinal parts): it's dried rhizome which harvested in autumn or winter.
Property and flavor: hot; pungent.
Main and collateral channels: kidney, liver and spleen meridians.
Administration and dosage: 3-10 g.

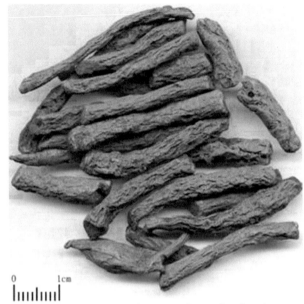

Indication: impotence, seminal emission, bones and muscles atrophy soft, diarrhea.
Precaution and warning: toxic.
(The picture is only for learning and identification the herb; the specific use of the herb please consult the herbalist or health professionals)

Cibot Rhizome (Gouji)
Chinese phonetic alphabet/pin yin: gǒu jǐ

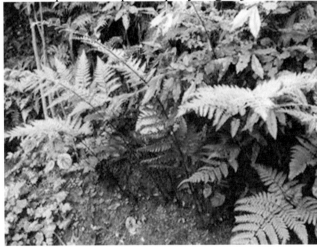

Chinese characters simplified/traditional:狗脊/ 狗脊
Chinese nickname's alphabet (Nickname's Chinese characters): Jinmaogouji/ Jingouji(金毛 狗脊/金狗脊)
Latin: Cibotii Rhizoma (Common name: Cibot Rhizome)
Plant: *Cibotium barometz* (L.) J. Sm.

TCM prepared in ready-to-use forms (medicinal parts): it's dried rhizome which harvested in autumn or winter.
Property and flavor: warm; bitter, sweet.
Main and collateral channels: liver and kidney meridians.

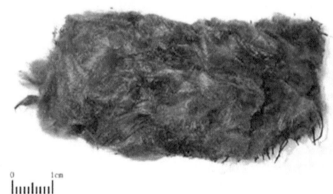

Administration and dosage: 6-12 g.

Indication: soreness and weakness of waist and knees, painful *bi* disorder and lack of strength in the limbs.

Attention: to protect the rare wild plant, please don't use the herb from wild plant.

(The picture is only for learning and identification the herb; the specific use of the herb please consult the herbalist or health professionals)

Sea Horse (Haima)

Chinese phonetic alphabet/pin yin: hǎi mǎ

Chinese characters simplified/traditional:海马/海馬

Chinese nickname's alphabet (Nickname's Chinese characters): Shuima/ Matouyu(水马/马头鱼)

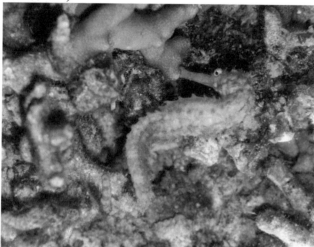

Latin: Hippocampus (Common name: Seahorse)
Animal: *Hippocampus histrix* Kaup. (or *Hippocampus kelloggi* Jordan. et Snyder., *Hippocampus kuda* Bleeker., *Hippocampus trimaculatus* Leach., *Hippocampus japonicus* Kaup., *Hippocampus coronatus* Temminck.)

TCM prepared in ready-to-use forms (medicinal parts): it's dried body (removed) internal organs.

Property and flavor: warm; sweet, salty.

Main and collateral channels: liver and kidney meridians.

Administration and dosage: 3-9 g. Topical application in appropriate amount, ground into powder and apply to the *pars affecta*.

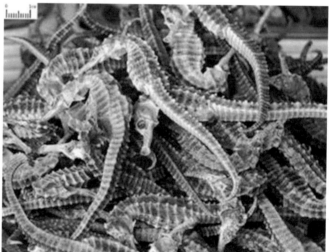

Indication: soreness and weakness of waist and knees, abdominal mass, scrofula, traumatic injury, impotence and enuresis; external use for carbuncle and sore.

Attention: to protect the rare wild animals, don't use it from wild animal.

(The picture is only for learning and identification the herb; the specific use of the herb please consult the herbalist or health professionals)

Chinese Angelica (Danggui)

Chinese phonetic alphabet/pin yin: dāng guī

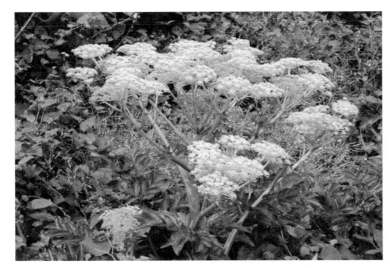

Chinese characters simplified/traditional: 当归/當歸
Chinese nickname's alphabet (Nickname's Chinese characters): Gangui(干归)

Latin: Angelicae Sinensis Radix (Common name: Chinese Angelica)
Plant:
Angelica sinensis (Oliv.) Diels.
TCM prepared in ready-to-use forms (medicinal parts) it's dried root which harvested in autumn.

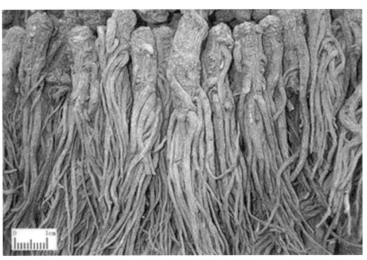

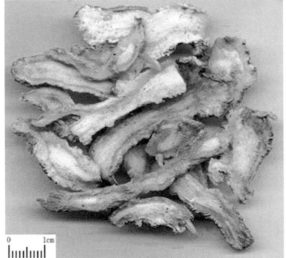

Property and flavor: warm; pungent, sweet.
Main and collateral channels: liver, heart and spleen meridians.
Administration and dosage: 6-12 g, it processed with wine or liquor could be used for painful *bi* disorder and traumatic injury.
Indication: blood deficiency, chlorosis, dizziness, palpitation, irregular menstruation, dysmenorrhea, amenorrhea, abdominal pain caused by cold/chill (*Hanliang*), constipation, painful *bi* disorder, traumatic injury, sore and ulcer.

It is taken as food in some part of China.
(The picture is only for learning and identification the herb; the specific use of the herb please consult the herbalist or health professionals)

Prepared Rehmannia Root (Shudihuang)

Chinese phonetic alphabet/pin yin: shú dì huáng
Chinese characters simplified/traditional:熟地黄/熟地黃

Chinese nickname's alphabet (Nickname's Chinese characters): Shudi(熟地)
Latin: Rehmanniae Radix Praeparata (Common name: Prepared Rehmannia Root)

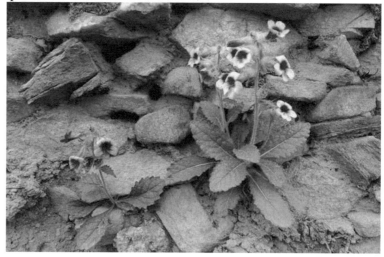

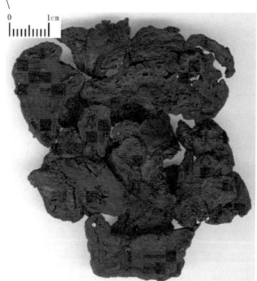

Plant: *Rehmannia glutinosa* (Gaetn.) Libosch. ex Fisch. et Mey.
TCM prepared in ready-to-use forms (medicinal parts): it's prepared dried root which harvested in winter.
Property and flavor: mild warm; sweet.
Main and collateral channels: liver and kidney meridians.
Administration and dosage: 9-15 g.
Indication: soreness and weakness of waist and knees, fever, night sweating, seminal emission, spermatorrhea, diabetes, blood deficiency, chlorosis, palpitation, irregular menstruation, hematuria, dizziness, tinnitus, premature graying hairs.

Procedure:
(Method 1) Stew the herb with the wine (30-50 kg yellow rice wine per 100 kg herb) until the wine is absorbed entirely, take out, sun-dry until the mucilage in bark is slightly dried, cut into thick slices, then dry thoroughly.
(Mehtod 2) Stew the herb with the wine (30-50 kg yellow rice wine per 100 kg herb) until it becomes blackish and shiny, take out, dry in the sun to be nearly dried, cut into thick slices or pieces, then dry thoroughly.
(The picture is only for learning and identification the herb; the specific use of the herb please consult the herbalist or health professionals)

Fleeceflower Root (Heshouwu)
Chinese phonetic alphabet/pin yin: hé shǒu wū
Chinese characters simplified/traditional:何首乌/何首烏
Chinese nickname's alphabet (Nickname's Chinese characters): Shouwu/ Duohualiao(首乌/多花蓼)
Latin: Polygoni Multiflori Radix (Common name: Fleeceflower Root)

Plant: *Polygonum multiflorum* Thunb. *(or Fallopia multiflora* (Thunb.) Harald.)
TCM prepared in ready-to-use forms (medicinal parts): it's dried tuber root which harvested in autumn or winter.

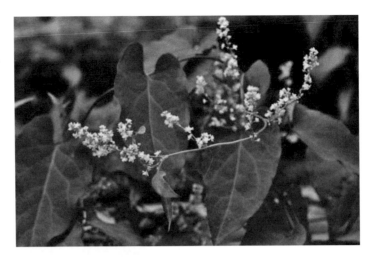

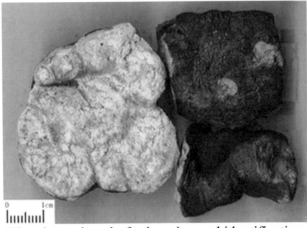

Property and flavor: mild warm; bitter, sweet and astringent.
Main and collateral channels: liver, heart and kidney meridians.
Administration and dosage: 3-6 g.
Indication: carbuncle, rubella itching, scrofula, constipation, malaria.

(The picture is only for learning and identification the herb; the specific use of the herb please consult the herbalist or health professionals)

Prepared Fleeceflower Root (Zhiheshouwu)
Chinese phonetic alphabet/pin yin: zhì hé shǒu wū
Chinese characters simplified/traditional:制何首乌/制何首烏

Latin: Polygoni Multiflori Radix Praeparata (Common name: Prepared Fleeceflower Root)
Plant: *Polygonum multiflorum* Thunb (See Fleeceflower Root).
TCM prepared in ready-to-use forms (medicinal parts): it's processed root.
Administration and dosage: 6-12 g.

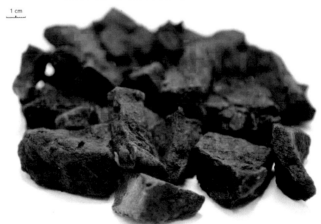

Procedure: Mix the slices or piece of Fleeceflower Root thoroughly with black bean juice (stew black bean with water for 4 hours to get it (10 kg black bean to get 15 kg juice)), stew until the juice is absorbed, then steam it after being mixed with black bean juice to brown color on all sides, dry. (For each 100 kg herb use 10 kg of black bean.)

Indication: dizziness, tinnitus, premature gray, soreness and weakness in the waist and knees, numbness of limbs, menstrual turbid, vaginal discharge and hyperlipidemia.

(The picture is only for learning and identification the herb; the specific use of the herb please consult the herbalist or health professionals)

White Peony Root (Baishao)

Chinese phonetic alphabet/pin yin: bái sháo

Chinese characters simplified/traditional:白芍/白芍

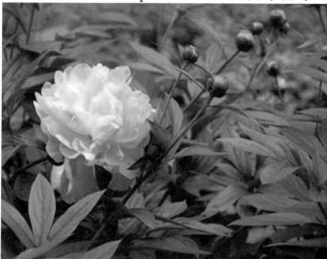

Chinese nickname's alphabet (Nickname's Chinese characters): Baishaoyao/Qingyangshen(白芍药/青羊参)

Latin: Paeoniae Radix Alba (Common name: White Peony Root)

Plant: *Paeonia lactiflora* Pall. TCM prepared in ready-to-use forms (medicinal parts): it's dried tuber root which harvested in summer or autumn.

Property and flavor: mild cold; bitter, acidity.

Main and collateral channels: liver and spleen meridians.

Administration and dosage: 6-15 g.

Indication: headache, dizziness, chest pain, abdominal pain, limb spasm pain, blood deficiency, chlorosis, irregular menstruation and night sweating.

Precaution and warning: incompatible with Black False Hellebore.

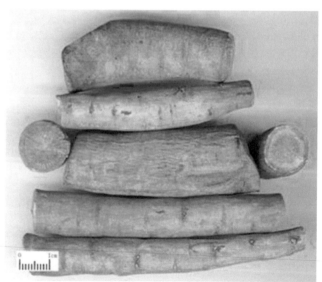

(The picture is only for learning and identification the herb; the specific use of the herb please consult the herbalist or health professionals)

Donkey-Hide Glue (Ejiao)

Chinese phonetic alphabet/pin yin: e jiāo

Chinese characters simplified/traditional:阿胶/阿膠

Chinese nickname's alphabet (Nickname's Chinese characters): Lvpijiao(驴皮胶)

Latin: Asini Corii Colla (Common name: Donkey-Hide Glue or Donkey-Hide Gelatin)

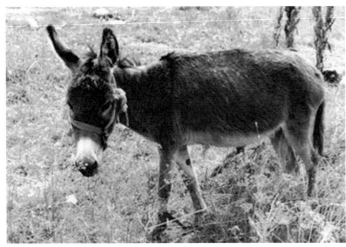

Animal: *Equus asinus* L.
TCM prepared in ready-to-use forms (medicinal parts): A solid gel made by boiling and concentrating the donkey skin.
Property and flavor: neutral; sweet.
Main and collateral channels: lung, liver and kidney meridians.

Administration and dosage: 3-9 g. Taken after dissolving in boiling decoction.
Indication: headache, dizziness, cough, muscle weakness, chest and abdominal pain, limb spasm pain, blood deficiency, chlorosis, vexation, palpitation, irregular menstruation, night sweating, hemoptysis, hematemesis and hematuria.
It is taken as food in some part of China.

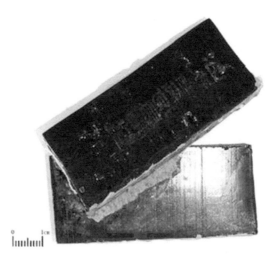

Attention: to protect the rare wild animals, please don't use it from wild animal. (The picture is only for learning and identification the herb; the specific use of the herb please consult the herbalist or health professionals)

Longan Aril (Longyanrou)
Chinese phonetic alphabet/pin yin: lóng yǎn ròu

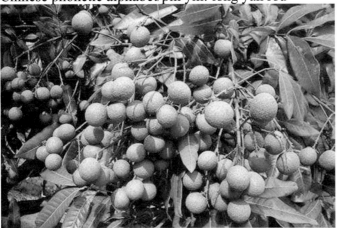

Chinese characters simplified/traditional:龙眼肉/龍眼肉
Chinese nickname's alphabet (Nickname's Chinese characters): Guiyuanrou/ Yalizhi(桂圆肉/亚荔枝)
Latin: Longan Arillus (Common name: Longan Aril or Cassia Pulp)

Plant: *Dimocarpus longan* Lour.
TCM prepared in ready-to-use forms (medicinal parts): it's dried aril of mature fruit.
Property and flavor: warm; sweet.

Main and collateral channels: heart and spleen meridians.
Administration and dosage: 9-15 g.
Indication: blood deficiency, palpitations, insomnia, forgetfulness and chlorosis.
It is taken as food in some part of China.
(The picture is only for learning and identification the herb; the specific use of the herb please consult the herbalist or health professionals)

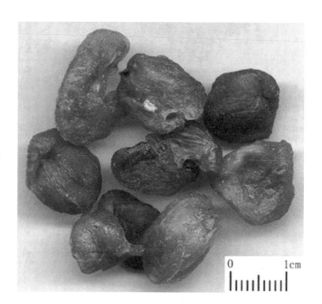

Fourleaf Ladybell Root (Nanshashen)
Chinese phonetic alphabet/pin yin: nán shā shēn
Chinese characters simplified/traditional:南沙参/南沙參
Chinese nickname's alphabet (Nickname's Chinese characters): Shashen/Paoshen(沙参/泡参)
Latin: Adenophorae Radix (Common name: Fourleaf Ladybell Root)

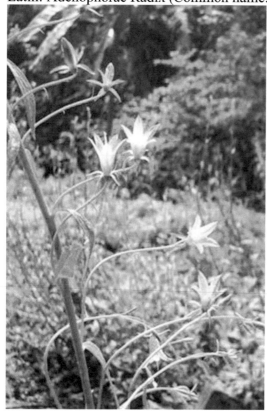

Plant: *Adenophora tetraphylla* (Thunb.) Fisch. (or *Adenophora stricta* Miq.)
TCM prepared in ready-to-use forms (medicinal parts): it's dried root which harvested between February and June.
Property and flavor: mild cold; sweet.
Main and collateral channels: lung and stomach meridians.
Administration and dosage: 9-15 g.
Indication: dry cough, phlegm sticky, irritated dry mouth, vomiting, less food intake and vexation.
Precaution and warning: incompatible with Black False Hellebore.

150

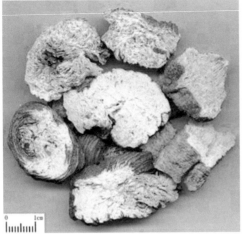
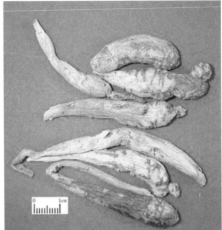

(The picture is only for learning and identification the herb; the specific use of the herb please consult the herbalist or health professionals)

Coastal Glehnia Root (Beishashen)
Chinese phonetic alphabet/pin yin: běi shā shēn
Chinese characters simplified/traditional:北沙参/北沙参
Chinese nickname's alphabet (Nickname's Chinese characters): Haishashen/
Yinshashen /Liaoshashen(海沙参/银沙参/辽沙参)

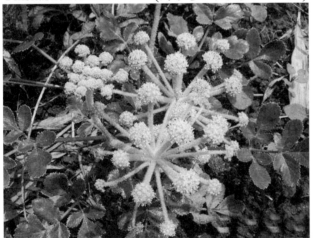

Latin: Glehniae Radix (Common name: Coastal Glehnia Root)
Plant: *Glehnia littoralis* Fr. Schmidt. ex Miq.
TCM prepared in ready-to-use forms (medicinal parts): it's dried root which harvested in summer or autumn.
Property and flavor: mild cold; sweet, mild bitter.

Main and collateral channels: lung and stomach meridians.
Administration and dosage: 5-12 g.
Indication: dry cough, phlegm with blood, fever, thirst.
Precaution and warning: incompatible with Black False Hellebore.
Attention: to protect the rare wild plant, please don't use the herb from wild plant.
(The picture is only for learning and identification the herb; the specific use of the herb please consult the herbalist or health professionals)

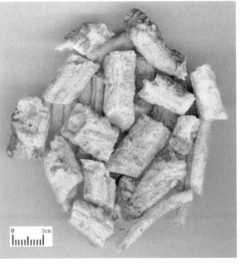

Dwarf Lilyturf Tuber (Maidong)

Chinese phonetic alphabet/pin yin: mài dōng
Chinese characters simplified/traditional:麦冬/麥冬

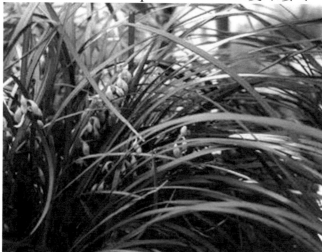

Chinese nickname's alphabet (Nickname's Chinese characters): Maimendong(麦门冬)
Latin: Ophiopogonis Radix (Common name: Dwarf Lilyturf Tuber)
Plant: *Ophiopogon japonicus* (Linn.f.) Ker-Gawl.
TCM prepared in ready-to-use forms (medicinal parts): it's dried tuber root which harvested in summer.

Property and flavor: mild cold; sweet, mild bitter.
Main and collateral channels: heart, lung and stomach meridians.
Administration and dosage: 6-12 g.
Indication: dry cough, sore throat, diarrhea, thirst, insomnia, constipation, vexation and diphtheria.
(The picture is only for learning and identification the herb; the specific use of the herb please consult the herbalist or health professionals)

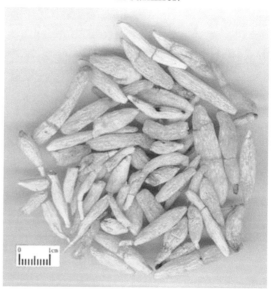

Liriope Root Tuber (Shanmaidong)

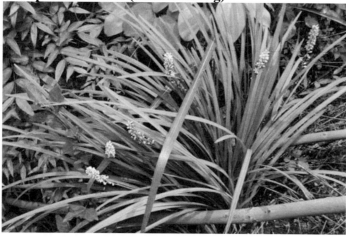

Chinese phonetic alphabet/pin yin: shān mài dōng
Chinese characters simplified/traditional: 山麦冬/山麥冬
Chinese nickname's alphabet (Nickname's Chinese characters): Damaidong/ Tumaidong(大麦冬/土麦冬)

Latin: Liriopes Radix (Common name: Liriope Root Tuber) Plant: *Liriope spicata* (Thunb.) Lour. var. *prolifera* Y. T. Ma. (or *Liriope muscari (*Decne.) Bailey.) TCM prepared in ready-to-use forms (medicinal parts): it's dried root tuber which harvested in summer.

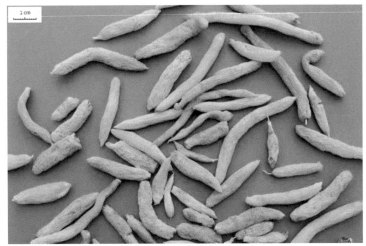

Property and flavor: mild cold; mild bitter, sweet.

Main and collateral channels: heart, lung and stomach meridians.

Administration and dosage: 9-15 g.

Indication: dry cough, sore throat, thirst, diarrhea, insomnia and constipation.

(The picture is only for learning and identification the herb; the specific use of the herb please consult the herbalist or health professionals)

Dendrobium (Shihu)

Chinese phonetic alphabet/pin yin: shí hú

Chinese characters simplified/traditional:石斛/石斛

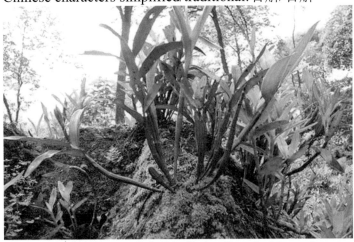

Chinese nickname's alphabet (Nickname's Chinese characters): Linlan/ Jinsheng/ Diaolan(林兰/禁生/吊兰)

Latin: Dendrobii Caulis (Common name: Dendrobium)

Plant: *Dendrobium nobile* Lindl. (or *Dendrobium chrysotoxum* Lindl., *Dendrobium fimbriatum* Hook., or other cultivates)

TCM prepared in ready-to-use forms (medicinal parts): it's dried stem which harvested in spring.

Property and flavor: mild cold; sweet.

Main and collateral channels: stomach and kidney meridians.

Administration and dosage: 6-12 g; or 15-30 g of the fresh one.

Indication: dry mouth, vexation, thirst, fever, dim vision and reduce food intake; build up a good physique and improve one's ealth.

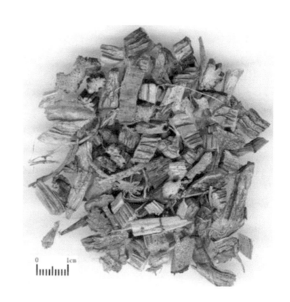

Attention:
to protect the rare wild plant, please don't use the herb from wild plant.
(The picture is only for learning and identification the herb; the specific use of the herb please consult the herbalist or health professionals)

Solomonseal Rhizome (Huangjing)
Chinese phonetic alphabet/pin yin: huáng jīng

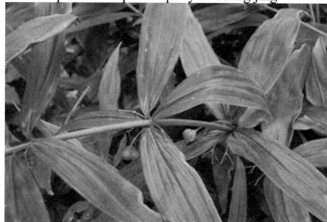

Chinese characters simplified/traditional:黄精/黄精
Chinese nickname's alphabet (Nickname's Chinese characters): Longxian/ Baiji(龙衔/白及)
Latin: Polygonati Rhizoma (Common name: Solomonseal Rhizome or Sealwort)

Plant: *Polygonatum sibiricum* Red. (or *Polygonatum kingianum* Coll. et Hemsl., *Polygonatum cyrtonema* Hua.)
TCM prepared in ready-to-use forms (medicinal parts): it's dried rhizome which harvested in autumn.
Property and flavor: neutral; sweet.
Main and collateral channels: spleen, lung and kidney meridians.
Administration and dosage: 9-15 g.

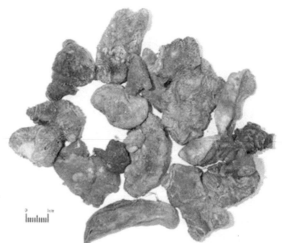

Indication: fatigue, lack of strength, dry mouth, dry cough, hemoptysis, blood deficiency, premature gray; appetizer.
It is taken as food in some part of China.
(The picture is only for learning and identification the herb; the specific use of the herb please consult the herbalist or health professionals)

Barbary Wolfberry Fruit (Gouqizi)
Chinese phonetic alphabet/pin yin: gǒu qǐ zǐ
Chinese characters simplified/traditional:枸杞子/枸杞子

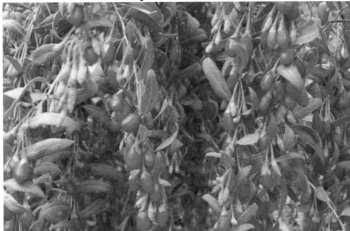

Chinese nickname's alphabet (Nickname's Chinese characters): Tiancaizi/ Diguzi(甜菜子/地骨子)
Latin: Lycii Fructus (Common name: Barbary Wolfberry Fruit or Chinese Wolfberry)
Plant: *Lycium barbarum* L. (or *Lycium chinense* Mill.)

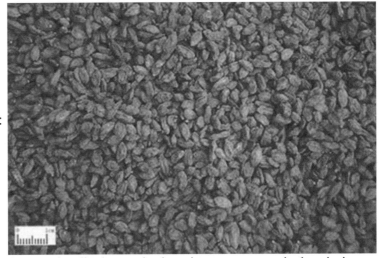

TCM prepared in ready-to-use forms (medicinal parts): it's dried mature fruit.
Property and flavor: neutral; sweet.
Main and collateral channels: liver and kidney meridians.
Administration and dosage: 6-12 g.

Indication: waist and knee pain, dizziness, tinnitus, impotence, seminal emission, blood deficiency, chlorosis and dim vision.
It is taken as food in some part of China.
(The picture is only for learning and identification the herb; the specific use of the herb please consult the herbalist or health professionals)

Tortoise Carapace and Plastron (Guijia)
Chinese phonetic alphabet/pin yin: guī jiǎ
Chinese characters simplified/traditional:龟甲/龜甲
Chinese nickname's alphabet (Nickname's Chinese characters): Guiban/ Guike(龟板/龟壳)
Latin: Testudinis Carapax et Plastrum (Common name: Tortoise Carapace and Plastron or Tortoise's Shell)
Animal: *Chinemys reevesii* (Gray.)
TCM prepared in ready-to-use forms (medicinal parts): it's dried shell.
Property and flavor: mild cold; salty, sweet.
Main and collateral channels: liver, kidney and heart meridians.

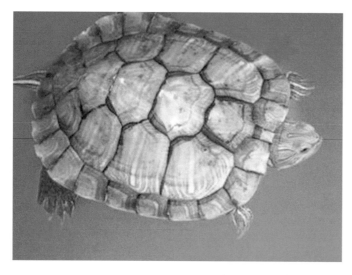

Administration and dosage: 9-24 g. It should be decocted first.
Indication: fever, night sweating, dizziness, flaccidity, amnesia, menstrual flooding and spotting.
Attention:
to protect the rare wild a nimals, don't use it from wild animal.

Attachment: procedure of Glue of Tortoise Shell. Immerse clean tortoise shell in water, decocted with water several times, filter and combine the filtrates (or add a little fine powder of alum), rest, filter, concentrate the glutinous filtrate (or add appropriate amount of yellow rice wine, crystal sugar and soybean oil) to thick glue, cool and congeal, cut into pieces and dry in the air.
(The picture is only for learning and identification the herb; the specific use of the herb please consult the herbalist or health professionals)

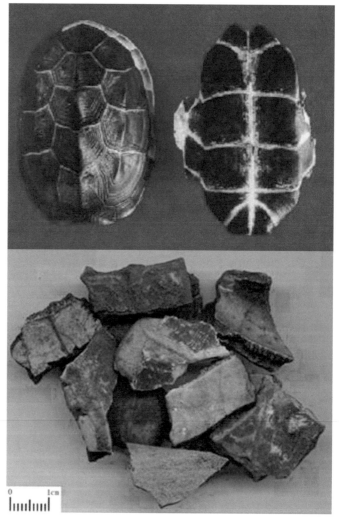

Turtle Carapace (Biejia)
Chinese phonetic alphabet/pin yin: biē jiǎ
Chinese characters simplified/traditional:鳖甲/鱉甲
Chinese nickname's alphabet (Nickname's Chinese characters): Shangjia/ Bieke/ Tuanyujian(上甲/鳖壳/团鱼甲)

156

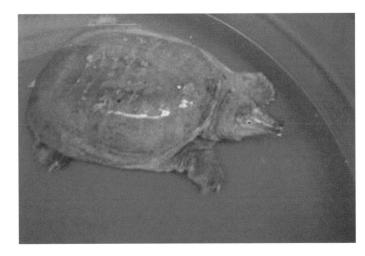

Latin: Trionycis Carapax (Common name: Turtle Carapace or Turtle's Shell) Animal: *Trionyx sinensis* Wiegmann. TCM prepared in ready-to-use forms (medicinal parts): it's dried shell.

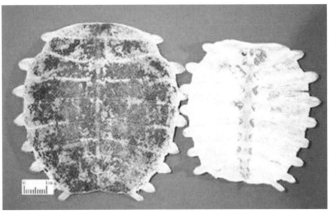

Property and flavor: mild cold; salty.
Main and collateral channels: liver and kidney meridians. Administration and dosage: 9-24 g. It should be decocted first.

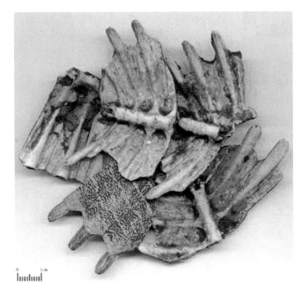

Indication: fever, night sweating, dizziness, convulsion, amenorrhea, abdominal mass, malaria.
Attention:
to protect the rare wild animals , don't use it from wild animal. (The picture is only for learning and identification the herb; the specific use of the herb please consult the herbalist or health professionals)

Cochinchinese Asparagus Root (Tiandong)
Chinese phonetic alphabet/pin yin: tiān dōng
Chinese characters simplified/traditional:天冬/天冬
Chinese nickname's alphabet (Nickname's Chinese characters): Tianmendong(天门冬)
Latin: Asparagi Radix (Common name: Cochinchinese Asparagus Root)

Plant: *Asparagus cochinchinensis* (Lour.) Merr.
TCM prepared in ready-to-use forms (medicinal parts): it's dried root which harvested in autumn or winter.
Property and flavor: cold; bitter, sweet.
Main and collateral channels: lung and kidney meridians.

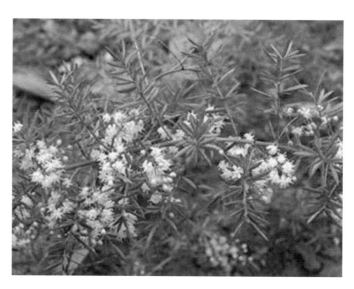

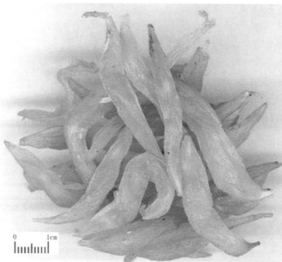

Administration and dosage: 6-12 g.
Indication: dry cough, phlegm sticky, fever, dry throat, thirsty, constipation.
(The picture is only for learning and identification the herb; the specific use of the herb please consult the herbalist or health professionals)

Fragrant Solomonseal Rhizome (Yuzhu)
Chinese phonetic alphabet/pin yin: yù zhú
Chinese characters simplified/traditional:玉竹/玉竹

Chinese nickname's alphabet (Nickname's Chinese characters): Wei/ Weishen(萎/尾参)
Latin: Polygonati Odorati Rhizoma (Common name: Fragrant Solomonseal Rhizome)
Plant: *Polygonatum odoratum* (Mill.) Druce.

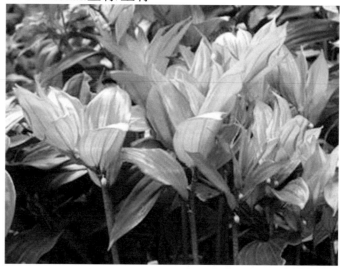

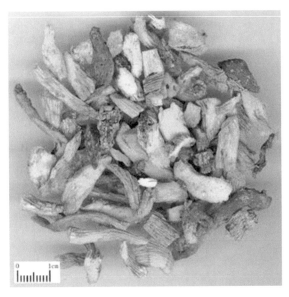

TCM prepared in ready-to-use forms (medicinal parts): it's dried rhizome which harvested in autumn.
Property and flavor: mild cold; sweet.
Main and collateral channels: lung and stomach meridians.
Administration and dosage: 6-12 g.
Indication: dry cough, dry throat, thirst, diabetes.
It is taken as food in some part of China.
(The picture is only for learning and identification the herb; the specific use of the herb please consult the herbalist or health professionals)

Lily Bulb (Baihe)
Chinese phonetic alphabet/pin yin: bǎi hé
Chinese characters simplified/traditional:百合/百合

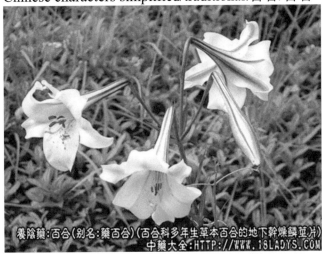

Chinese nickname's alphabet (Nickname's Chinese characters):Baibahe/ Baihesuan/ Yaobaihe(白百合/百合蒜/药百合)
Latin: Lilii Bulbus (Common name: Lily Bulb)
Plant: *Lilium brownii* F. E. Brown. var. *viridulum* Baker. (or *Lilium lancifolium* Thunb., *Lilium pumilum* DC.)

TCM prepared in ready-to-use forms (medicinal parts): it's dried fleshy bulb which harvested in autumn.
Property and flavor: cold; sweet.
Main and collateral channels: heart and lung meridians.
Administration and dosage: 6-12 g.
Indication: dry cough, phlegm with blood, hemoptysis, vexation, palpitation, insomnia.
It is taken as food in some part of China.

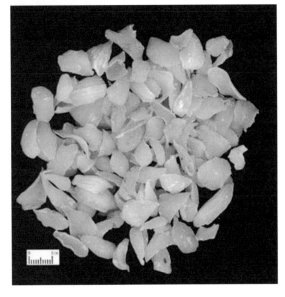

(The picture is only for learning and identification the herb; the specific use of the herb please consult the herbalist or health professionals)

Yerbadetajo Herb (Mohanlian)
Chinese phonetic alphabet/pin yin: mò hàn lián
Chinese characters simplified/traditional:墨旱莲/墨旱蓮

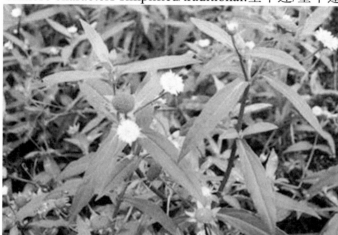

Chinese nickname's alphabet (Nickname's Chinese characters): Lichang/ Hanliancao(鳢肠/旱莲草)
Latin: Ecliptae Herba (Common name: Yerbadetajo Herb)
Plant: *Eclipta prostrata* L.

TCM prepared in ready-to-use forms (medicinal parts): it's dried up ground part which harvested when it is blooming.
Property and flavor: cold; sweet, acidity.
Main and collateral channels: kidney and liver meridians.
Administration and dosage: 6-12 g.
Indication: loose teeth, premature graying, dizziness, tinnitus, soreness and weakness of waist and knees, hematemesis, epistaxis, hematuria, bloody dysentery, metrorrhagia and metrostaxis; external use for bleeding.

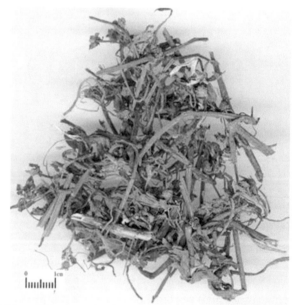

(The picture is only for learning and identification the herb; the specific use of the herb please consult the herbalist or health professionals)

Glossy Privet Fruit (Nyuzhenzi)
Chinese phonetic alphabet/pin yin: nǚ zhēn zǐ
Chinese characters simplified/traditional:女贞子/女貞子
Chinese nickname's alphabet (Nickname's Chinese characters): Dongqingzi/ Bailazi/ Shuzizi(冬青子/白蜡子/鼠梓子)
Latin: Ligustri Lucidi Fructus (Common name: Glossy Privet Fruit)

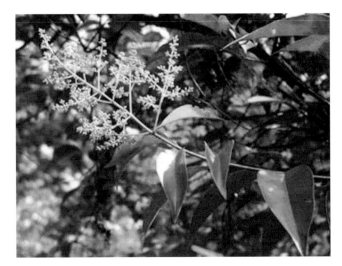

Plant: *Ligustrum lucidum* Ait.
TCM prepared in ready-to-use forms (medicinal parts): it's dried mature fruit.
Property and flavor: cool; sweet, bitter.
Main and collateral channels: liver and kidney meridians.
Administration and dosage: 6-12 g.

Indication: dizziness, tinnitus, soreness and weakness of waist and knees, early white beard and hair, dim vision and fever.
(The picture is only for learning and identification the herb; the specific use of the herb please consult the herbalist or health professionals)

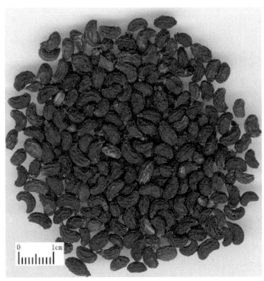

Mulberry Fruit (Sangshen)
Chinese phonetic alphabet/pin yin: sāng shèn
Chinese characters simplified/traditional:桑椹/桑椹

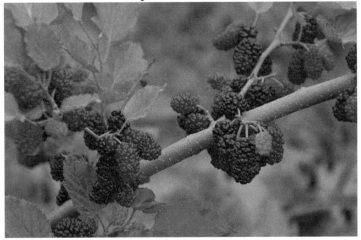

Chinese nickname's alphabet (Nickname's Chinese characters): Sangguo/ Sangshenzi(桑果/桑椹子)
Latin: Mori Fructus (Common name: Mulberry Fruit)

Plant: *Morus alba* L.
TCM prepared in ready-to-use forms (medicinal parts): it's dried mature fruit-spike/ ear fruit

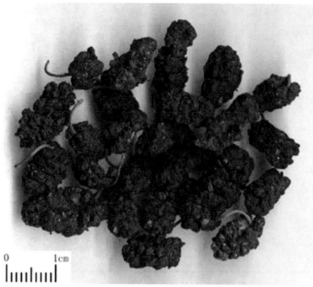

Property and flavor: cold; sweet, acidity.
Main and collateral channels: heart, liver and kidney meridians.
Administration and dosage: 9-15 g.
Indication: dizziness, tinnitus, palpitation, insomnia, early white beard and hair, thirst, blood deficiency, constipation. It is taken as food in some part of China.

(The picture is only for learning and identification the herb; the specific use of the herb please consult the herbalist or health professionals)

Forest Frog's Oviduct (Hamayou)

Chinese phonetic alphabet/pin yin: há ma yóu
Chinese characters simplified/traditional:蛤蟆油/蛤蟆油
Chinese nickname's alphabet (Nickname's Chinese characters): Hashimayou/ Xuehayou/ Linwayou(哈士蟆油/雪蛤油/林蛙油)

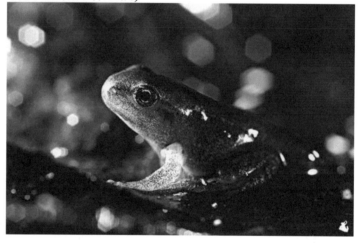

Latin: Ranae Oviductus (Common name: Forest Frog's Oviduct or Wood Frog Fallopian Tube)
Animal: *Rana temporaria chensinensis* David. (or *Rana amurensis* Boulenger.)

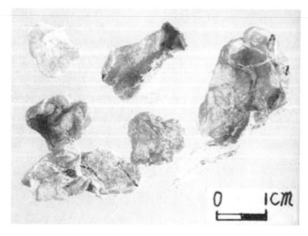

TCM prepared in ready-to-use forms (medicinal parts): it's dried female frog's fallopian tube/oviduct.
Property and flavor: neutral; sweet, salty.
Main and collateral channels: lung and kidney meridians.
Administration and dosage: 5-15 g, soaked in water, stewing or used in pills or powder.

162

Indication: lassitude, palpitations, insomnia, night sweating, cough, hemoptysis.
Attention: to protect the rare wild animals, please don't use it from wild animal.
(The picture is only for learning and identification the herb; the specific use of the herb please consult the herbalist or health professionals)

Papermulberry Fruit (Chushizi)
Chinese phonetic alphabet/pin yin: chǔ shí zǐ
Chinese characters simplified/traditional:楮实子/楮實子

Chinese nickname's alphabet (Nickname's Chinese characters): Goumuzi/ Shazhishu/ Goushuzi(榖木子/纱纸树/构树子)
Latin: Broussonetiae Fructus (Common name: Papermulberry Fruit)
Plant: *Broussonetia papyrifera* (L.) Vent.

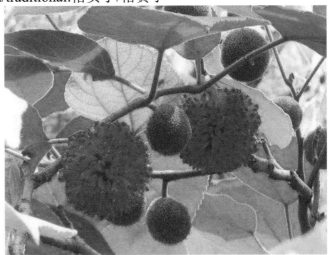

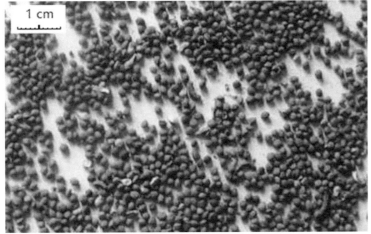

TCM prepared in ready-to-use forms (medicinal parts): it's dried mature fruit.
Property and flavor: cold; bitter.
Main and collateral channels: liver, heart, lung and stomach meridians.

Administration and dosage: 9-30 g. It should be decocted first.
Indication: soreness and weakness of waist and knees, dizziness, tinnitus, vomiting, belching, hematemesis, epistaxis, menstrual flooding and spotting, edema and swellings.
Precaution and warning: use with caution during pregnancy.
(The picture is only for learning and identification the herb; the specific use of the herb please consult the herbalist or health professionals)

Male Snake Genital (Shebian)
Chinese phonetic alphabet/pin yin: shé biān
Chinese characters simplified/traditional:蛇鞭/蛇鞭
Latin: Agkistrodon Testis et Penis (Common name: Male Snake Genital)
Property and flavor: warm; sweet, salty.
Main and collateral channels: liver, kidney and bladder meridians.

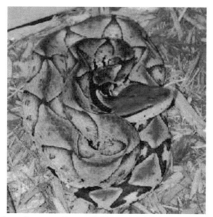

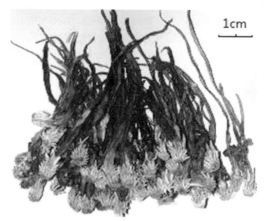

Animal: species of Serpentiformes   TCM prepared in ready-to-use forms (medicinal parts): it's male snake's genital organism.

Administration and dosage:6-15 g, or soaked in liquor.

Indication: build up a good physique and improve one's health; aphrodisiac.

Attention: to protect the rare wild animals, don't use it from wild animal.

(The picture is only for learning and identification the herb; the specific use of the herb please consult the herbalist or health professionals)

Common Fenugreek Seed (Huluba)

Chinese phonetic alphabet/pin yin: hú lu bā

Chinese characters simplified/traditional:葫芦巴/葫蘆巴

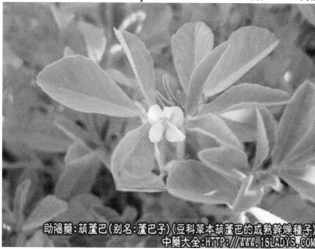

Chinese nickname's alphabet (Nickname's Chinese characters): Lubazi/ Xiangcao/ Xiangdou(芦巴子/香草/香豆)

Latin: Trigonellae Semen (Common name: Common Fenugreek Seed)

Plant: *Trigonella foenumgraecum* L.

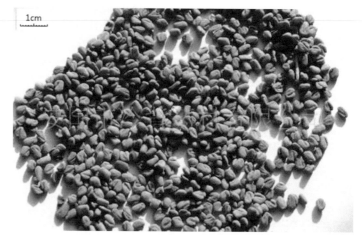

TCM prepared in ready-to-use forms (medicinal parts): it's dried mature seed.

Property and flavor: warm; bitter.

Main and collateral channels: kidney meridian.

Administration and dosage: 5-10 g.

Indication: abdomen pain caused by cold/chill (*Hanliang*), hernia, tinea pedis.
(The picture is only for learning and identification the herb; the specific use of the herb please consult the herbalist or health professionals)

Glossy Ganoderma (Lingzhi)
Chinese phonetic alphabet/pin yin: líng zhī
Chinese characters simplified/traditional:灵芝/靈芝
Chinese nickname's alphabet (Nickname's Chinese characters): Sanxiu/ Zhi/ Lingzhicao(三秀/芝/灵芝草)
Latin: Ganoderma (Common name: Glossy Ganoderma)

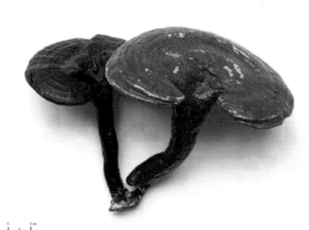

Fungus: *Ganoderma lucidum* (Leyss. ex Fr.) Karst. (or *Ganoderma sinensis* Zhao, Xu et Zhang.)
TCM prepared in ready-to-use forms (medicinal parts): it's (dried) sporophore.
Property and flavor: neutral; sweet.
Main and collateral channels: heart, lung, liver and kidney meridians.
Administration and dosage: 6-12 g.

Indication: dizziness, insomnia, wakefulness, palpitation, shortness of breath, cough and loss appetite.
(The picture is only for learning and identification the herb; the specific use of the herb please consult the herbalist or health professionals)

Leek Seed (Jiucaizi)
Chinese phonetic alphabet/pin yin: jiǔ cài zǐ

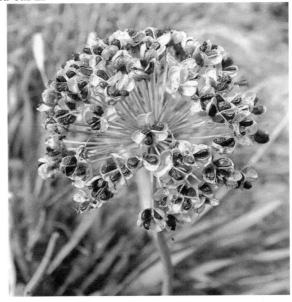

Chinese characters simplified/traditional:韭菜子/韭菜子
Chinese nickname's alphabet (Nickname's Chinese characters): Jiuzi(韭子)
Latin: Allii Tuberosi Semen (Common name: Leek Seed, Chinese Chive Seed or Tuber Onion Seed)
Plant: *Allium tuberosum* Rottle. ex Spreng.
TCM prepared in ready-to-use forms (medicinal parts): it's dried ripe seed.

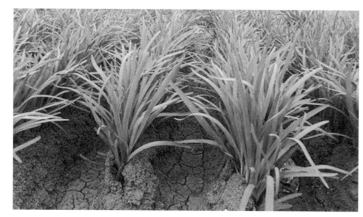

Property and flavor: warm; pungent, sweet. Main and collateral channels: liver and kidney meridians. Administration and dosage: 3-9 g.

1 cm

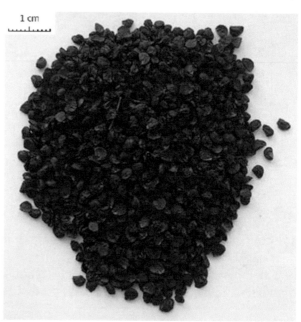

Indication: limp aching, impotence, seminal emission, enuresis, white and turbid vaginal discharge.
(The picture is only for learning and identification the herb; the specific use of the herb please consult the herbalist or health professionals)

Coriolus Versicolor Sporphore (Yunzhi)
Chinese phonetic alphabet/pin yin: yún zhī
Chinese characters simplified/traditional:云芝/云芝

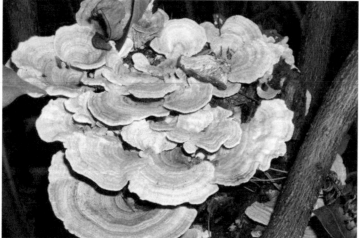

Chinese nickname's alphabet (Nickname's Chinese characters): Caiyungegaijun/ Wajun(彩云革盖菌/ 瓦菌)
Latin: Coriolus (Common name: Coriolus Versicolor Sporphore)
Fungus: *Coriolus versicolor* (L. ex Fr.) Quel.

TCM prepared in ready-to-use forms (medicinal parts): it's dried sporphore which harvested all year round.
Property and flavor: neutral; sweet.

Main and collateral channels: heart, spleen, liver and kidney meridians.
Administration and dosage: 9-27 g.
Indication: jaundice, hypochondriac pain, less intake, fatigue, lack of strength.
(The picture is only for learning and identification the herb; the specific use of the herb please consult the herbalist or health professionals)

Aleppo Arens Herb (Lanbuzheng)
Chinese phonetic alphabet/pin yin: lán bù zhèng

Chinese characters simplified/traditional:蓝布正/藍布正
Chinese nickname's alphabet (Nickname's Chinese characters): Lubianqing/ Zhuifengqi(路边青/追风七)
Latin: Gei Herba (Common name: Aleppo Arens Herb)

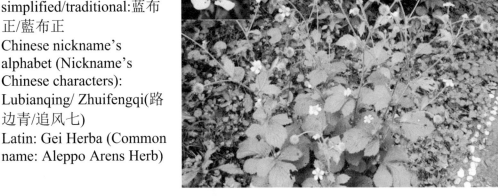

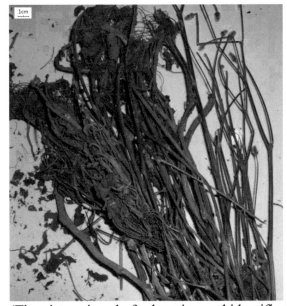

Plant: *Geum aleppicum* Jacq. (or *Geum japonicum* Thunb. var. *chinense* Bolle.)
TCM prepared in ready-to-use forms (medicinal parts): it's dried whole herb which harvested in summer or autumn.
Property and flavor: cool; mild bitter, sweet.
Main and collateral channels: liver, spleen and lung meridians.
Administration and dosage: 9-30 g.
Indication: consumptive disease with cough and vaginal discharge.

(The picture is only for learning and identification the herb; the specific use of the herb please consult the herbalist or health professionals)

Japanese Ginseng (Zhujieshen)
Chinese phonetic alphabet/pin yin: zhú jié shēn
Chinese characters simplified/traditional:竹节参/竹節參
Chinese nickname's alphabet (Nickname's Chinese characters): Renshenlu/ Baisanqi/ Mingqi/ Qiyezi(人参芦/白三七/明七/七叶子)
Latin: Panacis Japonici Rhizoma (Common name: Japanese Ginseng)
Plant: *Panax japonicus* C. A. Mey.

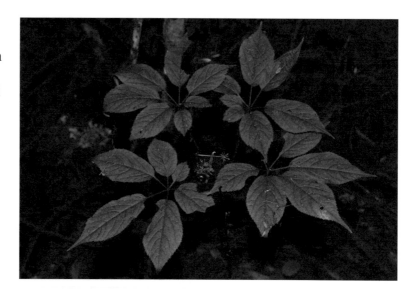

TCM prepared in ready-to-use forms (medicinal parts): it's dried rhizome which harvested in autumn. Property and flavor: warm; sweet, mild bitter.

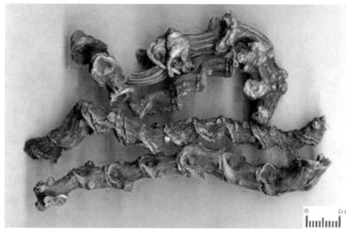

Main and collateral channels: liver, spleen and lung meridians. Administration and dosage: 6-9 g. Indication: hemoptysis, traumatic injuries, cough, excessive phlegm, weakness.

(The picture is only for learning and identification the herb; the specific use of the herb please consult the herbalist or health professionals)

Largeleaf Japanese Ginseng Rhizome (Zhuzishen)
Chinese phonetic alphabet/pin yin: zhū zǐ shēn
Chinese characters simplified/traditional: 珠子参/珠子參
Chinese nickname's alphabet (Nickname's Chinese characters): Qiuzishen/ Yuyesanqi/ Jiyaoshen(球子参/羽叶三七/鸡腰参)
Latin: Panacis Majoris Rhizoma (Common name: Largeleaf Japanese Ginseng Rhizome)

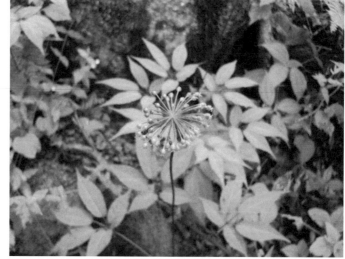

Plant: *Panax japonicus* C. A. Mey. var. *major* (Burk) C. Y. Wu et K. M. Feng. (or *Panax japonicus* C. A. Mey. var. *bipinnatifidus* (Seem.) C. Y. Wu. et K. M. Feng.)

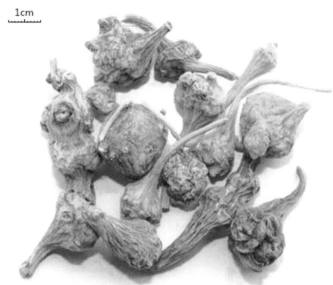

1cm

TCM prepared in ready-to-use forms (medicinal parts): it's dried rhizome which harvested in autumn. Property and flavor: mild cold; sweet, bitter. Main and collateral channels: liver, lung and stomach meridians. Administration and dosage: 3-9 g. Topical application in appropriate amount, ground into powder for application.

Indication: heat vexation, thrist, cough caused by consumptive disease, traumatic injuries, arthralgra, hemoptysis, hematemesis, external bleeding, epistaxis and metrorrhagia.

(The picture is only for learning and identification the herb; the specific use of the herb please consult the herbalist or health professionals)

Emblic Leafflower Fruit (Yuganzi)

Chinese phonetic alphabet/pin yin: yú gān zǐ
Chinese characters simplified/traditional:余甘子/余甘子

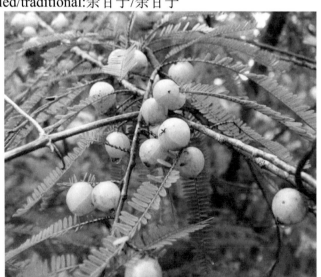

Chinese nickname's alphabet (Nickname's Chinese characters): Anmole/ Jiurula/ Maxiangbang(庵摩勒/ 久如拉/麻项邦)
Latin: Phyllanthi Fructus (Common name: Emblic Leafflower Fruit)
Plant: *Phyllanthus emblica* L.

TCM prepared in ready-to-use forms (medicinal parts): it's dried ripe fruit.
Property and flavor: cool; sweet, acidity and astringent.
Main and collateral channels: lung and stomach meridians.
Administration and dosage: 3-9 g, usually used in pills and powder.
Indication: blood stasis, dyspepsia, cough, sore throat and thirst.

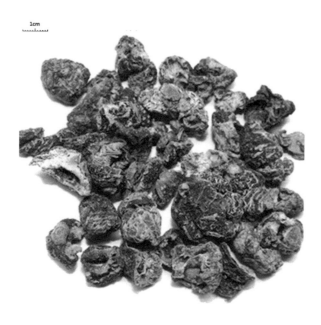

1cm

It is taken as food in some part of China. (The picture is only for learning and identification the herb; the specific use of the herb please consult the herbalist or health professionals)

Black Sesame (Heizhima)
Chinese phonetic alphabet/pin yin: hēi zhī má
Chinese characters simplified/traditional:黑芝麻/黑芝麻
Chinese nickname's alphabet (Nickname's Chinese characters): Youma/ Jusheng/ Zhima(油麻/巨胜/脂麻)
Latin: Sesami Semen Nigrum (Common name: Black Sesame)
Plant: *Sesamum indicum* L.

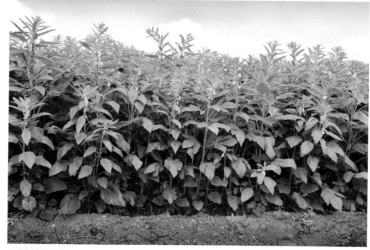

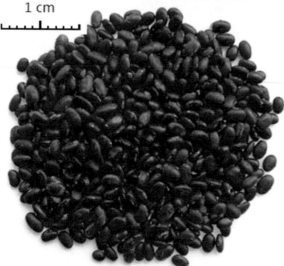

1 cm

TCM prepared in ready-to-use forms (medicinal parts): it's dried mature seed.
Property and flavor: neutral; sweet.
Main and collateral channels: liver, kidney and large intestine meridians.
Administration and dosage: 9-15 g.
Indication: dizziness, blurred vision, tinnitus, deafness, premature graying, hair loss and constipation.

It is taken as food in some part of China.
(The picture is only for learning and identification the herb; the specific use of the herb please consult the herbalist or health professionals)

Black Bean (Heidou)
Chinese phonetic alphabet/pin yin: hēi dòu
Chinese characters simplified/traditional:黑豆/黑豆

Chinese nickname's alphabet (Nickname's Chinese characters): Wudou/ Zhizidou(乌豆/枝仔豆)
Latin: Sojae Semen Nigrum (Common name: Black Bean)

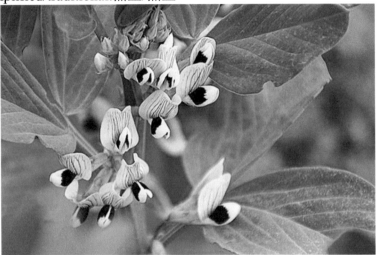

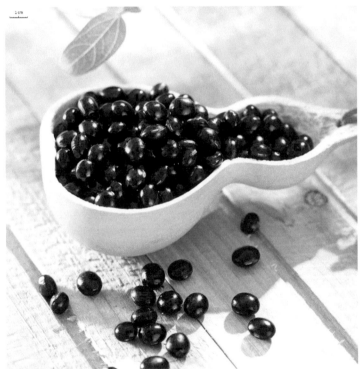

Plant: *Glycine max* (L.) Merr.
TCM prepared in ready-to-use forms (medicinal parts): it's dried ripe seed which harvested in autumn.
Property and flavor: neutral; sweet.
Main and collateral channels: spleen and kidney meridians.
Administration and dosage: 9-30 g.
Topical application in appropriate amount, decocted for bathing.

Indication: vexation and thirst, dizziness, blurred vision, weak constitution, night sweating, lumbago, edema, painful *bi* disorder, spasm, numbness, drug and food poisoning.
It is taken as food in some part of China.
(The picture is only for learning and identification the herb; the specific use of the herb please consult the herbalist or health professionals)

Shou Se Yao(收涩药)-astringent herbs

Shou Se Yao is a kind of herbs which's the major functions are to treat cough, chronic diarrhea, enuresis, night sweat, metrorrhagia.

Chinese Magnoliavine Fruit (Wuweizi)

Chinese phonetic alphabet/pin yin: wǔ wèi zǐ

Chinese characters simplified/traditional:五味子/五味子

Chinese nickname's alphabet (Nickname's Chinese characters): Xuanji/ Huiji/ Wumeizi(玄及/会及/五梅子)

Latin: Schisandrae Chinensis Fructus (Common name: Chinese Magnoliavine Fruit) Plant: *Schisandra chinensis* (Turcz) Barll.

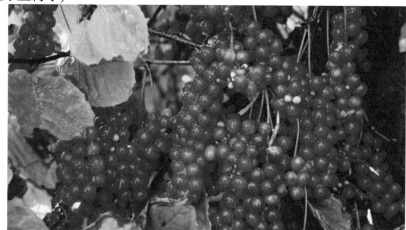

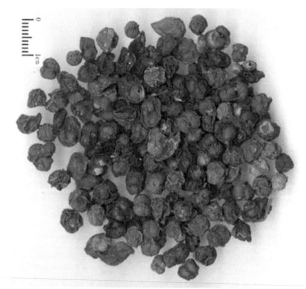

TCM prepared in ready-to-use forms (medicinal parts): it's dried mature fruit.

Property and flavor: warm; acidity, sweet.

Main and collateral channels: lung, heart and kidney meridians.

Administration and dosage: 2-6 g.

Indication: chronic cough and asthenia, dyspnea, spermatorrhea, enuresis, chronic diarrhea, night sweating, weak pulse, thirst, palpitation and insomnia.

(The picture is only for learning and identification the herb; the specific use of the herb please consult the herbalist or health professionals)

Southern Magnoliavine Fruit (Nanwuweizi)

Chinese phonetic alphabet/pin yin: nán wǔ wèi zǐ

Chinese characters simplified/traditional:南五味子/南五味子

Chinese nickname's alphabet (Nickname's Chinese characters): Huazhongwuweizi/ Xiangsu/ Honglingzi/ Hongmuxiang(华中五味子/香苏/红铃子/红木香)

Latin: Schisandrae Sphenantherae Fructus (Common name: Southern Magnoliavine Fruit)

Plant: *Schisandra Sphenanthera* Rehd. et Wils.
TCM prepared in ready-to-use forms (medicinal parts): it's dried ripe fruit.
Property and flavor: warm; acidity, sweet.
Main and collateral channels: lung, heart and kidney meridians.

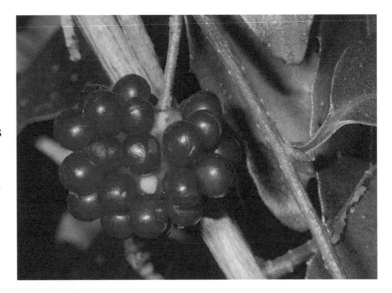

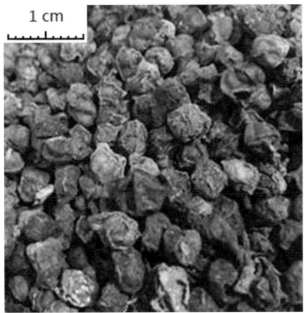

1 cm

Administration and dosage: 2-6 g.
Indication: chronic cough, emission, spermatorrhea, frequent urination, chronic diarrhea, night sweating, palpitation and insomnia.
(The picture is only for learning and identification the herb; the specific use of the herb please consult the herbalist or health professionals)

Smoked Plum (Wumei)
Chinese phonetic alphabet/pin yin: wū méi
Chinese characters simplified/traditional:乌梅/烏梅
Chinese nickname's alphabet (Nickname's Chinese characters): Meishi/ Heimei/ Xunmei(梅实/黑梅/熏梅)
Latin: Mume Fructus (Common name: Smoked Plum or Dark Plum)
Plant: *Prunus mume* Sieb. et Zuce.
TCM prepared in ready-to-use forms (medicinal parts): it's dried nearly mature fruit.
Property and flavor: neutral; acidity, astringent.
Main and collateral channels: liver, spleen, lung and large intestine meridians.
Administration and dosage: 6-12 g.

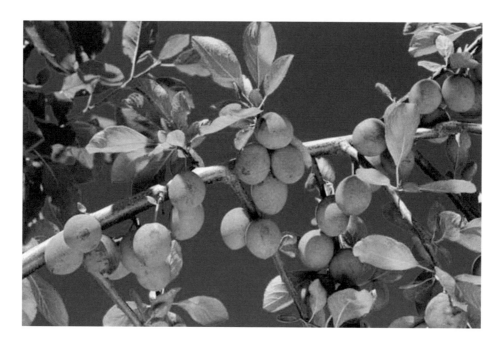

Indication: chronic cough, fever, diabetes, vomit, abdominal pain caused by ascaris and cestode, chronic dysentery and diarrhea. It is taken as food in some part of China. (The picture is only for learning and identification the herb; the specific use of the herb please consult the herbalist or health professionals)

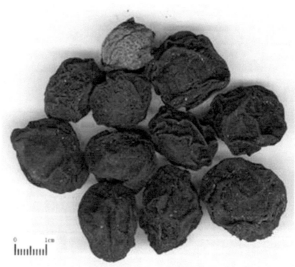

Gordon Euryale Seed (Qianshi)

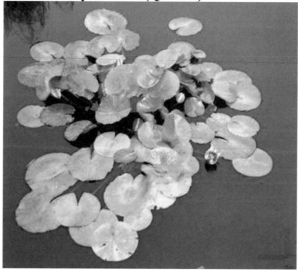

Chinese phonetic alphabet/pin yin: qiàn shí
Chinese characters simplified/traditional:芡实/芡實
Chinese nickname's alphabet (Nickname's Chinese characters): Jitoushi/ Suhuang/ Huangshi(鸡头实/苏黄/黄实)
Latin: Euryales Semen (Common name: Gordon Euryale Seed or Gorgon Fruit)
Plant: *Euryale ferox* Salisb.

TCM prepared in ready-to-use forms (medicinal parts): it's dried mature kernel/nuts. Property and flavor: neutral; sweet, astringent. Main and collateral channels: spleen and kidney meridians. Administration and dosage: 9-15 g. Indication: spermatorrhea, seminal emission, enuresis, frequent micturition, chronic dysentery, gonorrhea and leucorrhea with turbid.

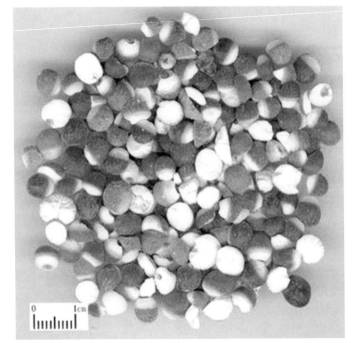

It is taken as food in some part of China.
(The picture is only for learning and identification the herb; the specific use of the herb please consult the herbalist or health professionals)

Palmleaf Raspberry Fruit (Fupenzi)
Chinese phonetic alphabet/pin yin: fù pén zi
Chinese characters simplified/traditional:覆盆子/覆盆子
Chinese nickname's alphabet (Nickname's Chinese characters): Fupen/ Xiaotuopan (覆盆/小托盘)

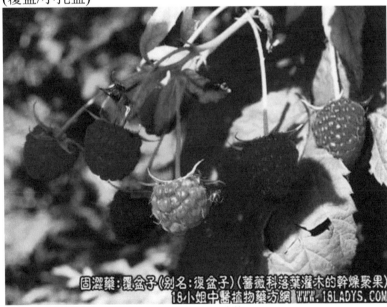

Latin: Rubi Fructus (Common name: Palmleaf Raspberry Fruit) Plant: *Rubus chingii* Hu. (or *Rubus' idaeus* L.) TCM prepared in ready-to-use forms (medicinal parts): it's dried mature fruit.

Property and flavor: warm; sweet, acidity.
Main and collateral channels: liver, kidney and bladder meridians.
Administration and dosage: 6-12 g.

Indication: frequent urination, impotence, seminal emission, spermatorrhea, enuresis, premature ejaculation and blurry vision.
It is taken as food in some part of China.
Precaution and warning: use with caution during pregnancy.
(The picture is only for learning and identification the herb; the specific use of the herb please consult the herbalist or health professionals)

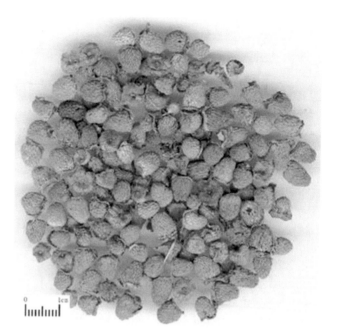

Tree-of-heaven Bark (Chunpi)
Chinese phonetic alphabet/pin yin: chūn pí
Chinese characters simplified/traditional:椿皮/椿皮
Chinese nickname's alphabet (Nickname's Chinese characters): Chouchun/ Chungenpi(臭椿/椿根皮)

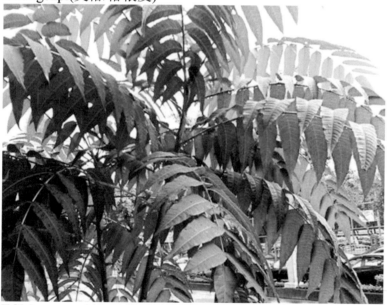

Latin: Ailanthi Cortex (Common name: Tree-of-heaven Bark)
Plant: *Ailanthus altissima* (Mill.) Swingle.

TCM prepared in ready-to-use forms (medicinal parts): it's dried stem bark or root bark which harvested all year round.
Property and flavor: cold; bitter, astringent.
Main and collateral channels: large intestine, stomach and liver meridians.
Administration and dosage: 6-9 g.

Indication: leucorrhea with blood, dysentery, chronic diarrhea, hematochezia, metrorrhagia and spotting.
(The picture is only for learning and identification the herb; the specific use of the herb please consult the herbalist or health professionals)

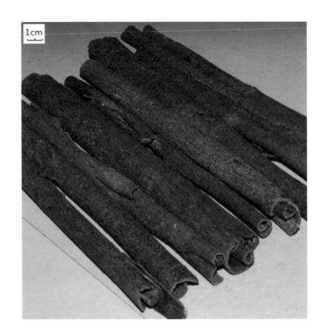

Red Halloysite (Chishizhi)
Chinese phonetic alphabet/pin yin: chì shí zhī
Chinese characters simplified/traditional:赤石脂/赤石脂

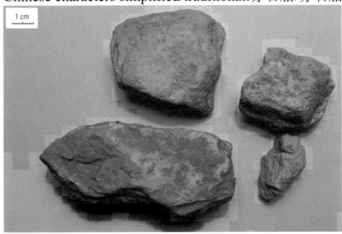

Chinese nickname's alphabet (Nickname's Chinese characters): Chifu/ Honggaoling(赤符/红高岭)
Latin: Halloysitum Rubrum (Common name: Red Halloysite)
Mineral: main component [Al$_4$(Si$_4$O$_{10}$)(OH)$_8$·4H$_2$O] with a little Fe$_2$O$_3$

TCM prepared in ready-to-use forms (medicinal parts): it's cleaned mineral (power).
Property and flavor: warm; sweet, acidity and astringent.
Main and collateral channels: large intestine and stomach meridians.
Administration and dosage: 9-12 g. It should be decocted first. Topical application in appropriate amount, ground into powder and apply to the *pars affecta*.
Indication: hematochezia, metrorrhagia, chlornic diarrhea and dysentery; external use for ulcer and eczema.

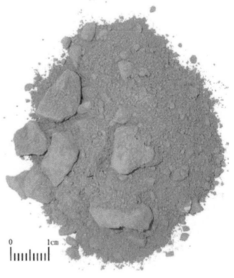

177

Precaution and warning: Incompatible with Cassia Bark.
(The picture is only for learning and identification the herb; the specific use of the herb please consult the herbalist or health professionals)

Wizened Wheat (Fuxiaomai)
Chinese phonetic alphabet/pin yin: fú xiǎo mài
Chinese characters simplified/traditional:浮小麦/浮小麥

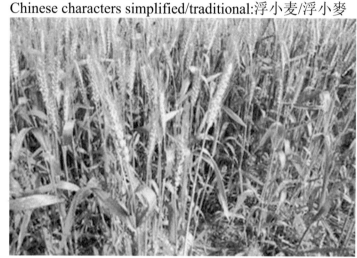

Chinese nickname's alphabet (Nickname's Chinese characters): Fumai(浮麦)
Latin: Tritici Levi Fructus seu Macie Tritii Semen (Common name: Wizened Wheat or Light Wheat)

Plant: *Triticum aestivum* L.
TCM prepared in ready-to-use forms (medicinal parts): it's dried light grain/immature caryopses.
Property and flavor: cool; sweet.
Main and collateral channels: heart meridian.
Administration and dosage: 3-10 g.
Indication: night sweating and fever.

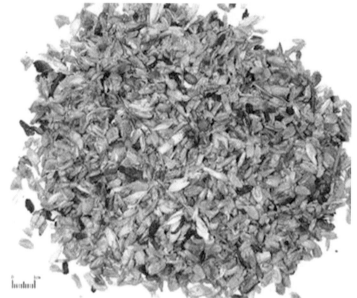

(The picture is only for learning and identification the herb; the specific use of the herb please consult the herbalist or health professionals)

Cherokee Rose Fruit (Jinyingzi)
Chinese phonetic alphabet/pin yin: jīn yīng zǐ
Chinese characters simplified/traditional:金樱子/金櫻子
Chinese nickname's alphabet (Nickname's Chinese characters): Shanshiliu/ Shanjitouzi (山石榴/山鸡头子)
Latin: Rosae Laevigatae Fructus (Common name: Cherokee Rose Fruit)
Plant: *Rosa laevigata* Michx.

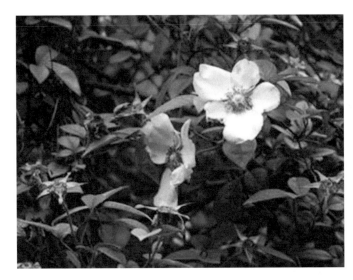

TCM prepared in ready-to-use forms (medicinal parts): it's dried mature fruit.
Property and flavor: neutral; acidity, sweet and astringent.
Main and collateral channels: kidney, bladder and large intestine meridians.
Administration and dosage: 6-12 g.

Indication: seminal emission, spermatorrhea, frequent urination, enuresis, metrorrhagi and metrostaxis, chlornic diarrhea and dysentery. (The picture is only for learning and identification the herb; the specific use of the herb please consult the herbalist or health professionals)

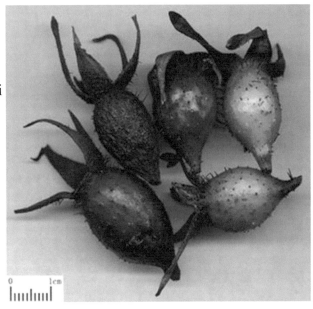

Lotus Seed (Lianzi)
Chinese phonetic alphabet/pin yin: lián zǐ
Chinese characters simplified/traditional:莲子/蓮子

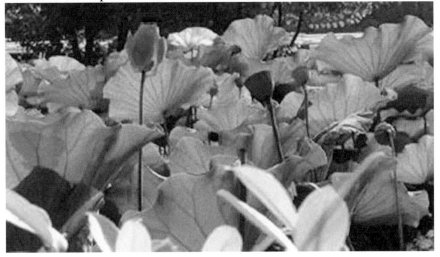

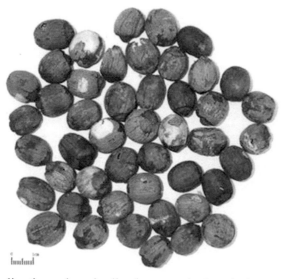

Chinese nickname's alphabet (Nickname's Chinese characters): Oushi/ Lianshi/ Lianpengzi(藕实/莲实/莲蓬子)
Latin: Nelumbinis Semen (Common name: Lotus Seed)
Plant: *Nelumbo nucifera* Gaertn.
TCM prepared in ready-to-use forms (medicinal parts): it's dried mature seeds.
Property and flavor: neutral; sweet, astringent.
Main and collateral channels: spleen, kidney and heart meridians.
Administration and dosage: 6-15 g.

Indication: chronic diarrhea, seminal emission, spermatorrhea, vaginal discharge, palpitation and insomnia.
It is taken as food in some part of China.
(The picture is only for learning and identification the herb; the specific use of the herb please consult the herbalist or health professionals)

Asiatic Cornelian Cherry Fruit (Shanzhuyu)

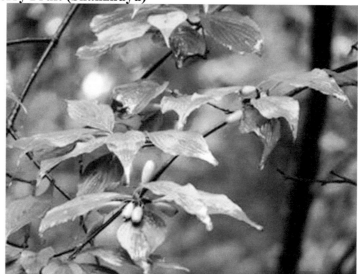

Chinese phonetic alphabet/pin yin: shān zhū yú
Chinese characters simplified/traditional: 山茱萸/山茱萸
Chinese nickname's alphabet (Nickname's Chinese characters): Rouzao/ Jizu/ Yurou(肉枣/鸡足/萸肉)

Latin: Corni Fructus (Common name: Asiatic Cornelian Cherry Fruit)
Plant: *Cornus officinalis* Sieb. et Zucc.
TCM prepared in ready-to-use forms (medicinal parts): it's dried mature fruit fresh/sarcocarp.
Property and flavor: mild warm; acidity, astringent.
Main and collateral channels: kidney and liver meridians.
Administration and dosage: 6-12 g.

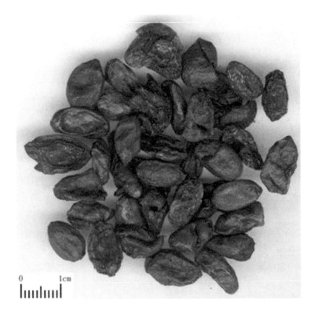

Indication: dizziness, tinnitus, waist and knee pain, impotence, seminal emission, spermatorrhea, sweating and collapse, internal heat dissipation. (The picture is only for learning and identification the herb; the specific use of the herb please consult the herbalist or health professionals)

Chinese Gall (Wubeizi)

Chinese phonetic alphabet/pin yin: wǔ bèi zǐ
Chinese characters simplified/ traditional: 五倍子/五倍子
Chinese nickname's alphabet (Nickname's Chinese characters): Wenge/ Baichongcang (文蛤/百虫仓)

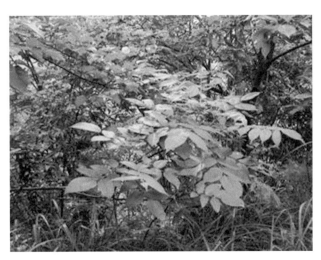

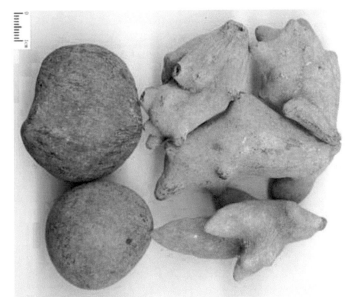

Latin: Galla Chinensis (Common name: Chinese Gall or Gallnut)
Cecidum: gall caused by *Rhus chinensis* Mill. (or *Rhus potaninii* Maxim, *Rhus punjabensis* Stew. var. *sinica* (Diels.) Rehd. et Wils.) parasitic by *Melaphis chinensis* Bell.

TCM prepared in ready-to-use forms (medicinal parts): it's the gall produced mainly by parasitic aphids of *Melaphis chinensis* (Bell.) Barker. on the leaf of *Rhus chinensis* Mill. (or *Rhus potaninii* Maxim., *Rhus punjabensis* Stew. var. *sinica* (Diels.) Rehd. et Wils.)

Property and flavor: cold; acidity, astringent.

Main and collateral channels: lung, large intestine and kidney meridians.

Administration and dosage: 3-6 g. Appropriate amount for topical application.

Indication: chronic cough, phlegm, chlornic diarrhea and dysentery, night sweating, thirst, hemorrhoids, traumatic with bleeding, bloody stool and carbuncle sore.

(The picture is only for learning and identification the herb; the specific use of the herb please consult the herbalist or health professionals)

Ephedra Root (Mahuanggen)

Chinese phonetic alphabet/pin yin: má huáng gēn

Chinese characters simplified/traditional:麻黄根/麻黄根

Chinese nickname's alphabet (Nickname's Chinese characters): Kuchuncai(苦椿菜)

Latin: Ephedrae Radix et Rhizoma (Common name: Ephedra Root)

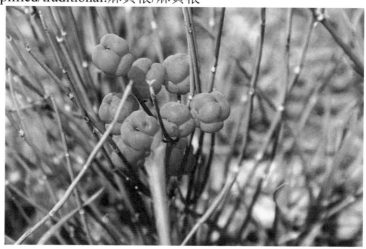

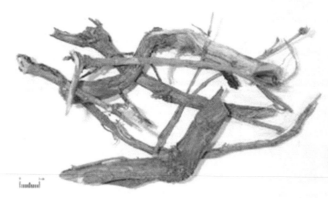

Plant: *Ephedra sinica* Stapf. (or *Ephedra intermedia* Schrenk. et C. A. Mey.) TCM prepared in ready-to-use forms (medicinal parts): it's dried root and rhizome which harvested in autumn.

Property and flavor: neutral; sweet, astringent.

Main and collateral channels: lung and heart meridians.

Administration and dosage: 3-9 g. Topical application in appropriate amount, ground into powder and apply to the *pars affecta*.

Indication: spontaneous sweating, night sweating.

(The picture is only for learning and identification the herb; the specific use of the herb please consult the herbalist or health professionals)

Mantis Egg-case (Sangpiaoxiao)

Chinese phonetic alphabet/pin yin: sāng piāo xiāo

Chinese characters simplified/traditional:桑螵蛸/桑螵蛸

Chinese nickname's alphabet (Nickname's Chinese characters): Tanglangzi(螳螂子)
Latin: Mantidis Oötheca (Common name: Mantis Egg-case)
Animal: *Tenodera sinensis* Saussure. (or *Statilia maculata* (Thurlberg.), *Hierodula patellifera* (Serville.))

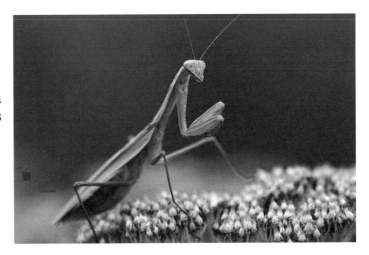

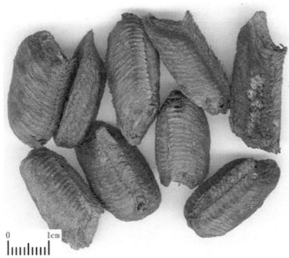

TCM prepared in ready-to-use forms (medicinal parts): it's dried egg sheath/capsule.
Property and flavor: neutral; sweet, salty.
Main and collateral channels: liver and kidney meridians.
Administration and dosage: 5-10 g.
Indication: spermatorrhea, seminal emission, enuresis, frequent micturition and turbid urine.

Attention: to protect the rare wild animals, don't use it from wild animal.
(The picture is only for learning and identification the herb; the specific use of the herb please consult the herbalist or health professionals)

Cuttlebone (Haipiaoxiao)
Chinese phonetic alphabet/pin yin: hǎi piāo xiāo
Chinese characters simplified/traditional: 海螵蛸/海螵蛸
Chinese nickname's alphabet (Nickname's Chinese characters): Wuzeigu/ Moyugai(乌贼骨/墨鱼盖)
Latin: Sepiae Endoconcha (Common name: Cuttlebone or Squidbone)

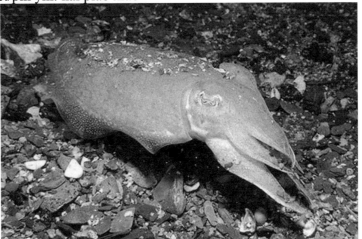

Animal: *Sepiella maindroni de* Roehebrune. (or *Sepia esculenta* Hoyle.)

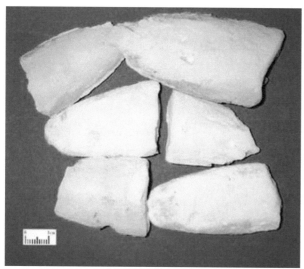

TCM prepared in ready-to-use forms (medicinal parts): it's dried the inner shell.
Property and flavor: warm; salty, astringent.
Main and collateral channels: spleen and kidney meridians.
Administration and dosage: 5-10 g. Topical application in appropriate amount, ground into powder and apply to the *pars affecta.*

Indication: acid regurgitation, epistaxis, hematemesis, hematochezia, metrorrhagia and spotting, spermatorrhoea ulcer disease, stomachache with acid reflux; external use for bleeding injury, sore and ulcer.
(The picture is only for learning and identification the herb; the specific use of the herb please consult the herbalist or health professionals)

Glutinous Rise Root (Nuodaogen)
Chinese phonetic alphabet/pin yin: nuò dào gēn
Chinese characters simplified/traditional:糯稻根/糯稻根
Chinese nickname's alphabet (Nickname's Chinese characters): Nuogugen/Daogenxu(糯谷根/稻根须)
Latin: Oryza Radix (Common name: Glutinous Rise Root)
Plant: *Oryza sativa* L. var. *glutinosa* Matsum.

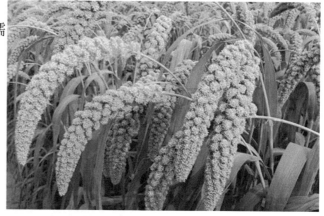

1cm

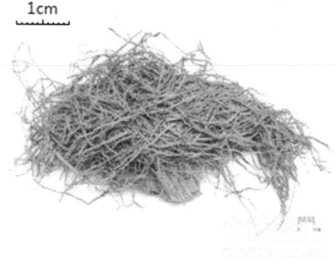

TCM prepared in ready-to-use forms (medicinal parts): it's dried root which harvested in autumn.
Property and flavor: neutral; sweet.
Main and collateral channels: heart and liver meridians.

Administration and dosage: 30-90 g.

Indication: spontaneous sweating, night sweating, hepatitis and chyluria.

(The picture is only for learning and identification the herb; the specific use of the herb please consult the herbalist or health professionals)

Poppy Capsule (Yingsuqiao)

Chinese phonetic alphabet/pin yin: yīng sù qiào

Chinese characters simplified/traditional:罂粟壳/罌粟殼

Chinese nickname's alphabet (Nickname's Chinese characters):Yumiqiao/Suqiao(御米壳/粟壳)

Latin: Papaveris Pericarpium (Common name: Poppy Capsule or Opium Poppy Shell)

Plant: *Papaver somniferum* L.

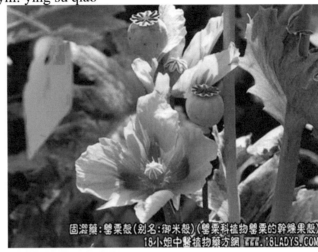

固澀藥：罌粟殼(別名：御米殼)(罌粟科植物罌粟的乾燥果殼) 18小姐中醫植物藥方網 WWW.18LADYS.COM

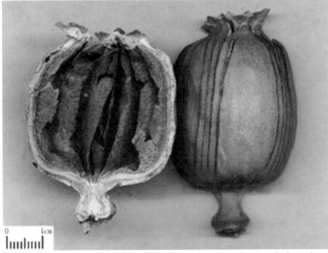

TCM prepared in ready-to-use forms (medicinal parts): it's dried mature fruit pericarp/capsule shell.

Property and flavor: neutral; acidity, astringent.

Main and collateral channels: lung, large intestine and kidney meridians.

Administration and dosage: 3-6 g.

Indication: chronic cough, chronic diarrhea, abdominal pain, archoptosis.

Precaution and warning: toxic. Additive, avoid frequent administration. Contraindicated during pregnancy and in child. Used cautiously for athletes.

(The picture is only for learning and identification the herb; the specific use of the herb please consult the herbalist or health professionals)

Medicine Terminalia Fruit (Hezi)

Chinese phonetic alphabet/pin yin: hē zǐ

Chinese characters simplified/traditional:诃子/訶子

Chinese nickname's alphabet (Nickname's Chinese characters): Helile/ Heli/ Suifengzi(诃黎勒/诃黎/随风子)

Latin: Chebulae Fructus (Common name: Medicine Terminalia Fruit)

Plant: *Terminalia chebula* Retz. (or *Terminalia chebula* Retz. var. *tomentella* Kurt.) TCM prepared in ready-to-use forms (medicinal parts): it's dried mature fruit.
Property and flavor: neutral; bitter, acidity and astringent.
Main and collateral channels: lung and large intestine meridians.

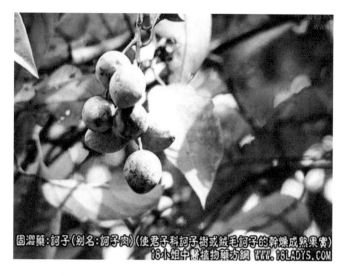

固澀藥:訶子(別名:訶子肉)(使君子科訶子樹或絨毛訶子的乾燥成熟果實)
16小姐中醫植物藥方網 WWW.16LADYS.COM

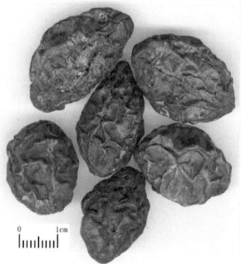

Administration and dosage: 3-10 g.
Indication: chronic diarrhea and dysentery, hematochezia, archoptosis, chronic cough, sore throat, hoarse.
(The picture is only for learning and identification the herb; the specific use of the herb please consult the herbalist or health professionals)

Western Fruit (Xiqingguo)

Chinese phonetic alphabet/pin yin: xī qīng guǒ
Chinese characters simplified/traditional:西青果/西青果
Chinese nickname's alphabet (Nickname's Chinese characters): Zhangqingguo(藏青果)

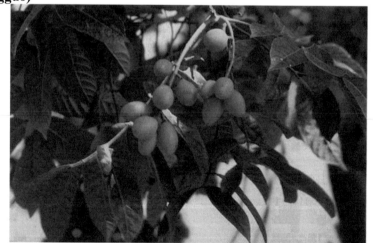

Latin: Chebulae Fructus Immaturus (Common name: Western Fruit)
Plant: *Terminalia chebula* Retz.

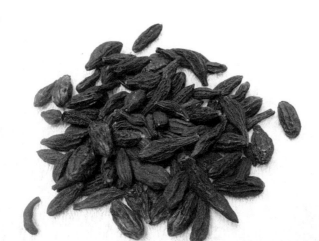

TCM prepared in ready-to-use forms (medicinal parts): it's dried fruit-let.
Property and flavor: neutral; bitter, acidity and astringent.
Main and collateral channels: lung and large intestine meridians.
Administration and dosage: 1.5-3 g.
Indication: diphtheria; clear heat; remove toxin.

(The picture is only for learning and identification the herb; the specific use of the herb please consult the herbalist or health professionals)

Nutmeg (Roudoukou)

Chinese phonetic alphabet/pin yin: ròu dòu kòu
Chinese characters simplified/traditional:肉豆蔻/肉豆蔻
Chinese nickname's alphabet (Nickname's Chinese characters): Doukou/ Rouguo(豆蔻/肉果)
Latin: Myristicae Semen (Common name: Nutmeg)
Plant: *Myristica fragrans* Houtt.
TCM prepared in ready-to-use forms (medicinal parts): it's dried mature kernel.
Property and flavor: warm; pungent.
Main and collateral channels: spleen, stomach and large intestine meridians.

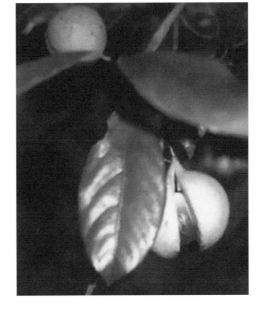

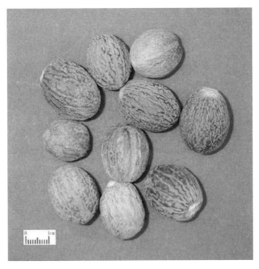

Administration and dosage: 3-10 g.
Indication: chronic diarrhea, epigastrium and abdominal pain, lack of appetite and vomiting.
It is taken as seasoning in some part of China.
(The picture is only for learning and identification the herb; the specific use of the herb please consult the herbalist or health professionals)

Pomegranate Rind (Shiliupi)

Chinese phonetic alphabet/pin yin: shí liù pí
Chinese characters simplified/traditional: 石榴皮/石榴皮
Chinese nickname's alphabet (Nickname's Chinese characters): Shiliuke/ Suanshiliupi(石榴壳/ 酸石榴皮)

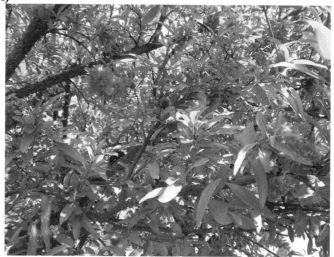

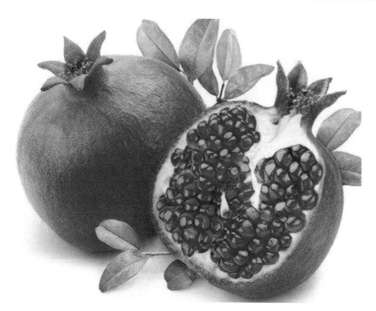

Latin: Granati Pericarpium (Common name: Pomegranate Rind)
Plant: *Punica granatum* L.
TCM prepared in ready-to-use forms (medicinal parts): it's dried mature peel/ pericarp.

Property and flavor: warm; acidity, astringent.
Main and collateral channels: large intestine meridian.
Administration and dosage: 3-9 g.
Indication: chronic diarrhea and dysentery, hematochezia, archoptosis, hematuria, leucorrhea turbidity, metrorrhagia, intestinal parasites.

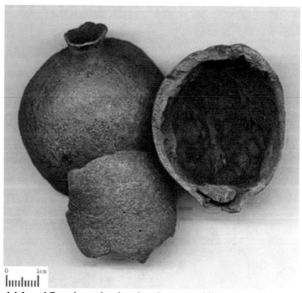

(The picture is only for learning and identification the herb; the specific use of the herb please consult the herbalist or health professionals)

Limonite (Yuyuliang)
Chinese phonetic alphabet/pin yin: yǔ yú liáng
Chinese characters simplified/traditional:禹余粮/禹餘糧
Chinese nickname's alphabet (Nickname's Chinese characters): Yuliangshi/ Baiyuyu/ Shinao(余粮石/白禹余/石脑)
Latin: Limonitum (Common name: Limonite)

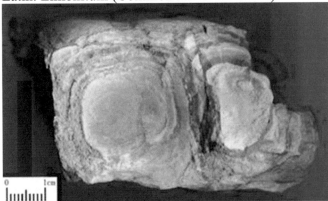

Mineral: main component FeO(OH)
TCM prepared in ready-to-use forms (medicinal parts): it's cleaned mineral.
Property and flavor: mild cold; sweet, astringent.
Main and collateral channels: stomach and large intestine meridians.

Administration and dosage: 9-15 g. It should be decocted first; or used in pills or powder.
Indication: chronic diarrhea and dysentery, uterine bleeding, metrorrhagia and bloody stool.
Precaution and warning: used with caution in pregnant women.
(The picture is only for learning and identification the herb; the specific use of the herb please consult the herbalist or health professionals)

Manyinflorescenced Sweetvetch Root (Hongqi)
Chinese phonetic alphabet/pin yin: hóng qi
Chinese characters simplified/traditional:红芪/紅芪
Chinese nickname's alphabet (Nickname's Chinese characters): Duoxuyanhuangqi(多序岩黄耆)
Latin: Hedysari Radix (Common name: Manyinflorescenced Sweetvetch Root)

Plant:
Hedysarum polybotrys Hand. -Mazz.
TCM prepared in ready-to-use forms (medicinal parts): it's dried root which harvested in spring or autumn.

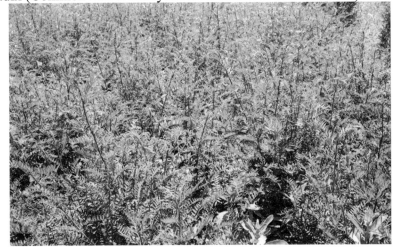

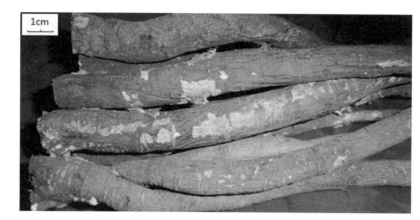

Property and flavor: mild warm; sweet. Main and collateral channels: lung and spleen meridians. Administration and dosage: 9-30 g.

Indication: lack of strength, less food intake, chronic diarrhea, bloody stool, edema, hemiplegia, arthrolgia, menstrual flooding and spotting.

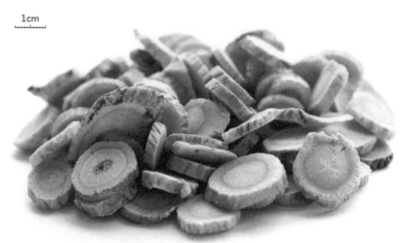

(The picture is only for learning and identification the herb; the specific use of the herb please consult the herbalist or health professionals)

Discolor Cinquefoil Herb (Fanbaicao)
Chinese phonetic alphabet/pin yin: fān bái cǎo

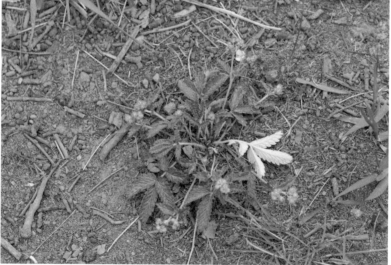

Chinese characters simplified/ traditional:翻白草/翻白草
Chinese nickname's alphabet (Nickname's Chinese characters): Jituigen/ Tian'ou(鸡腿根/天藕)

Latin: Potentillae Discoloris Herba (Common name: Discolor Cinquefoil Herb)
Plant: *Potentilla discolor* Bge.

TCM prepared in ready-to-use forms (medicinal parts): it's dried whole grass which harvested in summer or autumn.

Property and flavor: neutral; mild bitter, sweet.

Main and collateral channels: liver, large intestine and stomach meridians.

Administration and dosage: 9-15 g.

Indication: diarrhea, dysentery, swelling abscess, sore and toxin, hematemesis, hemafecia and metrorrhagia.

(The picture is only for learning and identification the herb; the specific use of the herb please consult the herbalist or health professionals)

Yong Tu Yao(涌吐药)-emetic herbs

Yong Tu Yao is a kind of herbs which's the major function is emetic.

Antifeverile Dichroa Root (Changshan)

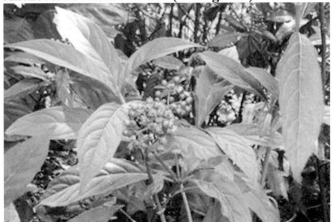

Chinese phonetic alphabet/pin yin: cháng shān

Chinese characters simplified/traditional:常山/常山

Chinese nickname's alphabet (Nickname's Chinese characters): Hucao/ Hengsha(互草/恒山)

Latin: Dichroae Radix (Common name: Antifeverile Dichroa Root)

Plant: *Dichroa febrifuga* Lour.

TCM prepared in ready-to-use forms (medicinal parts): it's dried root which harvested in autumn.

Property and flavor: cold; bitter, pungent.

Main and collateral channels: lung, liver and heart meridians.

Administration and dosage: 5-9 g.

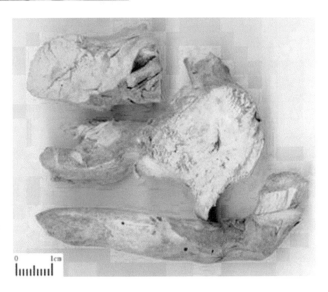

Indication: phlegm, malaria; induce vomiting.
Precaution and warning: toxic. Use with caution for pregnant women.
(The picture is only for learning and identification the herb; the specific use of the herb please consult the herbalist or health professionals)

Melon Pedicle (Guadi)
Chinese phonetic alphabet/pin yin: guā dì

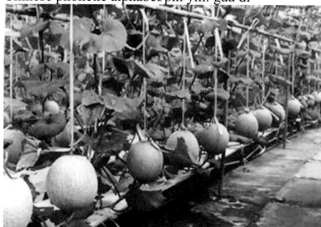

Chinese characters simplified/traditional:瓜蒂/瓜蒂
Chinese nickname's alphabet (Nickname's Chinese characters): Kudingxiang/ Tiangadi(苦丁香/甜瓜蒂)
Latin: Cucumis Calyx (Common name: Melon Pedicle or Melon Calyx)

Plant: *Cucumis melo* L.
TCM prepared in ready-to-use forms (medicinal parts): it's dried calyx of ripe fruit.
Property and flavor: cold; bitter.
Main and collateral channels: spleen and stomach meridians.
Administration and dosage: 3-5 g, or used for blowing into nose to sneeze.
Indication: excessive phlegm, indigestion, jaundice, stuffy nose and sore throat; induce vomiting.

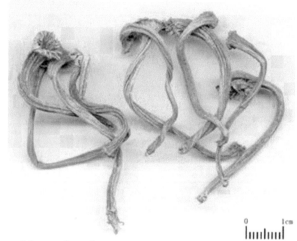

Precaution and warning: toxic. Use with caution for pregnant woman or patients with stomach disease.
(The picture is only for learning and identification the herb; the specific use of the herb please consult the herbalist or health professionals)

Black False Hellebore (Lilu)
Chinese phonetic alphabet/pin yin: lí lú
Chinese characters simplified/traditional:藜芦/藜蘆
Chinese nickname's alphabet (Nickname's Chinese characters): Shancong/ Duyaocao/Qilidan(山葱/毒药草/七厘丹)
Latin: Veratri Radix et Rhizoma (Common name: Black False Hellebore)
Plant: *Veratrum nigrum* L. (or *Veratrum schindleri* Loes. f., *Veratrum maackii* Regel., *Veratrum dahuricum* (Turcz.) Loes. f., *Veratrum grandiflorum* (Maxim.) Loes. f.)
TCM prepared in ready-to-use forms (medicinal parts): it's dried root which harvested in November or December.

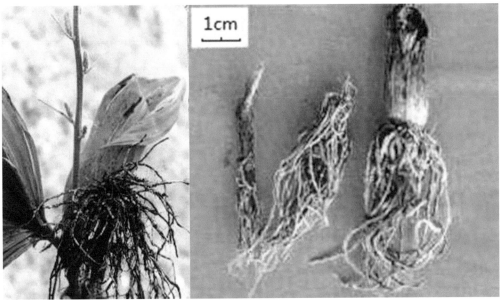

Property and flavor: cold; bitter, pungent.

Main and collateral channels: liver, stomach and stomach meridians.

Administration and dosage: 0.3-0.6 g. Topical application in appropriate amount, ground into powder for applyment.

Indication: epilepsy, apoplexy, sore throat, tinea and malara; induce vomitting.

Precaution and warning: highly toxic. Incompatible with Manchurian Wildginger Root, White Peony Root, Red Peony Root, Ginseng, Tangshen, American Ginseng, Lightyellow Sophora Root, Figwort, Asiatic Moonseed Rhizome, Danshen Root, Fourleaf Ladybell Root, Coastal Glehnia Root.

(The picture is only for learning and identification the herb; the specific use of the herb please consult the herbalist or health professionals)

Blue Vitriol (Danfan)

Chinese phonetic alphabet/pin yin: dǎn fán

Chinese characters simplified/traditional:胆矾/膽礬

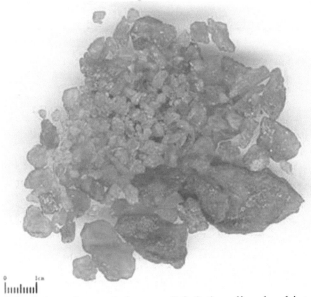

Chinese nickname's alphabet (Nickname's Chinese characters): Lanfan/ Wushuiliusuantong(蓝矾/五水硫酸铜)

Latin: Chalcanthitum (Common name: Blue Vitriol)

Mineral: main component $CuSO_4 \cdot 5H_2O$

TCM prepared in ready-to-use forms (medicinal parts): it's crystal powder.

Property and flavor: cold; acidity, pungent.

Main and collateral channels: liver and gallbladder meridians.

Administration and dosage: 0.3-0.6 g, dissolved into decoction or used in pill or powder. appropriate amount for topical application in, ground into powder for applyment or bathing.

Indication: phlegm, congestion, sore throat, epilepsy, red eye, ulcer, noma; induce vomiting.

Precaution and warning: toxic. Long-term oral administration is inadvisable.

(The picture is only for learning and identification the herb; the specific use of the herb please consult the herbalist or health professionals)

Melanterite (Zaofan)

Chinese phonetic alphabet/pin yin: zào fán

Chinese characters simplified/traditional:皂矾/皂礬

Chinese nickname's alphabet (Nickname's Chinese characters): Lvfan/ Qingfan(绿矾/青矾)

Latin: Melanteritum (Common name: Melanterite)

Mineral: main component $FeSO_4 \cdot 7H_2O$ TCM prepared in ready-to-use forms (medicinal parts): it's cleaned mineral.

Property and flavor: cool; acidity.

Main and collateral channels: liver and spleen meridians.

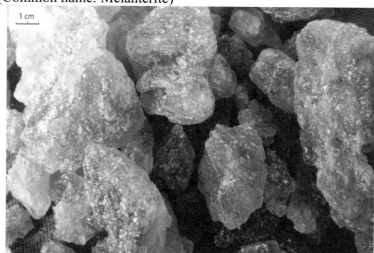

Administration and dosage: 0.8-1.6 g. Topical application in appropriate amount.

Indication: mild malnutrition with retention, chronic dysentery, hematochezia, sallow complexion, dampness sore, scabies and tinea; induce vomiting.

Precaution and warning: used with caution during pregnancy.

(The picture is only for learning and identification the herb; the specific use of the herb please consult the herbalist or health professionals)

Qu Chong Zhi Yang Yao(驱虫止痒药)-herbs for anthelmintic and antipruritic

Qu Chong Zhi Yang Yao is a kind of herbs which's the major functions are anthelmintic and antipruritic (they are usually for exterior use).

.

Calomel (Qingfen)

Chinese phonetic alphabet/pin yin: qīng fěn

Chinese characters simplified/traditional:轻粉/輕粉

Chinese nickname's alphabet (Nickname's Chinese characters): Gongfen/ Xiaofen/ Shuiyinfen(汞粉/峭粉/水银粉)

Latin: Calomelas (Common name: Calomel or Mercurous Chloride)

Mineral: main component Hg_2Cl_2 TCM prepared in ready-to-use forms (medicinal parts): it's crystal powder. Property and flavor: cold; pungent. Main and collateral channels: large intestine and small intestine meridians.

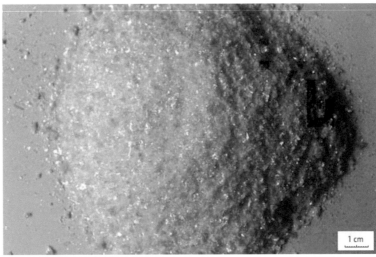

Administration and dosage: Topical application in appropriate amount, ground into powder for applyment. Oral administration: 0.1-0.2 g per time, 1-2 times a day, usually used in pills or capsules, gargling after oral administration.

Indication: excessive phlegm, constipations, tympanitis, edema and dysuria; external use for scabies, tinea, scrofula, chancre, skin ulcers and syphilis.

Precaution and warning: poisonous, avoid over-dosage. Be cautious for oral administration. Contraindicated for pregnant woman.

(The picture is only for learning and identification the herb; the specific use of the herb please consult the herbalist or health professionals)

Sulfur (Liuhuang)

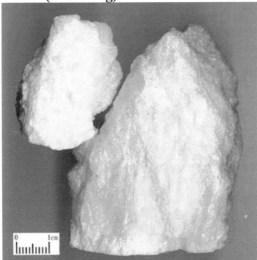

Chinese phonetic alphabet/pin yin: liú huáng

Chinese characters simplified/traditional:硫黄/硫磺

Chinese nickname's alphabet (Nickname's Chinese characters): Shiliuhuang(石硫磺)

Latin: Sulfur (Common name: Sulfur)

Mineral: main component S

TCM prepared in ready-to-use forms (medicinal parts): it's cleaned mineral (or powder).

Property and flavor: warm; acidity.

Main and collateral channels: kidney and large intestine meridians.

Administration and dosage: Topical application in appropriate amount, ground into powder for applyment. Oral administration: 1.5-3 g, usually used in pills or powder.

Indication: impotence, asthma, dyspnea and constipation; external use for scabies, tinea, favus, gangrene.

It is key herb to treat scabies.

Precaution and warning: toxic. Use cautiously for pregnant woman. Incompatible with Sodium Sulfate and Exsiccated Sodium Sulfate.

(The picture is only for learning and identification the herb; the specific use of the herb please consult the herbalist or health professionals)

Alum (Baifan)
Chinese phonetic alphabet/pin yin: bái fán
Chinese characters simplified/traditional:白矾/白礬
Chinese nickname's alphabet (Nickname's Chinese characters): Mingfan/ Lishi/ Baijun(明矾/理石/白君)
Latin: Alumen (Common name: Alum)

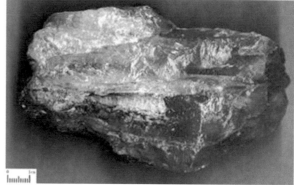

Mineral: main component $KAl(SO_4)_2 \cdot 12H_2O$
TCM prepared in ready-to-use forms (medicinal parts): it's cleaned mineral (or powder).
Property and flavor: cold; acidity and astringent.
Main and collateral channels: lung, spleen, liver and large intestine meridians.

Administration and dosage: Topical application in appropriate amount, ground into powder for applyment or dissolve in water for washing. Oral administration: 0.6-1.5 g.
Indication: metrorrhagia, diarrhea, hematochezia, epilepsy; external use for eczema, scabies, tinea, prolapse of the rectum, hemorrhoids, ear pus.
Precaution and warning: slightly toxic.
(The picture is only for learning and identification the herb; the specific use of the herb please consult the herbalist or health professionals)

Common Cnidium Fruit (Shechuangzi)

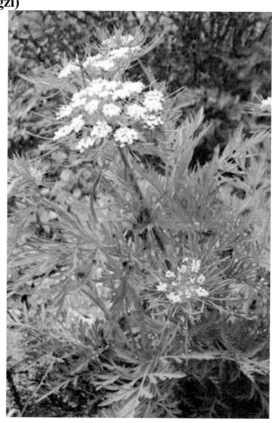

Chinese phonetic alphabet/pin yin: shé chuáng zǐ
Chinese characters simplified/traditional:蛇床子/蛇床子
Chinese nickname's alphabet (Nickname's Chinese characters): Shechuangren/ Shezhu/ Shemi(蛇床仁/蛇珠/蛇米)
Latin: Cnidii Fructus (Common name: Common Cnidium Fruit)
Plant: *Cnidium monnieri* (L.) Cuss.
TCM prepared in ready-to-use forms (medicinal parts): it's dried mature fruit.
Property and flavor: warm; pungent, bitter.
Main and collateral channels: kidney meridian.

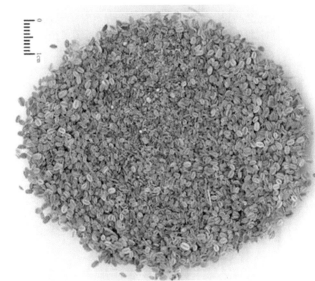

Administration and dosage: 3-10 g. Topical application in appropriate amount, usually decocted for fuming-wash therapy or ground into powder for application.
Indication: impotence, infertility; external use for eczema, pruritus vulvae, trichomonas vaginitis.
Precaution and warning: slightly toxic.

(The picture is only for learning and identification the herb; the specific use of the herb please consult the herbalist or health professionals)

Honeycomb (Lufengfang)
Chinese phonetic alphabet/pin yin: lù fēng fáng
Chinese characters simplified/traditional:露蜂房/露蜂房

Chinese nickname's alphabet (Nickname's Chinese characters): Fengfang/ Fengchang/ Baichuan/ Mafengwo(蜂房/蜂肠/百穿/马蜂窝)
Latin: Vespae Nidus (Common name: Honeycomb or The Hornet's Nest)

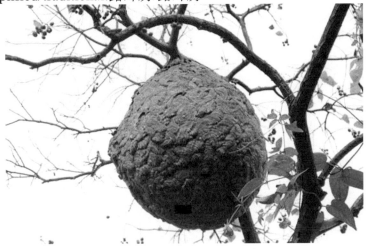

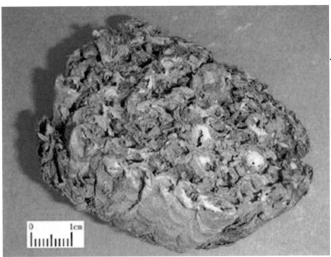

Animal: *Polistes olivaceous* (DeGeer.) (or *Polistes japonicus* Saussure., *Parapolybia varia* Fabricius., other species of *Vespidae*)
TCM prepared in ready-to-use forms (medicinal parts): it's dried nest/honeycomb.
Property and flavor: neutral; sweet.
Main and collateral channels: stomach meridian.

Administration and dosage: 3-5 g. Topical application in appropriate amount, ground into powder and mixed with oil for applying to *pars affecta*, or decocted for gargling or bathing.

Indication: acute mastits, tinea, toothache, painful *bi* disorder; external used for pruritus, swelling, sore and ulcer.

Precaution and warning: slightly toxic.

(The picture is only for learning and identification the herb; the specific use of the herb please consult the herbalist or health professionals)

Minium (Qiandan)

Chinese phonetic alphabet/pin yin: qiān dān

Chinese characters simplified/traditional:铅丹/鉛丹

Chinese nickname's alphabet (Nickname's Chinese characters): Huangdan/ Zhudan/ Zhangdan(黄丹/朱丹/章丹)

Latin: Plumbum Rubrum (Common name: Minium)
Mineral: main component Pb_3O_4
TCM prepared in ready-to-use forms (medicinal parts): it's cleaned mineral powder.
Property and flavor: mild cold; pungent.
Main and collateral channels: heart and liver meridians.

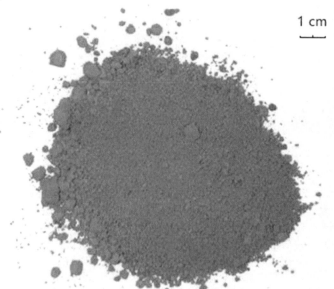

1 cm

Administration and dosage: 0.15-0.3 g, usually used in pills or powder. Topical application in appropriate amount, ground into powder for applying to *pars affecta*.

Indication: epilepsy, malaria; external use for skin ulcers, eczema.

Precaution and warning: toxic. Long-term and large quantity for topical application is inadvisable. Contraindicated with pregnant woman, breast-feeding women and child.

(The picture is only for learning and identification the herb; the specific use of the herb please consult the herbalist or health professionals)

Golden Larch Bark (Tujingpi)

Chinese phonetic alphabet/pin yin: tǔ jīng pí

Chinese characters simplified/traditional:土荆皮/土荊皮

Chinese nickname's alphabet (Nickname's Chinese characters): Jingshupi/ Jinqiansongpi(荆树皮/金钱松皮)

Latin: Pseudolaricis Cortex (Common name: Golden Larch Bark)

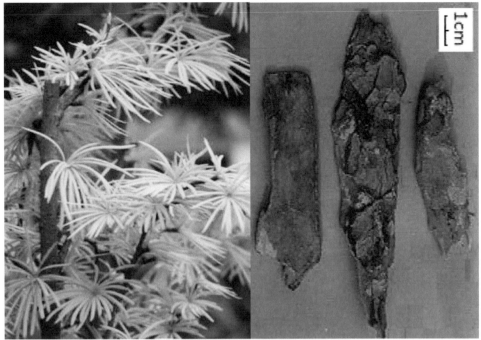

Plant: *Pseudolarix amabilis* (Nelson.)   TCM prepared in ready-to-use forms (
Rehd. (or *Pseudolarix kamepferi* Gord.)   medicinal parts): it's dried root bark
                                             or stem bark which harvested in summer.

Property and flavor: warm; pungent.
Main and collateral channels: lung and spleen meridians.
Administration and dosage: appropriate amount in vinegar or liquor preparation, or
ground into powder for topical application
Indication: external use for scabies, itching, tinea and external parasite.
Precaution and warning: toxic.
(The picture is only for learning and identification the herb; the specific use of the
herb please consult the herbalist or health professionals)

Orpiment (Cihuang)
Chinese phonetic alphabet/pin yin: cí huáng
Chinese characters simplified/traditional:雌黄/雌黃

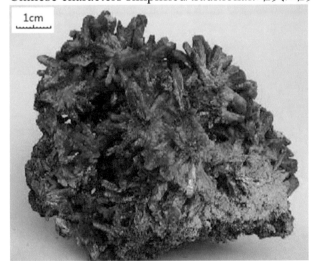

Chinese nickname's alphabet (Nickname's Chinese characters): Huangjinshi/ Shihuang/ Huangshi(黄金石/石黄/黄石)
Latin: Orpimentum (Common name: Orpiment)
Mineral: main component As$_2$S$_3$
TCM prepared in ready-to-use forms (medicinal parts): it's mineral crystal powder.
Property and flavor: warm; pungent.

Main and collateral channels: liver and large intestine meridians.

Administration and dosage: 0.05-0.1 g, used in pills or powder. Topical application in appropriate amount.

Indication: abdominal pain caused by inner parasite, epilepsy, malaria; external use for sore carbuncle, snake bites.

Precaution and warning: highly toxic. Used cautiously for oral administration. Avoid long-term administration. Contraindicated for pregnant women and weakness people.

(The picture is only for learning and identification the herb; the specific use of the herb please consult the herbalist or health professionals)

Realgar (Xionghuang)

Chinese phonetic alphabet/pin yin: xióng huáng

Chinese characters simplified/traditional:雄黄/雄黃

Chinese nickname's alphabet (Nickname's Chinese characters): Jiguanshi/Huangshishi(鸡冠石/黄食石)

Latin: Realgar (Common name: Realgar)

Mineral: main component As_2S_2
TCM prepared in ready-to-use forms (medicinal parts): it's mineral cleaned powder.
Property and flavor: warm; pungent.
Main and collateral channels: liver and large intestine meridians.

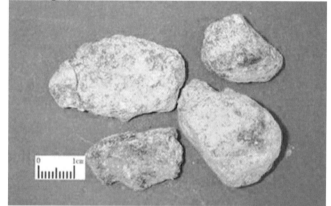

Administration and dosage: 0.05-0.1 g, used in pills or powder. Topical application in appropriate amount, ground into powder for applying to *pars affecta*.

Indication: swelling abscess, abdominal pain caused by parasite, fright epilepsy, malaria; external use for sore carbuncle, insect or snake bites.

Precaution and warning: highly toxic. Used cautiously for oral administration. Avoid long-term administration. Contraindicated for pregnant women.

(The picture is only for learning and identification the herb; the specific use of the herb please consult the herbalist or health professionals)

Lithargite (Mituoseng)

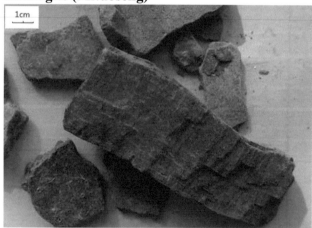

Chinese phonetic alphabet/pin yin: mì tuó sēng
Chinese characters simplified/traditional:密陀僧/密陀僧
Chinese nickname's alphabet (Nickname's Chinese characters): Qianhuang(铅黄)

Latin: Lithargyrum (Common name: Lithargite or Lead Oxide, Oxolead, Lead Monoxide)

Mineral: main component PbO

TCM prepared in ready-to-use forms (medicinal parts): it's cleaned mineral.

Property and flavor: neutral; salty, pungent.

Main and collateral channels: liver and spleen meridians.

Administration and dosage: 0.2-0.5 g, used in pills or powder. Topical application in appropriate amount, ground into powder or made into paste for applying to *pars affecta.*

Indication: external use for tinea, scabies, parasite.

Precaution and warning: highly toxic. Used cautiously for oral administration. Avoid long-term and large quantity administration. Contraindicated for pregnant women and child. Incompatible with Bracteole-lacked Euphorbia Root.

(The picture is only for learning and identification the herb; the specific use of the herb please consult the herbalist or health professionals)

Bracteole-lacked Euphorbia Root (Langdu)

Chinese phonetic alphabet/pin yin: láng dú

Chinese characters simplified/traditional:狼毒/狼毒

Chinese nickname's alphabet (Nickname's Chinese characters): Xudu/ Miandaji(续毒/绵大戟)

Latin: Euphorbiae Ebracteolatae Radix (Common name: Bracteole-lacked Euphorbia Root)

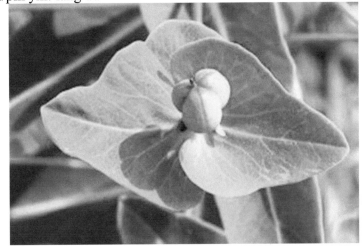

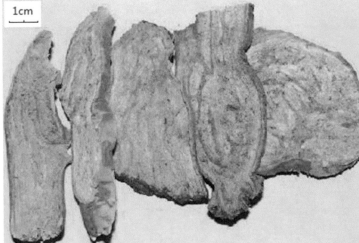

Plant: *Euphorbia ebracteolata* Hayata. (or *Euphorbia fischeriana* Steud.)

TCM prepared in ready-to-use forms (medicinal parts): it's dried root which harvested in spring or autumn.

Property and flavor: neutral; pungent.

Main and collateral channels: liver and spleen meridians.

Administration and dosage: boiled into paste or stir-baking with vinegar (30-50 kg vinegar per 100 kg herb) to dryness then ground into powder for topical application.

Indication: external use for lymphatic tuberculosis, tinea and maggot.

Precaution and warning: toxic. Incompatible with Lithargite.
(The picture is only for learning and identification the herb; the specific use of the herb please consult the herbalist or health professionals)

Mercury (Shuiyin)
Chinese phonetic alphabet/pin yin: shuǐ yín
Chinese characters simplified/traditional:水银/水銀
Chinese nickname's alphabet (Nickname's Chinese characters): Gong(汞)
Latin: Hydrargyrum (Common name: Mercury)
Mineral: main component Hg
TCM prepared in ready-to-use forms (medicinal parts): it's cleaned mineral.
Property and flavor: cold; pungent.
Main and collateral channels: heart, liver and spleen meridians.
Administration and dosage: topical application only. Topical application in appropriate amount.
Indication: external use for tinea, scabies, parasite.

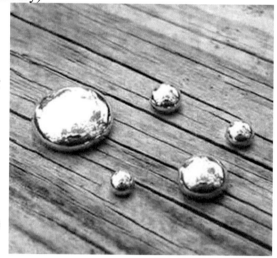

Precaution and warning: highly toxic, even its volatilization is toxic. Short time external use only. It's very rarely used now.

(The picture is only for learning and identification the herb; the specific use of the herb please consult the herbalist or health professionals)

Xiao Zhong Ba Du Lian Chuang Yao(消肿拔毒敛疮药)-herbs for detumescence, draw out poison, close sores
Xiao Zhong Ba Du Lian Chuang Yao is a kind of herbs which's the major functions are detumescence, draw out poison, close sores.

Blister Beetle (Banmao)
Chinese phonetic alphabet/pin yin: bān máo

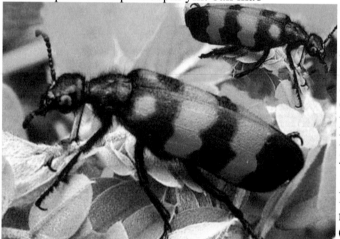

Chinese characters simplified/traditional:斑蝥/斑蝥
Chinese nickname's alphabet (Nickname's Chinese characters): Huakechong/Fangpichong/Zhangwa(花壳虫/放屁虫/章瓦)
Latin: Mylabris (Common name: Blister Beetle or Cantharis)

Animal: *Mylabris phalerate* Pallas. (or *Mylabris cichorii* L., *Lytta vesicatoria* L.)

TCM prepared in ready-to-use forms (medicinal parts): it's dried whole insect scalded by boiled water to death.
Property and flavor: hot; pungent.
Main and collateral channels: liver, stomach and kidney meridians.
Processing: stir-baked insect with rice (20 kg rice per 100 kg insect), taken out when the rice become light brown, removed the rice and cool.

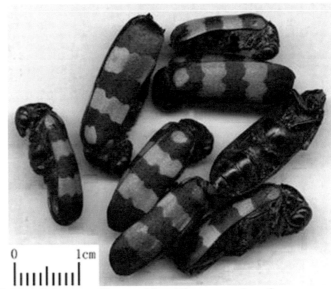

Administration and dosage: 0.03-0.06 g, usually used in pills or powder after processed. Topical application in appropriate amount, ground into powder or soaked in wine, liquor or vinegar, or made into balm for application. Large area topical application is inadvisable.

Indication: amenorrhea, mass and wart; external use for tinea, scrofula, ulcer and becrotic muscle.

Precaution and warning: highly toxic. Used cautiously for oral administration. Contraindicated during pregnancy.

(The picture is only for learning and identification the herb; the specific use of the herb please consult the herbalist or health professionals)

Toad Venom (Chansu)

Chinese phonetic alphabet/pin yin: chán sū

Chinese characters simplified/traditional:蟾酥/蟾酥

Chinese nickname's alphabet (Nickname's Chinese characters): Hamajiang(蛤蟆浆)

Latin: Bufonis Venenum (Common name: Toad Venom, Senso or Secretion of Toad)

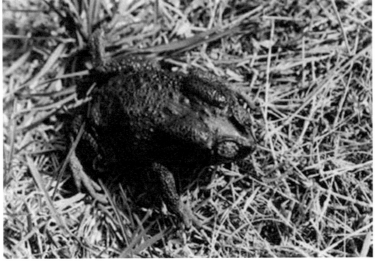

Animal: *Bufo bufo gargarizans* Cantor. (or *Bufo melanostictus* Schneider.)
TCM prepared in ready-to-use forms (medicinal parts): it's dried secretion of toad.
Property and flavor: warm; pungent.

Main and collateral channels: heart meridian.
Administration and dosage: 0.015-0.03 g, usually used in pills or powder. Topical application in appropriate amount.
Indication: abscesses and cellulitis, sore throat, vomiting, abdominal pain, diarrhea and coma; external used for carbuncle and furuncle.
Precaution and warning: poisonous.
Contraindicated during pregnancy.
(The picture is only for learning and identification the herb; the specific use of the herb please consult the herbalist or health professionals)

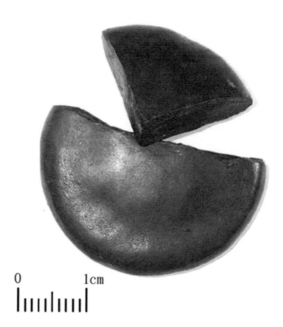

Nux Vomica (Maqianzi)
Chinese phonetic alphabet/pin yin: mǎ qián zǐ
Chinese characters simplified/traditional:马钱子/馬錢子

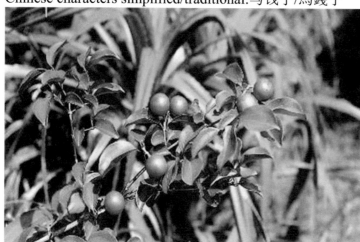

Chinese nickname's alphabet (Nickname's Chinese characters): Shidining/ Fanmubie/ Dafangba(士的宁/番木鳖/大方八)
Latin: Strychni Semen (Common name: Nux Vomic)
Plant: *Strychnos nux-vomica* L.

TCM prepared in ready-to-use forms (medicinal parts): it's dried mature seed.
Property and flavor: warm; bitter.
Main and collateral channels: lung and spleen meridians.
Administration and dosage: 0.3-0.6 g, usually used in pills or powder after processed.
Indication: stubborn painful *bi* disorder, hemiplegia, traumatic injury, numbness, ulcer pain, paralysis, sore and skin infection.
It is commonly used in dispersing blood stasis, easing the pain and spasm.

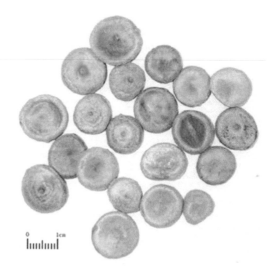

Precaution and warning: highly toxic. Contraindicated during pregnancy. Overdosage, long-term or unprocessed administration is inadvisable. Use cautiously in athletes. Large area topical application is inadvisable.

Attachment: processing of Nux Vomica Powder, pulverizes it to fine powder, then add a sufficient quantity of starch and mix, to make sure the powder contains 0.78-0.82 per cent strychnine ($C_{21}H_{22}N_2O_2$) and not less than 0.50 percent brucine ($C_{23}H_{26}N_2O_4$) of dried drug.

(The picture is only for learning and identification the herb; the specific use of the herb please consult the herbalist or health professionals)

Red Mercuric Oxide (Shengyao)

Chinese phonetic alphabet/pin yin: shēng yào

Chinese characters simplified/traditional:升药/升藥

Chinese nickname's alphabet (Nickname's Chinese characters): Hongfen/ Shengdan/ Sanxiandan/ Hongshengdan/ Huangshengdan(红粉/升丹/三仙丹/红升丹/黄升丹)

Latin: Hydrargyri Oxydum Rubrum seu Hydrargyrum Oxydatum Crudum (Common name: Red Mercuric Oxide)

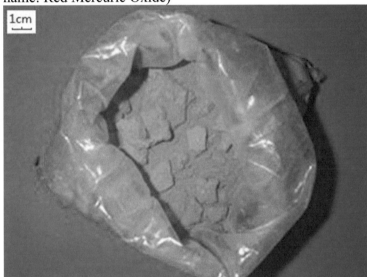

Its main component is HgO with a little $Hg(NO_3)_2$ and $HgSO_4$.

TCM prepared in ready-to-use forms (medicinal parts): it's crystal powder.

Property and flavor: hot; pungent.

Main and collateral channels: lung and spleen meridians.

Administration and dosage: appropriate amount for topical application, ground into extreme fine powder, applied alone or mixed with other drugs into powder or medicated thread.

Indication: external use for carbuncle, furuncle, syphilis, chancre and sore.

Precaution and warning: highly toxic. For topical application only, and should not last too long. Contraindicated during pregnancy.

(The picture is only for learning and identification the herb; the specific use of the herb please consult the herbalist or health professionals)

Calamine (Luganshi)

Chinese phonetic alphabet/pin yin: lú gān shí

Chinese characters simplified/traditional:炉甘石/爐甘石

Chinese nickname's alphabet (Nickname's Chinese characters): Ganshi(甘石)

Latin: Galamina (Common name: Calamine)

Mineral: main component $ZnCO_3$

TCM prepared in ready-to-use forms (medicinal parts): it's cleaned mineral.

Property and flavor: neutral; sweet.

Main and collateral channels: liver and spleen meridians.

Administration and dosage: appropriate amount for topical application.

Indication: external used for swollen eyes with pain, blepharitis, pterygium, ulcer not healing, eczema and pruritus.

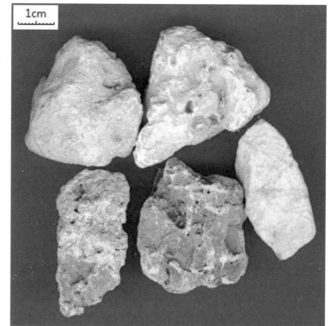

(The picture is only for learning and identification the herb; the specific use of the herb please consult the herbalist or health professionals)

Cutch (Ercha)

Chinese phonetic alphabet/pin yin: ér chá

Chinese characters simplified/traditional:儿茶/兒茶

Chinese nickname's alphabet (Nickname's Chinese characters): Hai'ercha/ Wudieni (孩儿茶/乌爹泥)

Latin: Catechu (Common name: Cutch or Black Catechu)

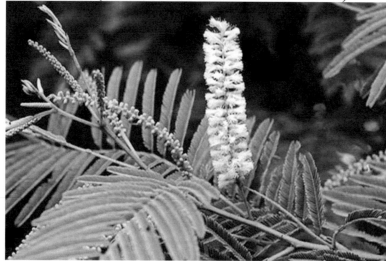

Plant: *Acacia catechu* (L. f.) Willd.
TCM prepared in ready-to-use forms (medicinal parts): it's dried concentrated decoction prepared from the peeled branch and stem.

Property and flavor: mild cold; bitter, astringent.

Main and collateral channels: spleen and stomach meridians.

Administration and dosage: 1-3 g, wrap-boiling. Usually used in pills or powder. Appropriate amount for topical application.

Indication: ulcers, eczema, sores, traunatic injuries, hematemesis, epistaxis, cough, trauma and bleeding.
(The picture is only for learning and identification the herb; the specific use of the herb please consult the herbalist or health professionals)

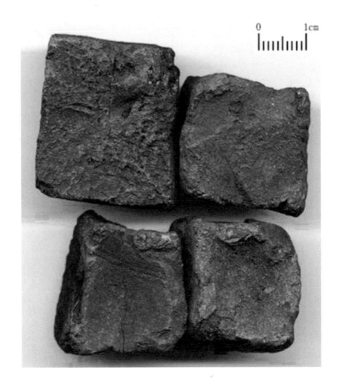

Arsenolite (Pishi)
Chinese phonetic alphabet/pin yin: pī shí
Chinese characters simplified/traditional:砒石/砒石
Chinese nickname's alphabet (Nickname's Chinese characters): Pihuang/ Renyan/ Xinshi(砒黄/人言/信石)
Latin: Aresenicum (Common name: Arsenolite)

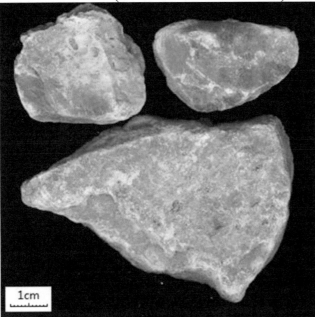

Mineral: main component As$_2$O$_3$
TCM prepared in ready-to-use forms (medicinal parts): it's refined mineral.
Property and flavor: hot; pungent, acidity.
Main and collateral channels: lung, spleen, stomach and large intestine meridians.
Administration and dosage: 0.001-0.003 g, used in pills or powder. Topical application in appropriate amount, ground into powder and mix with wheat powder for applying to *pars affecta.*

Indication: phlegm, asthma, malaria, scrofula, noma, dysentery, hemorrhoids, ulcer and tinea.
Precaution and warning: highly toxic. Used cautiously for oral administration. Avoid long-term and large area administration. Contraindicated for pregnant women and weakness people.

(The picture is only for learning and identification the herb; the specific use of the herb please consult the herbalist or health professionals)

Borax (Pengsha)

Chinese phonetic alphabet/pin yin: péng shā

Chinese characters simplified/traditional:硼砂/硼砂

Chinese nickname's alphabet (Nickname's Chinese characters): Yueshi(月石)

Latin: Borax (Common name: Borax or Sodium tetraborate decahydrate)

Mineral: main component $Na_2B_4O_7 \cdot 10H_2O$

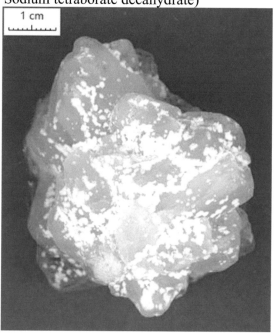

TCM prepared in ready-to-use forms (medicinal parts): it's refined mineral (powder).

Property and flavor: cool; sweet, salty.

Main and collateral channels: lung and stomach meridians.

Administration and dosage: 1.5-3 g, used in pills or powder. Topical application in appropriate amount, ground into powder or dissolved in boiled water for applying to *pars affecta*.

Indication: sore throat, red eyes, scales, phlegm heat stagnation and cough.

Precaution and warning: slightly toxic. Avoid long-term administration. Used cautiously for weakness people.

(The picture is only for learning and identification the herb; the specific use of the herb please consult the herbalist or health professionals)

Garlic Bulb (Dasuan)

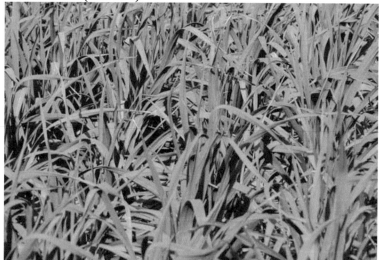

Chinese phonetic alphabet/pin yin: dà suàn
Chinese characters simplified/traditional:大蒜/大蒜
Chinese nickname's alphabet (Nickname's Chinese characters): Suantou(蒜头)

Latin: Allium Sativi Bulbus (Common name: Garlic Bulb)

Plant: *Allium sativum* L.

TCM prepared in ready-to-use forms (medicinal parts): it's bulb which harvested in summer.

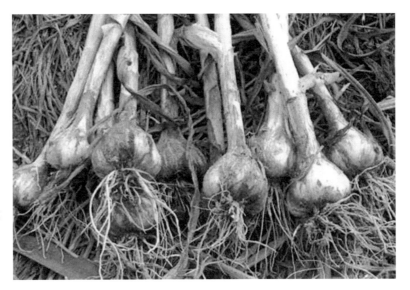

Property and flavor: warm; pungent.
Main and collateral channels: spleen, stomach and lung meridians.
Administration and dosage: 9-15 g.

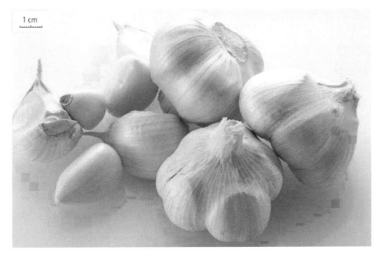

Indication: cough, scabies, dyspepsia, sore and ulcer, dysentery and diarrhea.
(The picture is only for learning and identification the herb; the specific use of the herb please consult the herbalist or health professionals)

Catclaw Buttercup Root (Maozhuacao)

Chinese phonetic alphabet/pin yin: māo zhuǎ cǎo
Chinese characters simplified/traditional:猫爪草/貓爪草
Chinese nickname's alphabet (Nickname's Chinese characters): Sansancao(三散草)

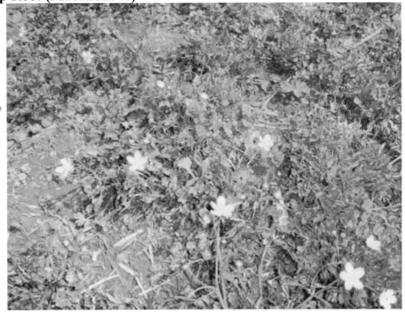

Latin: Ranunculi Ternati Radix (Common name: Catclaw Buttercup Root)

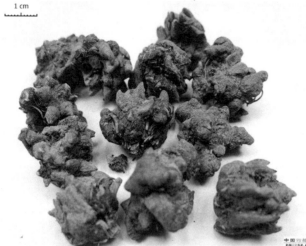

Plant: *Ranunculus ternatus* Thunb.
TCM prepared in ready-to-use forms (medicinal parts): it's dried tuber root which harvested in spring or autumn.
Property and flavor: warm; sweet, pungent.
Main and collateral channels: liver and lung meridians.
Administration and dosage:15-30 g; taken alone, the dosage can be up to 120 g.

Indication: scrofula, sore, pharyngitis, malaria, migraine, insect or snake bites.
(The picture is only for learning and identification the herb; the specific use of the herb please consult the herbalist or health professionals)

Chaulmoogra Seed (Dafengzi)

Chinese phonetic alphabet/pin yin: dà fēng zǐ
Chinese characters simplified/traditional:大风子/大風子

Chinese nickname's alphabet (Nickname's Chinese characters): Mafengzi(麻风子)
Latin: Hydnocarpi Semen (Common name: Chaulmoogra or Gynocardic)
Plant: *Hydnocarpus anthelmintica* Pierre. (or *Hydnocarpus hainanensis* (Merr.) Sleum., *Hydnocarpus wightianus*)

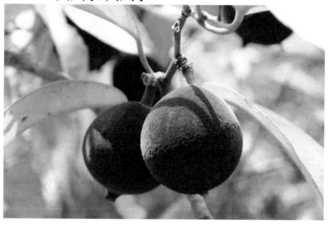

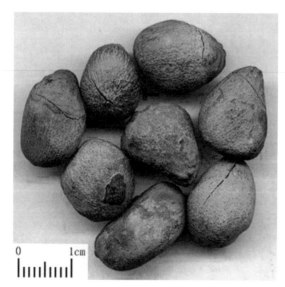

TCM prepared in ready-to-use forms (medicinal parts): it's dried mature fruit.
Property and flavor: hot; pungent.
Main and collateral channels: liver and spleen meridians.
Administration and dosage: 0.3-1 g, used in pills or powder. Topical application in appropriate amount, mashed for applying to *pars affecta*.
Indication: leprosy, syphilis, scabies and tinea.

210

Precaution and warning: toxic. Used cautiously for oral administration. Avoid long-term and large area administration. Contraindicated for pregnant women and weakness people.

(The picture is only for learning and identification the herb; the specific use of the herb please consult the herbalist or health professionals)

Insect Wax (Chongbaila)
Chinese phonetic alphabet/pin yin: chóng bái là

Chinese characters simplified/traditional:虫白蜡/蟲白蠟
Chinese nickname's alphabet (Nickname's Chinese characters): Baila/ Chongla/ Chonggao(白蜡/虫蜡/蜡膏)
Latin: Cera Chinensis (Common name: Insect Wax)

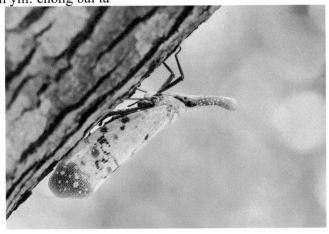

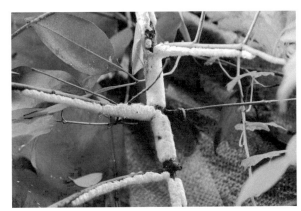

Animal: *Ericerus pela* (Chavannes.) Guerin
TCM prepared in ready-to-use forms (medicinal parts): it's purified wax secreted by male insect (*Ericerus pela* (Chavannes.) Guerin.) which dwelling gregariously at the stem and branch of *Fraxinus chinensis* Roxb. (or *Ligustrum lucidum* Ait.)

Usage: take it as excipient and lubricant to make pills and tablets.
Indication: external use for traumatic bleeding, unhealing sore and ulcer.
(The picture is only for learning and identification the herb; the specific use of the herb please consult the herbalist or health professionals)

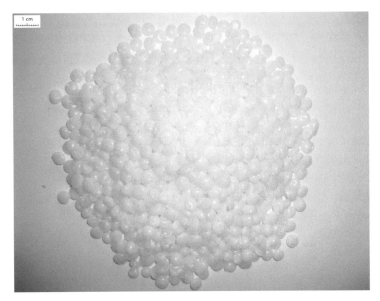

Beeswax (Fengla)

Chinese phonetic alphabet/pin yin: fēng là

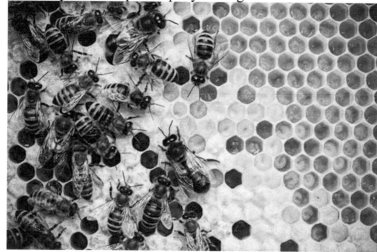

Chinese characters simplified/ traditional:蜂蜡/蜂蠟
Chinese nickname's alphabet (Nickname's Chinese characters): Mila/ Huangla(蜜蜡/黄蜡)
Latin: Cera Flava (Common name: Beeswax)

Animal: *Apis cerana* Fabricius. (or *Apis mellifera* Linnaeus.)
TCM prepared in ready-to-use forms (medicinal parts): it's wax secreted by bees.
Property and flavor: mild warm; sweet.
Main and collateral channels: spleen meridian.

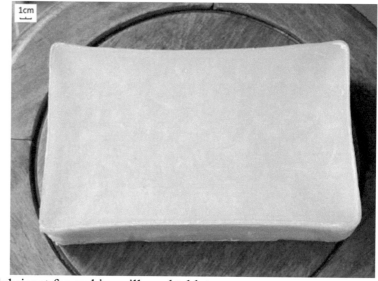

Usage: excipient and lubricant for making pills and tablets.
Administration and dosage: topical application in appropriate amount. Melted for applying to *pars affecta*.
Indication: remove toxin; promote wound healing and tissue regeneration; relieve pain.
(The picture is only for learning and identification the herb; the specific use of the herb please consult the herbalist or health professionals)

Pine Pollen (Songhuafen)

Chinese phonetic alphabet/pin yin: sōng huā fěn
Chinese characters simplified/traditional:松花粉/松花粉
Chinese nickname's alphabet (Nickname's Chinese characters): Songhuang(松黄)
Latin: Pini Pollen (Common name: Pine Pollen)

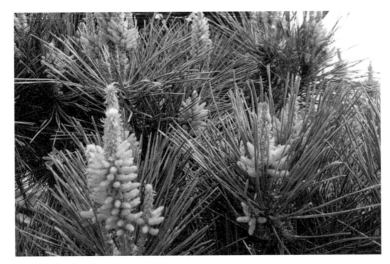

Plant: *Pinus massoniana* Lamb. (or *Pinus tabulaeformis* Carr.)
TCM prepared in ready-to-use forms (medicinal parts): it's dried pollen which harvested in spring.

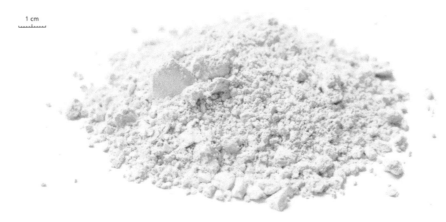

Property and flavor: warm; sweet.

Main and collateral channels: liver and spleen meridians.

Administration and dosage: 5-10 g. Topical application in appropriate amount, spreaded to the *pars affecta*.

Indication: wound bleeding, eczema, impetiginous sore, skin erosion and dripping pus.

It is taken as food in some part of China.

(The picture is only for learning and identification the herb; the specific use of the herb please consult the herbalist or health professionals)

Propolis (Fengjiao)

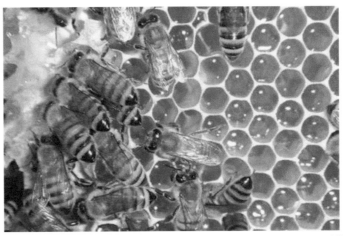

Chinese phonetic alphabet/pin yin: fēng jiāo
Chinese characters simplified/traditional:蜂胶/蜂膠
Latin: Propolis
(Common name: Propolis)
Animal: *Apis mellifera* L.

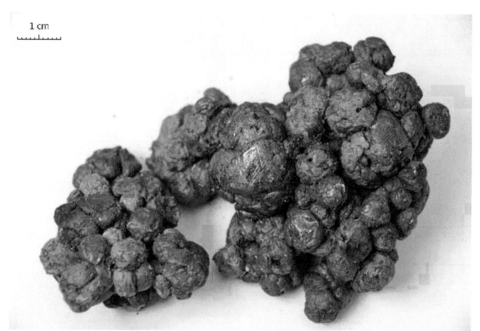

1 cm

TCM prepared in ready-to-use forms (medicinal parts): it's sticky gum mix with resin and bee's secretions of mandibular glands and wax glands.

Property and flavor: cold; bitter, pungent.

Main and collateral channels: spleen and stomach meridians.

Administration and dosage: 0.2-0.6 g. Topical application in appropriate amount. Usually used in pill or powder or being taken with some honey.

Indication: weak constitution, presenility, hyperlipidemia; external use for chapped skin, burns and scald.

Precaution and warning: used with caution in people liable to allergy.

(The picture is only for learning and identification the herb; the specific use of the herb please consult the herbalist or health professionals)

Part Ⅱ Commonly used Traditional Chinese Patent Medicine and Single Herb Preparation

Relieving Medicine(解表药)

Relieving Medicine is a kind of medicines, their major functions are to treat head and body pain, nasal obstruction, shed tears and sore throat caused by cold; some of them can treat fever relieve cough or induce perspiration.

Biaoshi Ganmao Granules (Biaoshi Ganmao Keli)

Chinese phonetic alphabet/pin yin: biǎo shí gǎn mào kē lì

Chinese characters simplified/traditional:表实感冒颗粒/表實感冒顆粒

Ingredients: Perilla leaf, Kudzuvine Root, Dahurian Angelica Root, Ephedra, Divaricate Saposhnikovia Root, Platycodon Root, Cassia Twig, Liquorice Root, Dried Tangerine Peel, Fresh Ginger, Bitter Apricot (stir-baked).

Indication: common cold, severe chills with mild fever and without sweating, headache, painful stiff nape and cough with phlegm.

Administration and dosage: take the medicine orally after mixing it with hot water, 1-2 packs per time, three times a day. Reduce the dosage in children.

Strength: 10 g per pack, 5 g per pack (without sucrose).

The specific strength and dosage are according to the medicine instruction.

Precaution and warning: use with caution in patients with hypertension or heart disease.

(The information is only for learning and identification the Chinese Patent Medicine; the specific use of the Medicine please consult the herbalist or health professionals)

Ganmao Qingre Granules (Capsules/Chewable Tablets/ Mixture) (Ganmao Qingre Keli (Jiaonang/Jujuepian/Koufuye))

Chinese phonetic alphabet/pin yin: gǎn mào qīng rè kē lì

Chinese characters simplified/traditional:感冒清热颗粒(胶囊/咀嚼片/口服液)/感冒清热颗粒(膠囊/咀嚼片/口服液)

Ingredients: Fineleaf Schizonepeta spike, Peppermint, Divaricate Saposhnikovia Root, Chinese Thorowax Root, Perilla leaf, Kudzuvine Root, Platycodon Root, Bitter Apricot, Dahurian Angelica Root, Bunge Corydalis Herb, Reed Rhizome.

The content of each ingredients may have a little variety due to different dosage forms.

Indication: headache, fever, chills (*Fenghan*) cold, generalized pain, nasal discharge, cough and dry throat.

Administration and dosage: (for oral administration) granule: take the medicine orally after mixing with hot water, 1 pack per time, twice a day; capsule: 3 capsules per time, twice a day; chew-able tablet: swallow the medicine after chewing, 2 tablets per time, twice a day; mixture: 10 ml per time, twice a day.

Strength: granule: 12 g per pack, 6 g per pack (without sucrose), 3 g per pack (with lactose); capsule: 0.45 g per capsule; chew-able tablet: 1.5 g per tablet; mixture: 10 ml per phial.

The specific strength and dosage are according to the medicine instruction.

(The information is only for learning and identification the Chinese Patent Medicine; the specific use of the Medicine please consult the herbalist or health professionals)

Zhengchaihuyin Granules (Zhengchaihuyin Keli)

Chinese phonetic alphabet/pin yin: zhèng chái hú yǐn kē lì
Chinese characters simplified/traditional:正柴胡饮颗粒/正柴胡飲顆粒
Ingredients: Chinese Thorowax Root, Dried Tangerine Peel, Divaricate
Saposhnikovia Root, Liquorice Root, Red Peony Root, Fresh Ginger.
Indication: fever and chills feeling, absence of sweating, headache, stuff nose,
sneezing, cough, early stage of influenza and low-grade upper respiratory tract
infection, throat itchy feeling.
Administration and dosage: take the medicine orally after mixing it with hot water, 1
pack per time, three times a day. Reduce the dosage in children or as advised by
health professionals.
Strength: 10 g per pack, 3 g (sucrose free) per pack.
The specific strength and dosage are according to the medicine instruction.
(The information is only for learning and identification the Chinese Patent Medicine;
the specific use of the Medicine please consult the herbalist or health professionals)

Yinqiao Powder (Yinqiao San)
Chinese phonetic alphabet/pin yin: yín qiào sǎn
Chinese characters simplified/traditional:银翘散/銀翹散
Ingredients: Japanese Honeysuckle Flower, Weeping Forsythia Capsule, Platycodon
Root, Peppermint, Fermented Soybean, Lophatherum Herb, Great Burdock Achene,
Fineleaf Schizonepeta Herb, Reed Rhizome, Liquorice Root.
Indication: fever, headache, dry mouth and throat, cough, sore throat, and short
voiding of deep-colored urine.
Administration and dosage: take the medicine orally after mixing it with hot water, 1
pack per time, two or three times a day.
Strength: 6 g per pack.
The specific strength and dosage are according to the medicine instruction.
(The information is only for learning and identification the Chinese Patent Medicine;
the specific use of the Medicine please consult the herbalist or health professionals)

Shuanghuanglian Mixture (Tablets/Granules/Capsules/Suppositories/Eye Drops) (Shuanghuanglian Koufuye (Pian/Keli/Jiaonang/Shuan/Diyanji))
Chinese phonetic alphabet/pin yin: shuāng huáng lián kǒu fú yè
Chinese characters simplified/ traditional 双黄连口服液(片/颗粒/胶囊/栓/滴眼剂)/
雙黃連口服液(片/顆粒/膠囊/栓/滴眼液)
Ingredients: Japanese Honeysuckle Flower, Baical Skullcap Root, Weeping Forsythia
Capsule.
The content of each ingredients may have a little variety due to different dosage
forms.
Indication: fever, cough and sore throat.
Administration and dosage: mixture: 20 ml [mixture strength (1) and (2)] or 10 ml
[mixture strength (3)] per time, three times a day for oral administration; tablet: 4 pills
per time, three times a day for oral administration; granule: take the medicine orally
after mixing it with hot water, 10 g per time, three times a day, for children under 6
months, 2-3 g per time, for between 6 month to 1 year, 3-4 g per time, for between 1
to 3, 4-5 g per time, for children above 3 years use appropriate dose advised by health
professionals, reduce the dose by half if it is sucrose-free granule; capsule: 4 capsules
per time, three times a day; suppositories: for rectal administration, 1 piece per time
for children, two or three times a day; eye drop: mix the powder with solvent and
shake fully prior to use as eye drops, apply 1-2 drops into eyelid each time, four times

a day, four weeks is one treatment course. Reduce the dosage in children.

Strength: mixture: (1) 10 ml per phial (equivalent to 1.5 g clean prepared slice per ml), (2) 20 ml per phial (equivalent to 1.5 g clean prepared slice per ml), (3) 10 ml per phial (equivalent to 3.0 g clean prepared slice per ml); tablet: 0.53 g per tablet; granule: 5 g per pack (1) granules without sucrose (equivalent to 30 g clean prepared slice), (2) granules with sucrose (equivalent to 15 g clean prepared slice); capsule: 0.4 g per capsule; suppositories: 1.5 g per suppository; eye drop: 60 mg per phial, 5 ml of the eye drop solvent per phial.

The specific strength and dosage are according to the medicine instruction.

Precaution and warning: contraindicated during pregnancy, for eye drop the prepared solution should be used within one month, avoid contamination during operation.

(The information is only for learning and identification the Chinese Patent Medicine; the specific use of the Medicine please consult the herbalist or health professionals)

Lianhuaqingwen Tablets (Granules/Capsules) (Lianhuaqingwen Pian (Keli/Jiaonang))

Chinese phonetic alphabet/pin yin: lián huā qīng wēn piàn

Chinese characters simplified/traditional:连花清瘟片(颗粒/胶囊)/連花清瘟片(顆粒/膠囊)

Ingredients: Weeping Forsythia Capsule, Japanese Honeysuckle Flower, Ephedra (processed with honey), Bitter Apricot (stir-baked), Gypsum, Isatis Root, Male Fern Rhizome, Heartleaf Houttuynia Herb, Cablin Patchouli Herb, Rhubarb, Bigflower Rhodiola Root, l-menthol, Liquorice Root.

The content of each ingredients may have a little variety due to different dosage forms.

Indication: fever, aversion to cold, stuffy nose, muscle pain, cough, headache, sore throat.

Administration and dosage: (for oral administration) tablet: 4 tablets per time, three times a day; granule: mixing it with hot water before usage, 6 g per time, three times a day; capsule: 4 capsules per time, three times a day.

Strength: tablet: 0.35 g per tablet; granule: 6 g per pack; capsule: 0.35 g per capsule.

The specific strength and dosage are according to the medicine instruction.

Precaution and warning: contraindicate for chill (*Fenghan*) cold.

(The information is only for learning and identification the Chinese Patent Medicine; the specific use of the Medicine please consult the herbalist or health professionals)

Jiuwei Qianghuo Pills (Granules/Mixture) (Jiuwei Qianghuo Wan (Keli/Koufuye))

Chinese phonetic alphabet/pin yin: jiǔ wèi qiāng huó wán

Chinese characters simplified/traditional:九味羌活丸(颗粒/口服液)/九味羌活丸(顆粒/口服液)

Ingredients: Incised Notopterygium Rhizome and Root, Divaricate Saposhnikovia Root, Atractylodes Rhizome, Manchurian Wildginger Root, Szechwan Lovage Rhizome, Dahurian Angelica Root, Baical Skullcap Root, Liquorice Root, Rehmannia Root.

The content of each ingredients may have a little variety due to different dosage forms.

Indication: fever, absence of sweating, headache and general body ache.

Administration and dosage: pill: take it orally with ginger spring onion soup or warm water, 6-9 g per time, two or three times a day; granule: take it orally after mixing it with ginger soup or warm water, 15 g per time, two or three times a day; mixture: 20 ml per time, two or three times a day.

Strength: granule: 15 g per pack; mixture: 10 ml per phial.

The specific strength and dosage are according to the medicine instruction.

(The information is only for learning and identification the Chinese Patent Medicine; the specific use of the Medicine please consult the herbalist or health professionals)

Wushicha Granules (Capsule) (Wushicha Keli (Jiaonang))

Chinese phonetic alphabet/pin yin: wǔ shí chá kē lì

Chinese characters simplified/traditional:午时茶颗粒(胶囊)/午時茶顆粒(膠囊)

Ingredients: Atractylodes Rhizome, Chinese Thorowax Root, Incised Notopterygium Rhizome and Root, Divaricate Saposhnikovia Root, Dahurian Angelica Root, Szechwan Lovage Rhizome, Cablin Patchouli Herb, Hogfennel Root, Weeping Forsythia Capsule, Dried Tangerine Peel, Hawthorn Fruit, Immature Orange Fruit, Germinated Barly (stir-baked), Liquorice Root, Platycodon Root, Perilla Leaf, Officinal Magnolia Bark, Black Tea, Medicated Leaven (stir-baked).

The content of each ingredients may have a little variety due to different dosage forms.

Indication: chill (*Fenghan*) cold, fever, headache, body pain, fullness and oppression in the chest and epigastrium, nausea, vomiting, diarrhea.

Administration and dosage: (for oral administration) granule: mixing it with hot water before usage, 1 pack per time, once or twice a day; capsule: 1.5 g per time, once or twice a day.

Strength: granule: 6 g per pack; capsules: 0.25g or 0.5 g per capsule.

The specific strength and dosage are according to the medicine instruction.

(The information is only for learning and identification the Chinese Patent Medicine; the specific use of the Medicine please consult the herbalist or health professionals)

Huoxiang Zhengqi Tincture (Oral Liquid/ Dripping Pills/ Soft Capsule) (Huoxiang Zhengqi Shui(Koufuye/ Diwan/ Ruanjiaonang))

Chinese phonetic alphabet/pin yin: huò xiāng zhèng qì shuǐ

Chinese characters simplified/traditional:藿香正气水(口服液/滴丸/软胶囊)/藿香正氣水(口服液/滴丸/軟膠囊)

Ingredients: Atractylodes Rhizome, Dried Tangerine Peel, Officinal Magnolia Bark (processed with ginger), Dahurian Angelica Root, Indian Bread, Areca Peel, Pinellia Tuber, Liquorice Root Extract, Cablin Patchouli Oil, Perilla Leaf Oil. (Tincture contain ethanol)

The content of each ingredients may have a little variety due to different dosage forms.

Indication: headache, dizziness, heavy sensation, vomiting, diarrhea, stomach flu.

Administration and dosage: (for oral administration) tincture: 5-10 ml per time, twice a day, shake fully before use; oral liquid: 5-10 ml per time, twice a day, shake fully before use; dripping pill: 1-2 pack per time, twice a day; capsule: 2-4 capsules per time, twice a day.

Strength: tincture: 10 ml per vial; capsules: 0.45 g per capsule.

The specific strength and dosage are according to the medicine instruction.

(The information is only for learning and identification the Chinese Patent Medicine; the specific use of the Medicine please consult the herbalist or health professionals)

Baoji Pills (Mixture) (Baoji Wan (Koufuye))

Chinese phonetic alphabet/pin yin: bǎo jì wán

Chinese characters simplified/traditional:保济丸(口服液)/保濟丸(口服液)

Ingredients: Gambir Plant, Chrysanthemum Flower, Puncturevine Caltrop Fruit, Official Magnolia Bark, Common Aucklandia Root, Atractylodes Rhizome, Snakegourd Root, Cablin Patchouli Herb, Kudzuvine Root, Pummelo Peel, Dahurian Angelica Root, Coix Seed, Rice Grain Sprout, Peppermint, Indian Bread, Medicated Leaven (Guangdong produced).

The content of each ingredients may have a little variety due to different dosage forms.

Indication: cold, fever, headache, abdominal pain, diarrhea, nausea, vomiting, gastrointestinal discomfort.

Administration and dosage: (for oral administration) pill: 1.85-3.7 g per time, three times a day; mixture: 10-20 ml per time, three times a day. Reduce the dosage in children.

Strength: pill: 1.85 g or 3.7 g per pill; mixture: 10 ml per phial.

The specific strength and dosage are according to the medicine instruction.

Precaution and warning: contraindicated during pregnancy and in patients with externally contracted dryness-heat.

(The information is only for learning and identification the Chinese Patent Medicine; the specific use of the Medicine please consult the herbalist or health professionals)

Zhuche Pills (Zhuche Wan)

Chinese phonetic alphabet/pin yin: zhù chē wán

Chinese characters simplified/traditional:驻车丸/駐車丸

Ingredients: Golden Thread, Prepared Dried Ginger, Chinese Angelica, Donkey-Hide Glue.

Indication: hemafecia with abdominal pain, tenesmus or recurrent dysentery.

Administration and dosage: 6-9 g per time, three times a day for oral administration.

Strength: 3 g per 50 pills.

The specific strength and dosage are according to the medicine instruction.

Precaution and warning: contraindicated in pattern of dampness-heat accumulation and stagnation or patients at onset of dysentery.

(The information is only for learning and identification the Chinese Patent Medicine; the specific use of the Medicine please consult the herbalist or health professionals)

Shensu Pills (Shensu Wan)

Chinese phonetic alphabet/pin yin: shēn sū wán

Chinese characters simplified/traditional:参苏丸/參蘇丸

Ingredients: Tangshen, Perilla leaf, Kudzuvine Root, Hogfennel Root, Indian Bread, Pinellia Tuber (processed), Dried Tangerine Peel, Orange Fruit (stir-baked), Platycodon Root, Liquorice Root, Common Aucklandia Root.

Indication: cold, fever, headache, nausea, cough with phlegm, shortness of breath, vomiting and hiccup, weakness.

Administration and dosage: 6-9 g per time, two or three times a day for oral administration.

The specific strength and dosage are according to the medicine instruction.

(The information is only for learning and identification the Chinese Patent Medicine; the specific use of the Medicine please consult the herbalist or health professionals)

Summer-heat clearing prescription(祛暑剂)

Summer-heat clearing prescription is a kind of medicines, their major functions are to treat headache, nausea, fainting, prickly heat and other symptoms caused by heat.

Liuyi Powder (Liuyi San)

Chinese phonetic alphabet/pin yin: liù yī sǎn

Chinese characters simplified/traditional:六一散/六一散

Ingredients: Talc powder, Liquorice Root.

Indication: fever, fatigue, thirst, diarrhea, prickly heat (external used).

Administration and dosage: for oral administration, take the medicine after mixing it with water, or decoct in a cotton bag with water, 6-9 g per time, once a day; for external application, apply the powder onto the *pars affecta*.

The specific strength and dosage are according to the medicine instruction.

(The information is only for learning and identification the Chinese Patent Medicine; the specific use of the Medicine please consult the herbalist or health professionals)

Ganlu Xiaodu Pills (Ganlu Xiaodu Wan)

Chinese phonetic alphabet/pin yin: gān lù xiāo dú wán

Chinese characters simplified/traditional:甘露消毒丸/甘露消毒丸

Ingredients: Talc, Virgate Wormwood Herb, Grassleaf Sweetflag Rhizome, Akebiae Stem, Blackberrylily Rhizome, Villous Amomum Fruit, Weeping Forsythia Capsule, Baical Skullcap Root, Tendrilleaf Fritilary Bulb, Ageratum Herb, Peppermint.

Indication: fever, limb weakness, oppression and distension in chest and abdomen, deep-coloured urine and jaundice.

Administration and dosage: 6-9 g per time, twice a day.

The specific strength and dosage are according to the medicine instruction.

Precaution and warning: avoid spicy, oil and greasy food during medication.

Attachment: Ageratum Herb (藿香, Latin name: Agastache Rugosa Herba) is the whole herb of *Agastache rugosa* (Fisch. et Mey.) O. Ktze.

(The information is only for learning and identification the Chinese Patent Medicine; the specific use of the Medicine please consult the herbalist or health professionals)

Zijin Troches (Zijin Ding)

Chinese phonetic alphabet/pin yin: zǐ jīn dìng

Chinese characters simplified/traditional:紫金锭/紫金錠

Ingredients: Appendiculate Cremastra Pseudobulb, Knoxia Root, Caper Euphorbia Seed Powder, Chinese Gall, Artificial Musk, Cinnabar, Realgar.

Indication: summer-heat stroke, tightness and pain in the epigastrium and abdomen, nausea, vomiting, dysentery, diarrhea, phlegm syncope in children, skin infection, mumps, erysipelas and sore throat.

Administration and dosage: 0.6-1.5 g per time, twice a day for oral administration; apply the medicine to the *pars affecta* after grinding and mixing it with vinegar for external use.

Strength: 0.3 g or 3 g per troche.

The specific strength and dosage are according to the medicine instruction.

Precaution and warning: contraindicated with pregnant woman, long-term oral administration is inadvisable.

(The information is only for learning and identification the Chinese Patent Medicine; the specific use of the Medicine please consult the herbalist or health professionals)

Liuhe Dingzhong Pills (Liuhe Dingzhong Wan)
Chinese phonetic alphabet/pin yin: liù hé dìng zhōng wán
Chinese characters simplified/traditional:六合定中丸/六合定中丸
Ingredients: Cablin Patchouli Herb, Perilla leaf, Chinese Mosla, Common Aucklandia Root, Sandalwood, Officinal Magnolia Bark (processed with ginger), Orange Fruit (stir-baked), Dried Tangerine Peel, Platycodon Root, Liquorice Root, Indian Bread, Papaya, White Hyacinth Bean (stir-baked), Hawthorn Fruit (stir-baked), Medicated Leaven (stir-baked), Germinated Barly (stir-baked), Rice Grain Sprout (stir-baked).
Indication: heat stroke, indigestion, headache with chills feeling and fever, oppression in the chest and nausea, vomiting, diarrhea and abdominal pain.
Administration and dosage: 3-6 g per time, two or three times a day for oral administration.
The specific strength and dosage are according to the medicine instruction.
(The information is only for learning and identification the Chinese Patent Medicine; the specific use of the Medicine please consult the herbalist or health professionals)

Shidi Tincture (Soft Capsule) (Shidi Shui (Ruanjiaonang))
Chinese phonetic alphabet/pin yin: shí dī shuǐ
Chinese characters simplified/traditional:十滴水(软胶囊)/十滴水(軟膠囊)
Ingredients: Camphor, Dried Ginger, Rhubarb, Fennel, Cassia Bark, Hot Pepper, Eucalyptus Oil.
The content of each ingredients may have a little variety due to different dosage forms.
Indication: summer heat-stroke, dizziness, nausea, abdominal pain, gastrointestinal discomfort.
Administration and dosage: (for oral administration) tincture: 2-5 ml per time; soft capsule: 1 or 2 capsules per time. Reduce the dosage in children.
Strength: capsule: 0.425 g per capsule.
The specific strength and dosage are according to the medicine instruction.
Precaution and warning: contraindicated during pregnancy. Use with caution before driving or operating at height.
Attachment: Camphor (樟脑, Its main component is $C_{10}H_{16}O$) is the extract which gets from *Cinnamomum camphora* (L.) Presl.
Eucalyptus Oil (桉油, Latin name: Eucalypti Oleum) is volatile oil which gets by steam distillate *Eucalyptus globulus* Labill.
(The information is only for learning and identification the Chinese Patent Medicine; the specific use of the Medicine please consult the herbalist or health professionals)

Qingshu Yiqi Pills (Qingshu Yiqi Wan)
Chinese phonetic alphabet/pin yin: qīng shǔ yì qì wán
Chinese characters simplified/traditional:清暑益气丸/清暑益氣丸
Ingredients: Ginseng, Milkvetch Root (processed with honey), Largehead Atractylodes Rhizome (stir-baked with bran), Atractylodes Rhizome (stir-baked with rice juice), Dwarf Lilyturf Tuber, Oriental Waterplantain Rhizome, Chinese Magnoliavine Fruit (processed with vinegar), Chinese Angelica, Chinese Cork-tree, Kudzuvine Root, Dried Immaturity Tangerine Peel (processed with vinegar), Dried Tangerine Peel, Medicated Leaven (stir-baked with bran), Largetrifoliolious Bugbane Rhizome, Liquorice Root.

Indication: summer heat-stroke with dizziness, fatigue and vexation, dry mouth and throat.

Administration and dosage: take the medicine orally with warm boiled water or ginger decoction. 1 pill per time, twice a day.

Strength: 9 g per pill.

The specific strength and dosage are according to the medicine instruction.

Precaution and warning: avoid spicy, greasy food.

(The information is only for learning and identification the Chinese Patent Medicine; the specific use of the Medicine please consult the herbalist or health professionals)

Formula for relieving both superficial and internal disorders(表里双解剂)

Formula for relieving both superficial and internal disorders is a kind of medicines which combine with purgating herbs, antipyretic herbs and warm herbs to treat some disease with both internal and external symptom.

Gegen Qinlian Pills (Tablets) (Gegen Qinlian Wan (Pian))

Chinese phonetic alphabet/pin yin: gě gēn qín lián wán

Chinese characters simplified/traditional:葛根芩连丸(片)/葛根芩連丸(片)

Ingredients: Kudzuvine Root, Baical Skullcap Root, Golden Thread, Prepared Liquorice Root.

The content of each ingredients may have a little variety due to different dosage forms.

Indication: fever, vexation, thirst, foul stool, diarrhea and dysentery.

Administration and dosage: (for oral administration) pill: 3 g per time, 1 g per time for children, three times a day; tablet: 3-4 pills per time, three times a day.

Strength: pill: 1 g per pack; tablet: (1) uncoated tablets (0.3 g per tablet), (2) uncoated tablets (0.5 g per tablet), (3) sugar coated tablets (0.3 g of the core per tablet), (4) film coated tablet (0.3 g per tablet).

The specific strength and dosage are according to the medicine instruction.

Precaution and warning: contraindicated during pregnancy.

(The information is only for learning and identification the Chinese Patent Medicine; the specific use of the Medicine please consult the herbalist or health professionals)

Fangfeng Tongsheng Pills (Granules) (Fangfeng Tongsheng Wan (Keli))

Chinese phonetic alphabet/pin yin: fáng fēng tōng shèng wán

Chinese characters simplified/traditional:防风通圣丸(颗粒)/防風通聖丸(顆粒)

Ingredients: Divaricate Saposhnikovia Root, Fineleaf Schizonepeta Spike, Peppermint, Ephedra, Rhubarb, Sodium Sulfate, Cape Jasmine Fruit, Talc, Platycodon Root, Gypsum, Szechwan Lovage Rhizome, Chinese Angelica, White Peony Root, Baical Skullcap Root, Weeping Forsythia Capsule, Liquorice Root, Largehead Atractylodes Rhizome (processed with bran).

The content of each ingredients may have a little variety due to different dosage forms.

Indication: cold and high fever, headache, dry mouth and throat, deep-colored urine, constipation, early onset of scrofula, rubella and eczema.

Administration and dosage: (for oral administration) pill: 6 g per time, twice a day; granule: 1 pack per time, twice a day.

Strength: pill: 1 g per 20 pills; granule: 3 g per pack.

The specific strength and dosage are according to the medicine instruction.

Precaution and warning: contraindicated during pregnancy.

Purging medicine(泻下药)

Purging medicine is a kind of medicines, their major functions are purgation, diuresis, detumescence.

Danggui Longhui Pills (Danggui Longhui Wan)

Chinese phonetic alphabet/pin yin: dāng guī lóng huì wán

Chinese characters simplified/traditional:当归龙荟丸/當歸龍薈丸

Ingredients: Chinese Angelica (stir-baked with wine), Chinese Gentian (stir-baked with wine), Aloes, Natural Indigo, Cape Jasmine Fruit, Golden Thread (stir-baked with wine), Baical Skullcap Root (stir-baked with wine), Chinese Cork-tree (stir-baked with salt), Rhubarb (stir-baked with wine), Common Aucklandia Root, Artificial Musk.

Indication: vexation, dizziness, vertigo, tinnitus and deafness, hypochondriac pain, tightness and pain in the epigastrium and abdomen, and constipation.

Administration and dosage: 6 g per time, twice a day for oral administration.

The specific strength and dosage are according to the medicine instruction.

Precaution and warning: contraindicated during pregnancy.

Jiuzhi Dahuang Pills (Jiuzhi Dahuang Wan)

Chinese phonetic alphabet/pin yin: jiǔ zhì dà huáng wán

Chinese characters simplified/traditional:九制大黄丸/九制大黃丸

Ingredients: Rhubarb, Rice Wine.

Indication: constipation, vexation, food stagnation and water retetion.

Administration and dosage: 6 g per time, once a day for oral administration.

Strength: 6 g per pill.

The specific strength and dosage are according to the medicine instruction.

Precaution and warning: contraindicated during pregnancy. Use with caution in patients with long-term illness and/or weakness. Long-term administration is inadvisable.

Maren Pills (Maren Wan)

Chinese phonetic alphabet/pin yin: má rén wán

Chinese characters simplified/traditional:麻仁丸/麻仁丸

Ingredients: Hemp Seed, Bitter Apricot, Rhubarb, Immature Orange Fruit (stir-baked), Official Magnolia Bark (processed with ginger), White Peony Root (stir-baked).

Indication: habitual constipation, dry faeces, abdominal distention and discomfort.

Administration and dosage: 6 g water-honeyed pill, 9 g small honeyed pill, or 1 big honeyed pill per time, once or twice a day for oral administration.

Strength: 9 g per big honeyed pill.

The specific strength and dosage are according to the medicine instruction.

Tongbianling Capsules (Tongbianling Jiaonang)
Chinese phonetic alphabet/pin yin: tōng biàn líng jiāo náng
Chinese characters simplified/traditional:通便灵胶囊/通便靈膠囊
Ingredients: Senna Leaf, Chinese Angelica, Desertliving Cistanche Herb.
Indication: constipation.
Administration and dosage: 5-6 pills per time, once a day for oral administration.
Strength: 0.25g per capsule.
The specific strength and dosage are according to the medicine instruction.
Precaution and warning: Use with caution in pregnant woman.
(The information is only for learning and identification the Chinese Patent Medicine;
the specific use of the Medicine please consult the herbalist or health professionals)

Zhouche Pills (Zhouche Wan)
Chinese phonetic alphabet/pin yin: zhōu chē wán
Chinese characters simplified/traditional:舟车丸/舟車丸
Ingredients: Pharbitis Seed (stir-baked), Rhubarb (processed with alcohol), Gansui
Root (processed with flour), Knoxia Root (processed with vinegar), Lilac Daphne
Flower Bud (processed with vinegar), Dried Immaturity Tangerines Peel (processed
with vinegar), Dried Tangerine Peel, Common Aucklandia Root, Calomel.
Indication: swelling of limbs, abdominal distention, constipation and inhibited
urination.
Administration and dosage: 1 pack per time, once a day for oral administration.
Strength: 3 g per pack.
The specific strength and dosage are according to the medicine instruction.
Precaution and warning: Use with caution in pregnant woman and patient with
weakness. Long-term administration is not advisable.
(The information is only for learning and identification the Chinese Patent Medicine;
the specific use of the Medicine please consult the herbalist or health professionals)

Antipyretic or heat-clearing formula(清热剂)
Antipyretic or heat-clearing formula is a kind of medicines, their major functions are
to treat fever, some of them can treat dysentery, carbuncle, abscess.

Longdan Xiegan Pills (Longdan Xiegan Wan)
Chinese phonetic alphabet/pin yin: lóng dǎn xiè gān wán
Chinese characters simplified/traditional:龙胆泻肝丸/龍膽瀉肝丸
Ingredients: Chinese Gentian, Chinese Thorowax Root, Baical Skullcap Root, Cape
Jasmine Fruit (stir-baked), Oriental Waterplantain Rhizome, Akebiae Stem, Plantain
Seed (stir-baked with salt), Chinese Angelica (stir-baked with wine), Rehmannia Root,
Prepared Liquorice Root.
Indication: dizziness, red eye, tinnitus, deafness, swelling and pain of ear,
hypochondriac pain and bitter taste in mouth, fluor vaginalis, dysuria and painful
urine.
Administration and dosage: 3-6 g for watered pills, 6-12 g for small honeyed pills, 1-2
pills for big honeyed pill per time, twice a day.
Strength: 20 g per 100 pills for small honeyed pill, 6 g per big honeyed pill.
The specific strength and dosage are according to the medicine instruction.
Precaution and warning: Use with caution in pregnant woman.
(The information is only for learning and identification the Chinese Patent Medicine;
the specific use of the Medicine please consult the herbalist or health professionals)

Huanglian Shangqing Tablets (Pills/Granules/Capsules) (Huanglian Shangqing Pian (Wan/Keli/Jiaonang))

Chinese phonetic alphabet/pin yin: huáng lián shàng qīng piàn

Chinese characters simplified/traditional:黄连上清片(丸/颗粒/胶囊)/黃連上清片(丸/顆粒/膠囊)

Ingredients: Golden Thread, Cape Jasmine Fruit (processed with ginger), Weeping Forsythia Capsule, Shrub Chastetree Fruit (stir-baked), Divaricate Saposhnikovia Root, Fineleaf Schizonepeta spike, Dahurian Angelica Root, Baical Skullcap Root, Chrysanthemum Flower, Peppermint, Rhubarb (processed with wine), Chinese Cork-tree, Platycodon Root, Szechwan Lovage Rhizome, Gypsum, Inula Flower, Liquorice Root.

The content of each ingredients may have a little variety due to different dosage forms.

Indication: dizziness and vertigo, epidemic conjunctivitis, toothache, mouth and tongue sores, swollen sore throat, ear pain and tinnitus, constipation and short voidings of reddish urine.

Administration and dosage: (for oral administration) tablet: 6 tablets per time, twice a day; pill: 3-6 g water pills or water-honeyed pills, or 1-2 big honeyed pills per time, twice a day; granule: 2 g per time, twice a day; capsule: 2 capsules per time, twice a day.

Strength: tablet: (1) 0.31 g per film coated tablet, (2) 0.3 g per core (sugar coated tablet); pill: 6 g per pack of watered pill, 3 g per forty water-honeyed pill, 6 g per big honeyed pill; granule: 2 g per pack; capsule: 0.4 g per capsule.

The specific strength and dosage are according to the medicine instruction.

Precaution and warning: avoid spicy food. Use with caution during pregnancy. Contraindicated in patients with spleen-stomach deficiency cold pattern.

(The information is only for learning and identification the Chinese Patent Medicine; the specific use of the Medicine please consult the herbalist or health professionals)

Yiqing Granules (Capsules) (Yiqing Keli (Jiaonang))

Chinese phonetic alphabet/pin yin: yī qīng kē lì

Chinese characters simplified/traditional:一清颗粒(胶囊)/一清顆粒(膠囊)

Ingredients: Golden Thread, Rhubarb, Baical Skullcap Root.

The content of each ingredients may have a little variety due to different dosage forms.

Indication: fever, vexation, reddened eyes, mouth sore, swollen sore throat and gum, constipation, hematemesis, hemoptysis, epistaxis or hemorrhoidal bleeding, pharyngitis, tonsillitis and gingivitis.

Administration and dosage: (for oral administration) granule: mixing the medicine with water before usage, 7.5 g per time, three or four times a day; capsule: 2 capusles per time, three times a day.

Strength: granule: 7.5 g pre-pack; capsule: 0.5 g per capsule.

The specific strength and dosage are according to the medicine instruction.

Precaution and warning: reduce the dosage if diarrhea occurs.

(The information is only for learning and identification the Chinese Patent Medicine; the specific use of the Medicine please consult the herbalist or health professionals)

Daige Powder (Daige San)

Chinese phonetic alphabet/pin yin: dài gě sǎn

Chinese characters simplified/traditional:黛蛤散/黛蛤散
Ingredients: Natural Indigo, Clam Shell.
Indication: dizziness, tinnitus, cough, hematemesis, epistaxis, profuse yellowish sticky phlegm, sore throat, dry mouth, thirst and vexation.
Administration and dosage: 6 g per time, once a day for oral administration, decoct with prescribed formula.
The specific strength and dosage are according to the medicine instruction.
(The information is only for learning and identification the Chinese Patent Medicine; the specific use of the Medicine please consult the herbalist or health professionals)

Niuhuang Shangqing Pills (Tablets/Capsules/Soft Capsules) (Niuhuang Shangqing Wan (Pian/Jiaonang/Ruanjiaonang))
Chinese phonetic alphabet/pin yin: niú huáng shàng qīng wán
Chinese characters simplified/traditional:牛黄上清丸(片/胶囊/软胶囊)/牛黄上清丸 (片/膠囊/軟膠囊)
Ingredients: Artificial Cow-bezoar, Peppermint, Chrysanthemum Flower, Fineleaf Schizonepeta Spike, Dahurian Angelica Root, Szechwan Lovage Rhizome, Cape Jasmine Fruit, Golden Thread, Chinese Cork-tree, Baical Skullcap Root, Rhubarb, Weeping Forsythia Capsule, Red Peony Root, Chinese Angelica, Rehmannia Root, Platycodon Root, Liquorice Root, Gypsum, Borneol.
The content of each ingredients may have a little variety due to different dosage forms.
Indication: headache, giddy, red eyes, tinnitus, sore throat, mouth and tongue sore, swelling painful gum and dry stool.
Administration and dosage: (for oral administration) pill: 3 g water pills, 6 g small honeyed pills, or 1 big honeyed pill per time, two times a day; tablet: 4 tablets per time, two times a day; capsule: 3 capsules per time, two times a day; soft capsule: 4 capsules per time, two times a day.
Strength: pill: 3 g per 16 pills for watered pills, 20 g per 100 small honeyed pills, 6 g for a big honeyed pill; tablet: 0.265 g per film coated tablet; capsule: 0.3 g per capsule; soft capsule: 0.6 g per capsule.
The specific strength and dosage are according to the medicine instruction.
Precaution and warning: use with caution in pregnant woman and lactation woman. Contraindicated in patients with spleen-stomach deficiency cold pattern.
(The information is only for learning and identification the Chinese Patent Medicine; the specific use of the Medicine please consult the herbalist or health professionals)

Qingwei Huanglian Pills (Tablets) (Qingwei Huanglian Wan (Pian))
Chinese phonetic alphabet/pin yin: qīng wèi huáng lián wán
Chinese characters simplified/traditional:清胃黄连丸(片)/清胃黄連丸(片)
Ingredients: Golden Thread, Gypsum, Platycodon Root, Liquorice Root, Common Anemarrhena Rhizome, Figwort, Rehmannia Root, Tree Peony Bark, Snakegourd Root, Weeping Forsythia Capsule, Cape Jasmine Fruit, Chinese Cork-tree, Baical Skullcap Root, Red Peony Root.
The content of each ingredients may have a little variety due to different dosage forms.
Indication: mouth and tongue sore, swelling and painful gum and throat.
Administration and dosage: (for oral administration) pill: 9 g water-honeyed pills or 1-2 big honeyed pills per time, twice a day; tablet: 8 tablets per time, twice a day.
Strength: pill: 9 g per pack for water-honeyed pills, 9 g for a big honeyed pill; tablet:

0.32 g per tablet core for sugar coated tablet, 0.33 g per tablet for film coated tablet. The specific strength and dosage are according to the medicine instruction.

Precaution and warning: use with caution in pregnant women.

(The information is only for learning and identification the Chinese Patent Medicine; the specific use of the Medicine please consult the herbalist or health professionals)

Niuhuang Jiedu Pills (Tablets/Capsules/Soft Capsules) (Niuhuang Jiedu Wan (Pian/Jiaonang/Ruanjiaonang))

Chinese phonetic alphabet/pin yin: niú huáng jiě dú wán

Chinese characters simplified/traditional:牛黄解毒丸(片/胶囊/软胶囊)/牛黃解毒丸(片/膠囊/軟膠囊)

Ingredients: Artificial Cow-bezoan, Realgar, Cypsum, Rhubarb, Baical Skullcap Root, Platycodon Root, Borneol, Liquorice Root.

The content of each ingredients may have a little variety due to different dosage forms.

Indication: sore throat, gum swelling and pain, sore in mouth and tongue and red painful eyes.

Administration and dosage: (for oral administration) pill: 2 g water-honeyed pills or 1 big honeyed pill per time, two or three times a day; tablet: 3 small tablets or 2 big tablets per time, two or three times a day; capsule: 2 pills [capsule strength (1)] or 3 pills [capsule strength (2)] per time, two or three times a day; soft capsule: 4 pills per time, two or three times a day.

Strength: pill: 5 g per 100 pills for water-honeyed pills, 3 g for a big honeyed pill; capsule: (1) capsule equivalent to 0.78 g of the prepared slice, 0.3, 0.4 or 0.5 g per capsule, (2) capsule equivalent to 0.52 g of the prepared slice, 0.3 g per capsule; soft capsule: 0.4 g per capsule.

The specific strength and dosage are according to the medicine instruction.

Precaution and warning: contraindicated in pregnant women.

(The information is only for learning and identification the Chinese Patent Medicine; the specific use of the Medicine please consult the herbalist or health professionals)

Niuhuang Zhibao Pills (Niuhuang Zhibao Wan)

Chinese phonetic alphabet/pin yin: niú huáng zhì bǎo wán

Chinese characters simplified/traditional:牛黄至宝丸/牛黃至寶丸

Ingredients: Weeping Forsythia Capsule, Cape Jasmine Fruit, Rhubarb, Sodium Sulfate, Gypsum, Sweet Wormwood Herb, Dried Tangerine Peel, Common Aucklandia Root, Cablin Patchouli Herb, Artificial Cow-bezoan, Borneol, Realgar.

Indication: headache, dizziness, red eyes, tinnitus, constipation, dry mouth and throat.

Administration and dosage: 1-2 pills per time, twice a day for oral administration. Reduce the dosage in children.

Strength: 6 g per pills.

The specific strength and dosage are according to the medicine instruction.

Precaution and warning: contraindicated in pregnant woman

(The information is only for learning and identification the Chinese Patent Medicine; the specific use of the Medicine please consult the herbalist or health professionals)

Xinxue Granules (Xinxue Keli)

Chinese phonetic alphabet/pin yin: xīn xuě kē lì

Chinese characters simplified/traditional:新雪颗粒/新雪顆粒

Ingredients: Magnetite, Gypsum, Talc, Calcitum, Saltpeter, Sodium Sulfate, Cape

Jasmine Fruit, White Powdery Bamboo Leaf, Cantonese Cohosh, Common Andrographis Herb, Nacreous Layer Powder, Chinese Eaglewood Wood, Artificial Cow-bezoan, Borneol.

Indication: high fever, vexation and agitation, tonsillitis, upper respiratory, tract infection, bronchitis and common cold.

Administration and dosage: 1 pack (bottle) per time, twice a day for oral administration.

Strength: 1.5 g per pack (bottle), or 1.53 g film coated granules per pack (bottle).

The specific strength and dosage are according to the medicine instruction.

Attachment: Saltpeter (硝石, Latin name: Nitrum) is Sodium nitrate and its chemical compound formula is $NaNO_3$.

White Powdery Bamboo Leaf (竹心, Latin name: Banbusae Folium) is dried leaf of *Bambusa chungii* Mc Clure.

Cantonese Cohosh (广升麻, Latin name: Serratulae Chinensis Radix) is dried tuber root of *Serratula chinensis* S. Moore.

(The information is only for learning and identification the Chinese Patent Medicine; the specific use of the Medicine please consult the herbalist or health professionals)

Qinlian Tablets (Qinlian Pian)

Chinese phonetic alphabet/pin yin: qín lián piàn

Chinese characters simplified/traditional:芩连片/芩連片

Ingredients: Baical Skullcap Root, Weeping Forsythia Capsule, Golden Thread, Chinese Cork-tree, Red Peony Root, Liquorice Root.

Indication: headache, red eyes, mouth and nose sore, dysentery, vaginal discharge.

Administration and dosage: 4 tablets per time, two or three times a day for oral administration.

Strength: 0.55 g per tablet.

The specific strength and dosage are according to the medicine instruction.

(The information is only for learning and identification the Chinese Patent Medicine; the specific use of the Medicine please consult the herbalist or health professionals)

Daochi Pills (Daochi Wan)

Chinese phonetic alphabet/pin yin: dǎo chì wán

Chinese characters simplified/traditional:导赤丸/導赤丸

Ingredients: Weeping Forsythia Capsule, Golden Thread, Cape Jasmine Fruit (stir-baked with ginger), Akebiae Stem, Figwort, Snakegourd Root, Red Peony Root, Rhubarb, Baical Skullcap Root, Talc.

Indication: throat pain, short voidings of reddish urine, constipation, mouth and tongue sore.

Administration and dosage: 2 g water-honeyed pill or 1 small honey pill per time, twice a day for oral administration. Reduce the dosage in children under 1 year old.

Strength: 1 g per ten water-honeyed pills, 3 g per pill.

The specific strength and dosage are according to the medicine instruction.

(The information is only for learning and identification the Chinese Patent Medicine; the specific use of the Medicine please consult the herbalist or health professionals)

Banlangen Granules (Tea) (Banlangen Keli (Cha))

Chinese phonetic alphabet/pin yin: bǎn lán gēn kē lì

Chinese characters simplified/traditional:板蓝根颗粒(茶)/板藍根顆粒(茶)

Ingredients: Isatis Root.

Indication: swollen and sore throat, dryness in mouth and throat, acute tonsillitis and parotitis.

Administration and dosage: tea: take the medicine orally after mixing it with hot water, 1 cube per time, three times a day; granule: mix it with boiled water 5-10 g [strengths (1) and (2)], or 1-2 pack [strengths (3) and (4)] per time, three to four times a day.

Strength: tea: 10 or 15 per piece; granule: (1) 5 g per pack, (2) 10 g per pack, (3) 3 g per pack (without sucrose), (4) 1 g per pack (without sucrose).

The specific strength and dosage are according to the medicine instruction.

(The information is only for learning and identification the Chinese Patent Medicine; the specific use of the Medicine please consult the herbalist or health professionals)

Qingre Jiedu Mixture (Tablets) (Qingre Jiedu Koufuye (Pian))

Chinese phonetic alphabet/pin yin: qīng rè jiě dú kǒu fú yè

Chinese characters simplified/traditional:清热解毒口服液(片)/清熱解毒口服液(片)

Ingredients: Gypsum, Japanese Honeysuckle Flower, Figwort, Rehmannia Root, Weeping Forsythia Capsule, Cape Jasmine Fruit, Gueldenstaedtia Herb, Baical Skullcap Root, Chinese Gentian, Isatis Root, Common Anemarrhena Rhizome, Dwarf Lilyturf Tuber.

The content of each ingredients may have a little variety due to different dosage forms.

Indication: influenza, upper respiratory tract infection with fever, vexation, agitation, thirst and sore throat.

Administration and dosage: mixture: 10-20 ml per time, three times a day; tablet: 4 tablets per time, three times a day. Reduce the dosage in children.

Strength: mixture: 10 ml per phial; 0.52 or 0.37 g per film-coated tablet, 0.35 g per tablet core for file coated tablet.

The specific strength and dosage are according to the medicine instruction.

Attachment: Gueldenstaedtia Herb (甜地丁, Latin name: Gueldenstaedtiae Herba) is dried whole herb of *Gueldenstaedtia multifora* Bunge., *Gueldenstaedtia verna* (Georgi) Boriss., *Gueldenstaedtia stenophylla* Bunge., or *Gueldenstaedtia coelestis* (Diels) Simpson.

(The information is only for learning and identification the Chinese Patent Medicine; the specific use of the Medicine please consult the herbalist or health professionals)

Xihuang Pills (Xihuang Wan)

Chinese phonetic alphabet/pin yin: xī huáng wán

Chinese characters simplified/traditional:西黄丸/西黃丸

Ingredients: Cow-bezoar (or Sativus Cow-bezoar), Musk (or Artificial Musk), Olibanum (processed with vinegar), Myrrh (processed with vinegar).

Indication: abscesses, cellulitis, scrofula and tumor swelling.

Administration and dosage: 3 g per day, twice a day for oral administration.

Strength: 1 g per 20 pills.

The specific strength and dosage are according to the medicine instruction.

Precaution and warning: contraindicated during pregnancy.

(The information is only for learning and identification the Chinese Patent Medicine; the specific use of the Medicine please consult the herbalist or health professionals)

Prescriptions for dispelling internal cold(温里剂)

Prescriptions for dispelling internal cold is a kind of medicines, their major functions are dispelling cold, abdominal pain or stomachache caused by cold/chill; some of them can antiemetic, cardiac, treat excessive phlegm.

Lizhong Pills (Lizhong Wan)

Chinese phonetic alphabet/pin yin: lǐ zhōng wán
Chinese characters simplified/traditional:理中丸/理中丸
Ingredients: Tangshen, Largehead Atractylodes Rhizome (processed with terra), Prepared Liquorice Root, Prepared Dried Ginger.
Indication: vomiting, diarrhea, fullness and pain in chest and abdominal, and indigestion.
Administration and dosage: 1 pill per day, twice a day for oral administration. Reduce the dosage in children.
Strength: 9 g per pill.
The specific strength and dosage are according to the medicine instruction.
Precaution and warning: avoid row, cold, greasy and indigestible food.
(The information is only for learning and identification the Chinese Patent Medicine; the specific use of the Medicine please consult the herbalist or health professionals)

Xiaojianzhong Mixture (Granules/Tablets) (Xiaojianzhong Heji (Keli/Wan))

Chinese phonetic alphabet/pin yin: xiǎo jiàn zhōng hé jì
Chinese characters simplified/traditional:小建中合剂(颗粒/片)/小建中合劑(顆粒/片)
Ingredients: Cassia Twig, White Peony Root, Prepared Liquorice Root, Fresh Ginger, Chinese Date.
The content of each ingredients may have a little variety due to different dosage forms.
Indication: pain in the epigastrium and abdomen, preference for warmth and pressing, gastric upset, acid regurgitation, less food intake and gastroduodenal ulcer.
Administration and dosage: (for oral administration) mixture: 20-30 ml per time, three times a day, shake well before use; granule: 1 pack per time, three time a day; tablet: 2-3 tablets per time, three times a day.
Strength: granule: 15 g per pack; tablet: 0.6 g per file coated tablet.
The specific strength and dosage are according to the medicine instruction.
Precaution and warning: used with caution in patient with stomach or gastrointestinal bleeding.
(The information is only for learning and identification the Chinese Patent Medicine; the specific use of the Medicine please consult the herbalist or health professionals)

Liangfu Pills (Liangfu Wan)

Chinese phonetic alphabet/pin yin: liáng fù wán
Chinese characters simplified/traditional:良附丸/良附丸
Ingredients: Lesser Galangal Rhizome, Nutgrass Galingale Rhizome (processed with vinegar).
Indication: stomachache and acid reflux, distension and fullness in the chest and abdomen.
Administration and dosage: 3 to 6 g per time, twice a day for oral administration.
The specific strength and dosage are according to the medicine instruction.
(The information is only for learning and identification the Chinese Patent Medicine; the specific use of the Medicine please consult the herbalist or health professionals)

Xiangsha Yangwei Pills (Xiangsha Yangwei Wan)

Chinese phonetic alphabet/pin yin: xiāng shā yǎng wèi wán

Chinese characters simplified/traditional:香砂养胃丸/香砂養胃丸

Ingredients: Common Aucklandia Root, Villous Amomum Fruit, Largehead Atractylodes Rhizome, Dried Tangerine Peel, Indian Bread, Pinellia Tuber (baked with ginger), Nutgrass Galingale Rhizome (processed with vinegar), Immature Orange Fruit (stir-baked), Round Cardamon Fruit (peeled), Officinal Magnolia Bark (processed with ginger), Cablin Patchouli Herb, Liquorice Root, Fresh Ginger, Chinese Date.

Indication: stomachache and stuffiness, discomfort in epigastrium, acid regurgitation, vomiting and no desire for food and drink.

Administration and dosage: 8 pills of concentrated pill or 9 g honeyed pill per time, twice a day for oral administration.

Strength: 8 pills equivalent to 3 g of prepared slice for concentrated pill.

The specific strength and dosage are according to the medicine instruction.

(The information is only for learning and identification the Chinese Patent Medicine; the specific use of the Medicine please consult the herbalist or health professionals)

Fuzi Lizhong Pills (Tablets) (Fuzi Lizhong Wan (Pian))

Chinese phonetic alphabet/pin yin: fù zǐ lǐ zhōng wán

Chinese characters simplified/traditional:附子理中丸(片)/附子理中丸(片)

Ingredients: Prepared Common Monkshood Daugher Root, Tangshen, Largehead Atractylodes Rhizome (stir-baked), Dried Ginger, Liquorice Root.

The content of each ingredients may have a little variety due to different dosage forms.

Indication: cold pain in the epigastrium and abdomen, vomiting, diarrhea and cold limbs.

Administration and dosage: (for oral administration) pill: 6 g water-honeyed pill per time, 9 g small honeyed pills, or 1 big honey pill per time, twice or three times a day; tablet: 6-8 tablets per time, once to three times a day.

Strength: pill: 20 g per 100 small honeyed pill, 9 g per big honeyed pill; tablet: 0.25 g of the core per tablet.

The specific strength and dosage are according to the medicine instruction.

Precaution and warning: use with caution during pregnancy

(The information is only for learning and identification the Chinese Patent Medicine; the specific use of the Medicine please consult the herbalist or health professionals)

Xiangsha Pingwei Pills (Xiangsha Pingwei Wan)

Chinese phonetic alphabet/pin yin: xiāng shā píng wèi wán

Chinese characters simplified/traditional:香砂平胃丸/香砂平胃丸

Ingredients: Atractylodes Rhizome, Dried Tangerine Peel, Officinal Magnolia Bark (stir-baked with ginger), Common Aucklandia Root, Villous Amomum Fruit, Liquorice Root.

Indication: indigestion, distention and oppression in the chest and diaphragm, stomachache and vomiting.

Administration and dosage: 6-9 g per time, one or two times a day for oral administration.

Strength: 6 g or 60 g per bottle.

The specific strength and dosage are according to the medicine instruction.

(The information is only for learning and identification the Chinese Patent Medicine; the specific use of the Medicine please consult the herbalist or health professionals)

Sini Mixture (Sini Tang)

Chinese phonetic alphabet/pin yin: sì nì tāng

Chinese characters simplified/traditional:四逆汤/四逆湯

Ingredients: Prepared Common Monkshood Daughter Root, Dried Ginger, Prepared Liquorice Root.

Indication: cold limbs, diarrhea with undigested food, spontaneous or night sweating and feeble pulse.

Administration and dosage: 10-20 ml per time, three times a day for oral administration.

Strength: 10 ml per phial.

The specific strength and dosage are according to the medicine instruction.

(The information is only for learning and identification the Chinese Patent Medicine; the specific use of the Medicine please consult the herbalist or health professionals)

Expectorant(祛痰剂)

Expectorant is a kind of medicines, which can remove the phlegm.

Erchen Pills (Erchen Wan)

Chinese phonetic alphabet/pin yin: èr chén wán

Chinese characters simplified/traditional:二陈丸/二陳丸

Ingredients: Dried Tangerine Peel, Pinellia Tuber (processed), Indian Bread, Liquorice Root.

Indication: cough with excessive phlegm, distension and oppression in chest and epigastrium, nausea and vomiting.

Administration and dosage: 9-15 g per time, twice a day for oral administration.

The specific strength and dosage are according to the medicine instruction.

(The information is only for learning and identification the Chinese Patent Medicine; the specific use of the Medicine please consult the herbalist or health professionals)

Mengshi Guntan Pills (Mengshi Guntan Wan)

Chinese phonetic alphabet/pin yin: méng shí gǔn tán wán

Chinese characters simplified/traditional:礞石滚痰丸/礞石滾痰丸

Ingredients: Mica-Schist (calcined)，Chinese Eaglewood Wood, Baical Skullcap Root, Rhubarb (steamed).

Indication: fright palpitation, cough with purulent phlegm and constipation.

Administration and dosage: 6-12 g per time, once a day for oral administration.

The specific strength and dosage are according to the medicine instruction.

Precaution and warning: contraindicated with pregnant woman.

(The information is only for learning and identification the Chinese Patent Medicine; the specific use of the Medicine please consult the herbalist or health professionals)

Qingqi Huatan Pills (Qingqi Huatan Wan)

Chinese phonetic alphabet/pin yin: qīng qì huà tán wán

Chinese characters simplified/traditional:清气化痰丸/清氣化痰丸

Ingredients: Baical Skullcap Root (stir-baked with wine), Prepared Snakegourd Seed Powder, Pinellia Tuber (processed), Bile Arisaema, Dried Tangerine Peel, Bitter

Apricot, Immature Orange Fruit, Indian Bread.

Indication: excessive phlegm, yellow thick greasy sputum, fullness and tightness in the chest and abdomen.

Administration and dosage: 6-9 g per time, twice a day for oral administration. Reduce the dosage in children.

The specific strength and dosage are according to the medicine instruction.

(The information is only for learning and identification the Chinese Patent Medicine; the specific use of the Medicine please consult the herbalist or health professionals)

Fufang Xianzhuli Mixture (Fufang Xianzhuli Ye)

Chinese phonetic alphabet/pin yin: fù fāng xiān zhú lì yè

Chinese characters simplified/traditional:复方鲜竹沥液/複方鮮竹瀝液

Ingredients: Bamboo Juice, Heartleaf Houttuynia Herb, Pinellia Tuber (processed with Ginger and Alum), Fresh Ginger, Loquat Leaf, Platycodon Root, Peppermint Oil.

Indication: cough with yellow thick sticky sputum.

Administration and dosage: 20 ml per time, twice or three times a day for oral administration.

Strength: 10 ml, 20 ml, 30 ml, 100ml, 120ml, 20ml (without sucrose) per bottle.

The specific strength and dosage are according to the medicine instruction.

(The information is only for learning and identification the Chinese Patent Medicine; the specific use of the Medicine please consult the herbalist or health professionals)

Banxia Tianma Pills (Banxia Tianma Wan)

Chinese phonetic alphabet/pin yin: bàn xià tiān má wán

Chinese characters simplified/traditional:半夏天麻丸/半夏天麻丸

Ingredients: Prepared Pinellia Tuber, Tall Gastrodia Tuber, Prepared Milkvetch Root, Ginseng, Atractylodes Rhizome (processed with rice water), Largehead Atractylodes Rhizome (stir-baked), Indian Bread, Dried Tangerine Peel, Oriental Waterplantain Rhizome, Medicated Leaven (stir-baked with bran), Germinated Barly (stir-baked), Chinese Cork-tree.

Indication: dizziness, headache, fullness and oppression in the chest and epigastrium.

Administration and dosage: 6 g per time, twice or three times per day for oral administration.

Strength: 6 g per 100 pills.

The specific strength and dosage are according to the medicine instruction.

Precaution and warning: avoid raw, cold and oily food.

(The information is only for learning and identification the Chinese Patent Medicine; the specific use of the Medicine please consult the herbalist or health professionals)

Xiaoying Pills (Xiaoying Wan)

Chinese phonetic alphabet/pin yin: xiāo yīng wán

Chinese characters simplified/traditional:消瘿丸/消瘿丸

Ingredients: Kelp, Seaweed, Clam Shell, Thunberg Fritillary Bulb, Platycodon Root, Common Selfheal Fruit-Spike, Dried Tangerine Peel, Areca Seed.

Indication: initial onset of goiter and tumor, and simple endemic goiter.

Administration and dosage: 1pill g per time, three times a day for oral administration before meals. Reduce the dosage in children.

Strength: 3 g per pill.

The specific strength and dosage are according to the medicine instruction.

(The information is only for learning and identification the Chinese Patent Medicine;

the specific use of the Medicine please consult the herbalist or health professionals)

Antitussive and antiasthmatic prescription(止咳平喘剂)

Antitussive and antiasthmatic prescription is a kind of medicines, which are usually used to relieve cough and asthma.

Tongxuan Lifei Pills (Tablets/Capsules/Granules) (Tongxuan Lifei Wan (Pian/Jiaonang/Keli))

Chinese phonetic alphabet/pin yin: tōng xuān lǐ fèi wán

Chinese characters simplified/traditional:通宣理肺丸(片/胶囊/颗粒)/通宣理肺丸(片/膠囊/顆粒)

Ingredients: Perilla Leaf, Hogfennel Root, Platycodon Root, Bitter Apricot, Ephedra, Liquorice Root, Dried Tangerine Peel, Pinellia Tuber (processed), Indian Bread, Orange Fruit (stir-baked), Baical Skullcap Root.

The content of each ingredients may have a little variety due to different dosage forms.

Indication: fever, chills feeling, cough, stuffy and runny nose, headache, absence of sweating and pain in limbs.

Administration and dosage: (for oral administration) pill: 7 g water-honeyed pills, or 2 big honeyed pills per time, two or three times a day; tablet: 4 tablets per time, two or three times a day; capsule: 2 capsules per time, two or three times a day; granule: mixing the medicine with hot water before usage, 9 g per time, twice a day.

Strength: pill: 10 g per 100 water-honeyed pills, 6 g per big honeyed pill; tablet: 0.3 g per file-coated tablet, 0.29 g core per sugar-coated tablet; capsule: 0.36 g per capsule; granule: 9 g per pack or 3 g per pack (without sucrose).

The specific strength and dosage are according to the medicine instruction.

Precaution and warning: use with caution in patients with hypertension, epilepsy, wind-stroke and arrhythmia.

(The information is only for learning and identification the Chinese Patent Medicine; the specific use of the Medicine please consult the herbalist or health professionals)

San'ao Tablets (San'ao Pian)

Chinese phonetic alphabet/pin yin: sān ǎo piàn

Chinese characters simplified/traditional:三拗片/三拗片

Ingredients: Ephedra, Bitter Apricot, Liquorice Root, Fresh Ginger.

Indication: cough, hoarse voice, excessive white clear phlegm and acute bronchitis.

Administration and dosage: 2 tablets per time, three times a day for oral administration.

Strength: 0.5 g per tablet.

The specific strength and dosage are according to the medicine instruction.

(The information is only for learning and identification the Chinese Patent Medicine; the specific use of the Medicine please consult the herbalist or health professionals)

Qingfei Yihuo Pills (Qingfei Yihuo Wan)

Chinese phonetic alphabet/pin yin: qīng fèi yì huǒ wán

Chinese characters simplified/traditional:清肺抑火丸/清肺抑火丸

Ingredients: Baical Skullcap Root, Cape Jasmine Fruit, Common Anemarrhena Rhizome, Thunberg Fritillary Bulb, Chinese Cork-tree, Lightyellow Sophora Root, Platycodon Root, Hogfennel Root, Snakegourd Root, Rhubarb.

Indication: cough, profuse sputum, yellow thick phlegm, dry mouth and throat, sore throat and dry stool.

Administration and dosage: 6 g water-honeyed pills or 1 big honeyed pill per time, two or three times a day for oral administration.

Strength: 9 g per big honeyed pill.

The specific strength and dosage are according to the medicine instruction.

Precaution and warning: use with caution during pregnancy.

(The information is only for learning and identification the Chinese Patent Medicine; the specific use of the Medicine please consult the herbalist or health professionals)

Shedan Chuanbei Powder (Capules/Soft Capsules) (Shedan Chuanbei San (Jiaonang/Ruanjiaonang))

Chinese phonetic alphabet/pin yin: shé dǎn chuān bèi sǎn

Chinese characters simplified/traditional:蛇胆川贝散(胶囊/软胶囊)/蛇膽川貝散(膠囊/軟膠囊)

Ingredients: Snake Gallbladder, Tendrilleaf Fritilary Bulb.

The content of each ingredients may have a little variety due to different dosage forms.

Indication: cough with excessive phlegm.

Administration and dosage: (for oral administration) powder: 0.3-0.6 g per time, two or three times a day; capsule: 1-2 capsules per time, two or three times a day; soft capsule: 2-4 capsules per time, two or three times a day.

Strength: powder: 0.3 or 0.6 g per bottle; capsule: 0.3 g per capsule; soft capsule: 0.3 g per capsule.

The specific strength and dosage are according to the medicine instruction.

Attachment: Snake Gallbladder (蛇胆, Latin name: Serpentis Fel) is the gallbladder of snake. **Attention**: to protect the rare wild animals, don't use it from wild animal.

(The information is only for learning and identification the Chinese Patent Medicine; the specific use of the Medicine please consult the herbalist or health professionals)

Juhong Tablets (Capules/Granules) (Juhong Pian (Jiaonang/Keli))

Chinese phonetic alphabet/pin yin: jú hóng piàn

Chinese characters simplified/traditional:橘红片(胶囊/颗粒)/橘紅片(膠囊/顆粒)

Ingredients: Pummelo Peel, Dried Tangerine Peel, Prepared Pinellia Tuber, Indian Bread, Liquorice Root, Platycodon Root, Bitter Apricot, Perilla Fruit (stir-baked), Tatarian Aster Root, Common Coltsfoot Flower, Snakegourd peel, Thunberg Fritillary Bulb, Rehmannia Root, Dwarf Lilyturf Tuber, Gypsum.

The content of each ingredients may have a little variety due to different dosage forms.

Indication: cough with profuse yellow thick greasy sputum, dry mouth, oppression in chest and hypochondrium.

Administration and dosage: tablet: 6 tablets per time, twice a day for oral administration; capsule: 5 capsules per time, twice a day; granule: take medicine after mixing it with boiled water, 1 pack per time, twice a day.

Strength: tablet: 0.6 g per tablet; capsule: 0.5 g per capsule; granule: 11 g per pack.

The specific strength and dosage are according to the medicine instruction.

(The information is only for learning and identification the Chinese Patent Medicine; the specific use of the Medicine please consult the herbalist or health professionals)

Jizhi Syrup (Jizhi Tangjiang)

Chinese phonetic alphabet/pin yin: jí zhī táng jiāng

Chinese characters simplified/traditional:急支糖浆/急支糖漿

Ingredients: Heartleaf Houttuynia Herb, Golden Buckwheat Rhizome, Ilex Chinese Leaf, Ephedra, Tatarian Aster Root, Hogfennel Root, Orange Fruit, Liquorice Root.

Indication: fever, chills feeling, fullness and oppression in the chest and the diaphragm, cough and sore throat, acute and chronic bronchitis.

Administration and dosage: 20-30 ml per time, three or four times a day for oral administration. 5 ml per time for children under one year old, 7 ml for between 1 and 3, 10 ml for between 3 and 7, 15 ml for above 7, 3-4 times a day.

Strength: 100 or 200 ml per vial.

The specific strength and dosage are according to the medicine instruction.

(The information is only for learning and identification the Chinese Patent Medicine; the specific use of the Medicine please consult the herbalist or health professionals)

Qiangli Pipa Concentrated Decoction (refined with honey) (Qiangli Pipa Gao (Milian))

Chinese phonetic alphabet/pin yin: qiáng lì pí pá gāo

Chinese characters simplified/traditional:强力枇杷膏/強力枇杷膏

Ingredients: Loquat Leaf, Poppy Capsule, Stemona Root, Willowleaf Swallowwort Rhizome, White Mulberry Root-bark, Platycodon Root, Menthol.

Indication: cough, phlegm and chronic cough in brochitis.

Administration and dosage: 20 g per time, three times a day for oral administration. Reduce the dose in children.

Strength: 180, 240 or 300 ml per bottle. The specific strength and dosage are according to the medicine instruction.

Precaution and warning: used with caution in diabetic.

(The information is only for learning and identification the Chinese Patent Medicine; the specific use of the Medicine please consult the herbalist or health professionals)

Chuanbei Zhike Syrup or Chuanbei Pipa Syrup (Chuanbei Zhike Lu or Chuanbei Pipa Lu)

Chinese phonetic alphabet/pin yin: chuān bèi zhǐ ké lù, chuān bèi pí pá lù

Chinese characters simplified/traditional:川贝止咳露,川贝枇杷露/川貝止咳露, 川貝枇杷露

Ingredients: Tendrilleaf Fritilary Bulb, Loquat Leaf, Stemona Root, Hogfennel Root, Platycodon Root, White Mulberry Root-bark, Menthol.

Indication: cough with sputum, shortness of breath and dry cough and throat.

Administration and dosage: 15 ml per time, three times a day for oral administration. The dosage can be lowered by half in pediatric use.

Strength: 100, 120 or 150 ml per bottle.

The specific strength and dosage are according to the medicine instruction.

(The information is only for learning and identification the Chinese Patent Medicine; the specific use of the Medicine please consult the herbalist or health professionals)

Yangyin Qingfei Concentrated Decoction (Mixture/Pilla) (Yangyin Qingfei Gao (Koufuye/Wan))

Chinese phonetic alphabet/pin yin: yǎng yīn qīng fèi gāo

Chinese characters simplified/traditional:养阴清肺膏(口服液/丸)/養陰清肺膏(口服液/丸)

Ingredients: Rehmannia Root, Dwarf Lilyturf Tuber, Figwort, Tendrilleaf Fritilary Bulb, White Peony Root, Tree Peony Bark, Peppermint, Liquorice Root.
The content of each ingredients may have a little variety due to different dosage forms.
Indication: dry and sore throat, dry cough and scanty phlegm and bloody sputum.
Administration and dosage: (for oral administration) concentrated decoction: 10-20 ml per time, two or three times a day; mixture: 10 ml per time, two or three times a day; pill: 6 g water-honeyed pill or 1 big honeyed pill per time, twice a day.
Strength: mixture: 10 ml per bottle; pill: 10 g per 100 pills for water-honeyed pills or 9 g per big honeyed pill.
The specific strength and dosage are according to the medicine instruction.
(The information is only for learning and identification the Chinese Patent Medicine; the specific use of the Medicine please consult the herbalist or health professionals)

Ermu Ningsou Pills (Ermu Ningsou Wan)
Chinese phonetic alphabet/pin yin: èr mǔ níng sòu wán
Chinese characters simplified/traditional:二母宁嗽丸/二母寧咳丸
Ingredients: Tendrilleaf Fritilary Bulb, Common Anemarrhena Rhizome, Gypsum, Cape Jasmine Fruit (stir-baked), Baical Skullcap Root, White Mulberry Root-bark (processed with honey), Indian Bread, Snakegourd Seed (stir-baked), Dried Tangerine Peel, Immature Orange Fruit (stir-baked with bran), Prepared Liquorice Root, Chinese Magnoliavine Fruit (steamed).
Indication: cough with yellow thick greasy sputum, oppression in the chest, wheezing, persistent cough, hoarse voice and sore throat.
Administration and dosage: 6 g water-honeyed pills or 1 big honey pill per time, twice a day for oral administration.
Strength: 9 g per big honeyed pill, 10 g per 100 pills for water-honeyed pill.
The specific strength and dosage are according to the medicine instruction.
(The information is only for learning and identification the Chinese Patent Medicine; the specific use of the Medicine please consult the herbalist or health professionals)

(Refined with honey) Chuanbei Pipa Syrup or Pei Pa Syrup ((Milian) Chuanbei Pipa Gao or Pei Pa Koa)
Chinese phonetic alphabet/pin yin: mì liān chuān bèi pí pá gāo
Chinese characters simplified/traditional:蜜炼川贝枇杷膏/蜜煉川貝枇杷膏
Ingredients: Tendrilleaf Fritillary Bulb, Loquat Leaf, Fourleaf Ladybell Root, Indian Bread, Pummelo Peel, Platycodon Root, Prepared Pinellia Tuber, Chinese Magnoliavine Fruit, Snakegourd Seed, Common Coltsfoot Flower, Thinleaf Milkwort Root, Bitter Apricot, Fresh Ginger, Liquorice Root, Almond Extract, Menthol, Honey, Maltose, Syrup.
Indication: cough, profuse and thick sputum, sore throat and hoarse voice.
Administration and dosage: 1 tablespoon per time, three times a day. Reduce the dosage for children according to age.
Strength: 75ml, 150 ml or 200 ml per bottle.
The specific strength and dosage are according to the medicine instruction.
Precaution and warning: use with caution in diabetics and the patients with liver or kidney disease. Avoid spicy, cold and greasy food, and avoid cigarettes.
(The information is only for learning and identification the Chinese Patent Medicine; the specific use of the Medicine please consult the herbalist or health professionals)

Xiaoqinglong Granules (Mixture) (Xiaoqinglong Keli (Mixture))

Chinese phonetic alphabet/pin yin: xiǎo qīng lóng kē lì

Chinese characters simplified/traditional:小青龙颗粒(合剂)/小青龍顆粒(合劑)

Ingredients: Ephedra, Cassia Twig, White Peony Root, Dired Ginger, Manchurian Wildginger Root, Prepared Liquorice Root, Prepared Pinellia Tuber, Chinese Magnoliavine Fruit.

The content of each ingredients may have a little variety due to different dosage forms.

Indication: chills feeling, fever, absence of sweating, wheezing, cough with watery sputum and chill (*Fenghan*) cold.

Administration and dosage: granule: take the medicine orally after mixing with hot water, 1 pack per time, three times a day; mixture: 10-20 ml per time, three times a day, shake well before oral administration.

Strength: granule: 6 g per pack (sucrose free), or 13 g per pack; mixture: 10 ml per phial, 100 ml per bottle, or 120 ml per bottle.

The specific strength and dosage are according to the medicine instruction.

Precaution and warning: long-term and over dosage administration is not advisable.

(The information is only for learning and identification the Chinese Patent Medicine; the specific use of the Medicine please consult the herbalist or health professionals)

Guilong Kechuanning Granules (Capsules) (Guilong Kechuanning Keli (Jiaonang))

Chinese phonetic alphabet/pin yin: guì lóng ké chuǎn níng kē lì

Chinese characters simplified/traditional:桂龙咳喘宁颗粒(胶囊)/桂龍咳喘寧顆粒(膠囊)

Ingredients: Cassia Twig, Skeleton Fossil, White Peony Root, Fresh Ginger, Chinese Date, Prepared Liquorice Root, Oysters Shell, Golden Thread, Prepared Pinellia Tuber, Snakegourd Peel, Bitter Apricot (stir-baked).

The content of each ingredients may have a little variety due to different dosage forms.

Indication: cough, wheezing, profuse sputum, drooling and chronic bronchitis.

Administration and dosage: granule: take the medicine orally after mixing with hot water, 1 pack per time, three times a day; capsule: 3 capsules per time, three times a day for oral administration.

Strength: 6 g granule per pack, 0.5 g per capsule (equivalent to 1.67 g of crude drug).

The specific strength and dosage are according to the medicine instruction.

Precaution and warning: avoid smoking, alcohol, pork, raw and cold food during medication

(The information is only for learning and identification the Chinese Patent Medicine; the specific use of the Medicine please consult the herbalist or health professionals)

Juanxiao Tablets (Juanxiao Pian)

Chinese phonetic alphabet/pin yin: juān xiào piàn

Chinese characters simplified/traditional:蠲哮片/蠲哮片

Ingredients: Pepperweed Seed, Dried Immaturity Tangerines Peel, Dried Tangerine Peel, Hempleaf Negundo Chastetree Fruit, Areca Seed, Rhubarb, Fresh Ginger.

Indication: asthma, rough breathing, excessive sputum, roaring wheezing, severe cough with yellow thick sputum.

Administration and dosage: 8 tablets per time, three times a day for oral administration after meals. 7 days is a treatment course.

Strength: 0.3 g per tablet.

The specific strength and dosage are according to the medicine instruction.

Precaution and warning: contraindicated during pregnancy, and patients with weak constitution, and spleen-stomach weakness and sloppy stool.

Attachment: Hempleaf Negundo Chastetree Fruit (黄荆子, Latin name: Viticis Negundo Fructus) is dried fruit of *Vitex negundo* L.

(The information is only for learning and identification the Chinese Patent Medicine; the specific use of the Medicine please consult the herbalist or health professionals)

Suzi Jiangqi Pills (Suzi Jiangqi Wan)

Chinese phonetic alphabet/pin yin: sū zǐ jiàng qì wán

Chinese characters simplified/traditional:苏子降气丸/蘇子降氣丸

Ingredients: Perilla Fruit (stir-baked), Officinal Magnolia Bark, Hogfennel Root，Liquorice Root, Prepared Pinellia Tuber (processed with Ginger and Alum), Dried Tangerine Peel, Chinese Eaglewood Wood, Chinese Angelica.

Indication: cough and wheezing, obstruction and oppression in the chest and the diaphragm.

Administration and dosage: 6 g per time, once or twice a day for oral administration.

Strength: 1 g per 13 pills.

The specific strength and dosage are according to the medicine instruction.

Precaution and warning: contraindicated in patients with *yin* deficiency and red tongue with coating.

(The information is only for learning and identification the Chinese Patent Medicine; the specific use of the Medicine please consult the herbalist or health professionals)

Qiwei Duqi Pills (Qiwei Duqi Wan)

Chinese phonetic alphabet/pin yin: qī wèi dū qì wán

Chinese characters simplified/traditional:七味都气丸/七味都氣丸

Ingredients: Chinese Magnoliavine Fruit (processed with vinegar), Asiatic Cornelian Cherry Fruit (processed), Indian Bread, Tree Peony Bark, Prepared Rehmannia Root, Common Yam Rhizome, Oriental Waterplantain Rhizome.

Indication: wheezing, panting, persistent cough, shortness of breath, dry throat, seminal emission, night sweating and frequent urination.

Administration and dosage: 9 g per time, twice a day for oral administration.

Strength: 3 g per 40 pills.

The specific strength and dosage are according to the medicine instruction.

Precaution and warning: contraindicated in patients with infection of pathogens.

(The information is only for learning and identification the Chinese Patent Medicine; the specific use of the Medicine please consult the herbalist or health professionals)

Guben Kechuan Tablet (Guben Kechuan Pian)

Chinese phonetic alphabet/pin yin: gù běn ké chuǎn piàn

Chinese characters simplified/traditional:固本咳喘片/固本咳喘片

Ingredients: Tangshen, Largehead Atractylodes Rhizome (stir-baked with bran), Indian Bread, Dwarf Lilyturf Tuber, Malaytea Scurfpea Fruit (processed with salt), Prepared Liquorice Root, Chinese Magnoliavine Fruit (processed with vinegar).

Indication: cough, excessive phlegm, chronic bronchitis, pulmonary, emphysema, and borchial asthma.

Administration and dosage: 3 tablets per time, three times a day.

Strength: 0.4 g per tablet.

The specific strength and dosage are according to the medicine instruction.

(The information is only for learning and identification the Chinese Patent Medicine; the specific use of the Medicine please consult the herbalist or health professionals)

Gejie Dingchuan Pills (Capsules) (Gejie Dingchuan Wan (Jiaonang))

Chinese phonetic alphabet/pin yin: gě jiè dìng chuǎn wán

Chinese characters simplified/traditional:蛤蚧定喘丸(胶囊)/蛤蚧定喘丸(膠囊)

Ingredients: Tokay Gecko, Snakegourd seed, Tatarian Aster Root, Ephedra, Turtle Carapace (processed with vinegar), Baical Skullcap Root, Liquorice Root, Dwarf Lilyturf Tuber, Golden Thread, Lily Bulb, Perilla Fruit (stir-baked), Gypsum, Bitter Apricot (stir-baked), Gypsum (calcined).

The content of each ingredients may have a little variety due to different dosage forms.

Indication: asthma, shortness of breath, heat vexation, fullness and oppression in the chest, spontaneous and night sweating.

Administration and dosage: (for oral administration) pill: 5-6 g water-honeyed pills, 9 g small honeyed pills, or 1 big honeyed pill per time, twice a day; capsule: 3 capsules per time, twice a day, or as advised by health professionals.

Strength: pill: 9 g per 60 pills for small honeyed pills, 9 g per big honeyed pill; capsule: 0.5 g per capsule.

The specific strength and dosage are according to the medicine instruction.

(The information is only for learning and identification the Chinese Patent Medicine; the specific use of the Medicine please consult the herbalist or health professionals)

Medicine for inducing resuscitation(开窍药)

Medicine for inducing resuscitation is a kind of medicines, their major functions are to treat coma, epilepsy, hemiplegia, apoplexy.

Angong Niuhuang Powder (Pills) (Angong Niuhuang San (Wan))

Chinese phonetic alphabet/pin yin: ān gōng niú huáng sǎn

Chinese characters simplified/traditional:安宫牛黄散(丸)/安宫牛黄散(丸)

Ingredients: Cow-bezoar, Powder of Buffalo Horn Concentratus, Artificial Musk, Pearl, Cinnabar, Realgar, Golden Thread, etc.

The content of each ingredients may have a little variety due to different dosage forms.

Indication: fever, loss of conscious, apoplexy with coma, encephalitis, meningitis, toxic encephalopathy, cerebral hemorrhage and septicemia.

Administration and dosage: (for oral administration) powder: 1.6 g per time, once a day, 0.4 g per time for children under 3 years old, 0.8 g for between 4-6, once a day or as advised by health professionals; pills: 3 g per time, once a day, 0.75 g/d for children under 3 years, 1.5 g/d for 4-6 years children, once a day; or as advised by health professionals.

Strength: 1.6 g per bottle for powder, 1.5 g or 3 g per pill.

The specific strength and dosage are according to the medicine instruction.

Precaution and warning: use with caution during pregnancy. Long-term administration is not advisable.

(The information is only for learning and identification the Chinese Patent Medicine; the specific use of the Medicine please consult the herbalist or health professionals)

Zixue Powder (Zixue San)
Chinese phonetic alphabet/pin yin: zǐ xuě sǎn
Chinese characters simplified/traditional:紫雪散/紫雪散
Ingredients: Gypsum, Calcitum, Talc, Magnetite, Figwort, Common Aucklandia Root, Chinese Eaglewood Wood, Largetrifoliolious Bugbane Rhizome, Liquorice Root, Clove, Exsiccated Sodium Sulfate, Saltpeter (refined), Powdered Buffalo Horn Extract, Antelope Horn, Artificial Musk, Cinnabar.
Indication: high fever, vexation and agitation, loss of consciousness, infantile convulsion, skin rashes, vomiting, apostaxis, reddish urine and constipation.
Administration and dosage: 1.5-3 g per time, twice a day. 0.3 g for children under 1 year old, add 0.3g/year per time for children within 5 years old, once a day; alter the dosage in children above 5 years old for oral administrating, or take it as advise of health professionals.
Strength: 1.5 g per bottle or 1.5 g per pack.
The specific strength and dosage are according to the medicine instruction.
Precaution and warning: contraindicated during pregnancy. Long-term administration is not advisable.
(The information is only for learning and identification the Chinese Patent Medicine; the specific use of the Medicine please consult the herbalist or health professionals)

Jufang Zhibao Powder (Jufang Zhibao San)
Chinese phonetic alphabet/pin yin: jú fāng zhì bǎo sǎn
Chinese characters simplified/traditional:局方至宝散/局方至寶散
Ingredients: Powdered Buffalo Horn Extract, Cow-bezoar, Hawksbill Turtle Shell, Artificial Musk, Cinnabar, Realgar, Lamber, Benzoin, Borneol.
Indication: high fever, seizure, coma, delirium and febrile convulsion.
Administration and dosage: 2 g per time, once a day. 0.5 g for children under 3 years old, 1 g for children between 4 to 6 years old per time. Take it by oral administration.
Strength: 2 g per bottle.
The specific strength and dosage are according to the medicine instruction.
Precaution and warning: long-term administration is not advisable.
Attachment: Hawksbill Turtle Shell (玳瑁, Latin namen: Eretmochelydis Carapx) is shell of *Eretmochelys imbricate*. **Attention**: to protect the rare wild animals, don't use it from wild animal.
(The information is only for learning and identification the Chinese Patent Medicine; the specific use of the Medicine please consult the herbalist or health professionals)

Niuhuang Qingxin Pills (Niuhuang Qingxin Wan)
Chinese phonetic alphabet/pin yin: niú huáng qīng xīn wán
Chinese characters simplified/traditional:牛黄清心丸/牛黄清心丸
Ingredients: Cow-bezoar, Chinese Angelica, Szechwan Lovage Rhizome, Liquorice Root, Common Yam Rhizome, Baical Skullcap, Bitter Apricot (stir-baked), Soybean Yellow Germination, Chinese Date (cored), Largehead Atractylodes Rhizome (stir-baked), Indian Bread, Platycodon Root, Divaricate Saposhnikovia Root, Chinese Thorowax Root, Donkey-Hide Glue, Dired Ginger, White Peony Root, Ginseng, Medicated Leaven (stir-baked), Cassia Bark, Dwarf Lilyturf Tuber, Japanese Ampelopsis Root, Cattail Pollen (stir-baked), Artificial Musk, Borneol, Powdered Buffalo Horn Extract, Antelope Horn, Cinnabar, Realgar.
Indication: high fever, vexation, coma and seizures in children.
Administration and dosage: 1.5 g for water-honeyed pill or 1 pill for big honeyed pill

per time, once or twice a day.

Strength: 1.5 g per 20 pills for water-honeyed pill, 3 g per big honeyed pill.

The specific strength and dosage are according to the medicine instruction.

Precaution and warning: use with caution in pregnant woman, long-term administration is not advisable.

(The information is only for learning and identification the Chinese Patent Medicine; the specific use of the Medicine please consult the herbalist or health professionals)

Wanshi Niuhuang Qingxin Pills (Wanshi Niuhuang Qingxin Wan)

Chinese phonetic alphabet/pin yin: wàn shì niú huáng qīng xīn wán

Chinese characters simplified/traditional:万氏牛黄清心丸/萬氏牛黄清心丸

Ingredients: Cow-bezoar, Cinnabar, Golden Thread, Baical Skullcap Root, Turmeric Root Tuber, Cape Jasmine Fruit.

Indication: vexation and restlessness in high fever, loss of consciousness and delirious speech, and seizures in children.

Administration and dosage: 3 g per time, two or three times a day for oral administration.

Strength: 1.5 g per small pill, 3 g per big pill.

The specific strength and dosage are according to the medicine instruction.

Precaution and warning: used with caution in pregnant woman. long-term administration is not advisable.

(The information is only for learning and identification the Chinese Patent Medicine; the specific use of the Medicine please consult the herbalist or health professionals)

Qingkailing Mixture (Granules/Capsules/Soft Capsules/Tablets/ Effervescent Tablets) (Qingkailing Koufuye (Keli/Jiaonang/ Ruanjiaonang/ Pian/ Paotengpian))

Chinese phonetic alphabet/pin yin: qīng kāi líng kǒu fú yè

Chinese characters simplified/traditional:清开灵口服液(颗粒/胶囊/软胶囊/片/泡腾片)/清開靈口服液(顆粒/膠囊/軟膠囊/片/泡騰片)

Ingredients: Cholic acid (胆酸), Nacre Powder, Hyodeoxycholic acid (猪去氧胆酸), Cape Jasmine Fruit, Buffalo Horn powder, Isatis Root, Baicalin (黄芩苷), Japanese Honeysuckle Flower.

The content of each ingredients may have a little variety due to different dosage forms.

Indication: upper respiratory tract infection, acute suppuration tonsillitis, acute pharyngitis, acute tracheitis, vexation, agitation, sore throat and high fever.

Administration and dosage: (for oral administration) mixture: 20-30 ml per time, twice a day; granule: mixing it with warm boiled water before usage, 1-2 pack per time, two or three times a day; capsule and soft capsule: 0.4 g-1 g per time, three times a day; tablet: 1-2 tablets per time, three times a day; effervescent tablet: take the medicine after effervesced it to dissolve in hot water, 2-4 tablets per time, three times a day. Reduce the dosage in children.

Strength: mixture: 10 ml per phial; granule: 1.5 g per pack (contain 20 mg baicalin, without sucrose), 3 g per pack or 10 g per pack (both of strength contain 20 mg baicalin); capsule: 0.25 g per capsule (contain 10 mg baicalin), 0.4 g per capsule (contain 20 mg baicalin); soft capsule: 0.2 g per capsule (contain 10 mg baicalin) , 0.4 g per capsule (contain 20 mg baicalin); tablet: 0.5 g per tablet (contain 20 mg baicalin); effervescent tablet: 1 g per tablet (contain 10 mg baicalin).

The specific strength and dosage are according to the medicine instruction.

Precaution and warning: use with caution when diarrhea occurs in patients with weak constitution due to long-term illness.

(The information is only for learning and identification the Chinese Patent Medicine; the specific use of the Medicine please consult the herbalist or health professionals)

Suhexiang Pills (Suhexiang Wan)

Chinese phonetic alphabet/pin yin: sū hé xiāng wán

Chinese characters simplified/traditional:苏合香丸/蘇合香丸

Ingredients: Storax, Benzoin, Borneol, Powdered Buffalo Horn Extract, Artificial Musk, Sandalwood, Chinese Eaglewood Wood, Clove, Nutgrass Galingale Rhizome, Common Aucklandia Root, Olibanum (processed), Long Pepper, Largehead Atractylodes Rhizome, Medicine Terminalia Fruit, Cinnabar.

Indication: summer-heat stroke and pain, syncope and hemiplegia in apolexy.

Administration and dosage: 1 pill per time, once or twice a day for oral administration.

Strength: 2.4 g per water-honeyed pill, 3 g per big honeyed pill.

The specific strength and dosage are according to the medicine instruction.

Precaution and warning: used with caution in pregnant woman.

(The information is only for learning and identification the Chinese Patent Medicine; the specific use of the Medicine please consult the herbalist or health professionals)

Astringent prescription(固涩药)

Astringent prescription is a kind of medicines, which are usually used to treat spermatorrhea and premature ejaculation, spontaneous and night sweating, dysentery and diarrhea, uterine bleeding and morbid leukorrhea.

Yupingfeng Capsules (Mixture/Granules/Tea Bags) (Yupingfeng Jiaonang (Koufuye/Keli/Daipaocha))

Chinese phonetic alphabet/pin yin: yù píng fēng jiāo náng

Chinese characters simplified/traditional:玉屏风胶囊(口服液/颗粒/袋泡茶)/玉屏風膠囊(口服液/顆粒/袋泡茶)

Ingredients: Milkvetch Root, Divaricate Saposhnikovia Root, Largehead Atractylodes Rhizome (processed with bran).

The content of each ingredients may have a little variety due to different dosage forms.

Indication: spontaneous and night sweating, aversion to wind, bright pale complexion and weak constitution susceptible.

Administration and dosage: (for oral administration) capsule: 2 capsules per time, three times a day; mixture: 10 ml per time, three times a day; granule: mix the medicine with hot water before usage, 1 pack per time, three times a day; tea bag: drink the herbal tea after steeping the medicine bag into boiling water for 15 minutes, 2 packs per time, two to three times a day.

Strength: capsule: 0.5 g per capsule; mixture: 10 ml per phial; granule: 5 g per pack; tea bag: 5 g per tea bag.

The specific strength and dosage are according to the medicine instruction.

(The information is only for learning and identification the Chinese Patent Medicine; the specific use of the Medicine please consult the herbalist or health professionals)

Suoquan Pills (Suoquan Wan)

Chinese phonetic alphabet/pin yin: suō quán wán

Chinese characters simplified/traditional:缩泉丸/縮泉丸

Ingredients: Common Yam Rhizome, Sharpleaf Glangal Fruit (roasted with salt), Combined Spicebush Root.

Indication: urinary frequency and enuresis during the night.

Administration and dosage: 3-6 g per time, three times a day for oral administration.

Strength: 1 g per 20 pills.

The specific strength and dosage are according to medicine instruction.

(The information is only for learning and identification the Chinese Patent Medicine; the specific use of the Medicine please consult the herbalist or health professionals)

Sishen Pills (Tablets) (Sishen Wan (Pian))

Chinese phonetic alphabet/pin yin: sì shén wán

Chinese characters simplified/traditional:四神丸(片)/四神丸(片)

Ingredients: Nutmeg (stir-baked with gentle heat), Malaytea Scurfpea Fruit (processed with salt), Chinese Magnoliavine Fruit (processed with vinegar), Medicinal Evodia Fruit (prepared), Chinese Date (kernel removed), Dried Ginger.

The content of each ingredients may have a little variety due to different dosage forms.

Indication: borborygmus, diarrhea before dawn, less food intake and undigested food in the stool, protracted diarrhea and cold limbs.

Administration and dosage: (for oral administration) pill: 9 g per time, once or twice a day; tablet: 4 tablets per time, twice a day.

Strength: tablet: uncoated tablet 0.6 g per tablets, film coated tablet 0.3 g per tablets.

The specific strength and dosage are according to the the medicine instruction.

(The information is only for learning and identification the Chinese Patent Medicine; the specific use of the Medicine please consult the herbalist or health professionals)

Guben Yichang Tablets (Guben Yichang Pian)

Chinese phonetic alphabet/pin yin: gù běn yì cháng piàn

Chinese characters simplified/traditional:固本益肠片/固本益腸片

Ingredients: Tangshen, Largehead Atractylodes Rhizome (stir-baked), Malaytea Scurfpea Fruit, Common Yam Rhizome (stir-baked with bran), Milkvetch Root, Prepared Dried Ginger, Chinese Angelica (stir-baked with wine), White Peony Root (stir-baked), Yanhusuo (processed with vinegar), Common Aucklandia Root (roasted), Carbonized Garden Burnet Root, Red Halloysite (calcined), Cutch, Prepared Liquorice Root.

Indication: dull abdominal pain, loose stool with mucus and blood, reduce food intake, coldness of the body and limbs, weakness, pale tongue and its coating, weak pulse and chronic enteritis.

Administration and dosage: 8 small or 4 large tablets per time, three times a day for oral administration.

Strength: (1) uncoated tablets, 0.32 g per small tablet, (2) uncoated tablets, 0.60 g per large tablet, (3) 0.62 g per file coated tablet (large tablet).

The specific strength and dosage are according to the medicine instruction.

Precaution and warning: avoid raw, cold, spicy and greasy food during medication. It is not indicated for dampness-heat dysentery.

(The information is only for learning and identification the Chinese Patent Medicine; the specific use of the Medicine please consult the herbalist or health professionals)

Tonifying medicine (补虚药)

Tonifying medicine is a kind of medicines, their major functions are tonic, build up a good physique and improve one's health.

Sijunzi Pills (Granules) (Sijunzi Wan (Keli))

Chinese phonetic alphabet/pin yin: sì jūn zǐ wán

Chinese characters simplified/traditional:四君子丸(颗粒)/四君子丸(顆粒)

Ingredients: Tangshen, Largehead Atractylodes Rhizome (stir-baked with bran), Indian Bread, Prepared Liquorice Root.

The content of each ingredients may have a little variety due to different dosage forms.

Indication: poor appetite, less food intake and loose stool.

Administration and dosage: (for oral administration) pill: 3-6 g per time, three times a day; granule: 1 pack per time, three times a day.

Strength: 15 g per pack for granule.

The specific strength and dosage are according to the medicine instruction.

(The information is only for learning and identification the Chinese Patent Medicine; the specific use of the Medicine please consult the herbalist or health professionals)

Buzhong Yiqi Pills (Granules/Mixture) (Buzhong Yiqi Wan (Keli/Heji))

Chinese phonetic alphabet/pin yin: bǔ zhōng yì qì wán

Chinese characters simplified/traditional:补中益气丸(颗粒/合剂)/補中益氣丸(顆粒/合劑)

Ingredients: Prepared Milkvetch Root, Tangshen, Prepared Liquorice Root, Largehead Atractylodes Rhizome (stir-baked), Chinese Angelica, Largetrifoliolious Bugbane Rhizome, Chinese Thorowax Root, Dried Tangerine Peel.

The content of each ingredients may have a little variety due to different dosage forms.

Indication: diarrhea, prolapse of the rectum and uterus, fatigue, lack of strength, poor appetite and abdominal distension.

Administration and dosage: (for oral administration) pill: 9 g small honeyed pills or 1 big honeyed pill per time, twice or three times a day, 6 g for watered pill per time, twice or three times a day; granule: 3 g per time, twice or three times a day; mixture: 10-15 ml per time, three times a day.

Strength: 3 g per pack for granule.

The specific strength and dosage are according to the medicine instruction.

(The information is only for learning and identification the Chinese Patent Medicine; the specific use of the Medicine please consult the herbalist or health professionals)

Shenling Baizhu Powder (Pills) (Shenling Baizhu San (Wan))

Chinese phonetic alphabet/pin yin: shēn líng bái zhù sǎn

Chinese characters simplified/traditional:参苓白术散(丸)/参苓白尤散(丸)

Ingredients: Ginseng, Indian Bread, Largehead Atractylodes Rhizome (stir-baked), Common Yam Rhizome, White Hyacinth Bean (stir-baked), Lotus Seed, Coix Seed (stir-baked), Villous Amomum Fruit, Platycodon Root, Liquorice Root.

The content of each ingredients may have a little variety due to different dosage forms.

Indication: poor appetite, sloppy stool, shortness of breath, cough, fatigue and lack of strength.

Administration and dosage: (for oral administration) powder: 6-9 g per time, two or three times a day; pill: 6 g per time, three times a day.
Strength: pill: 6 g per 100 pills.
The specific strength and dosage are according to the medicine instruction.
(The information is only for learning and identification the Chinese Patent Medicine; the specific use of the Medicine please consult the herbalist or health professionals)

Liujunzi Pills (Liujunzi Wan)
Chinese phonetic alphabet/pin yin: liù jūn zǐ wán
Chinese characters simplified/traditional:六君子丸/六君子丸
Ingredients: Tangshen, Largehead Atractylodes Rhizome (stir-baked with bran), Indian Bread, Prepared Pinellia Tube (processed with Ginger and Alum), Dried Tangerine Peel, Prepared Liquorice Root.
Indication: less food intake, excessive phlegm, abdominal distention and sloppy stool.
Administration and dosage: 9 g per time, twice a day for oral administration.
Strength: 9 g per pack.
The specific strength and dosage are according to the medicine instruction.
(The information is only for learning and identification the Chinese Patent Medicine; the specific use of the Medicine please consult the herbalist or health professionals)

Xiangsha Liujun Pills (Xiangsha Liujun Wan)
Chinese phonetic alphabet/pin yin: xiāng shā liū jūn wán
Chinese characters simplified/traditional:香砂六君丸/香砂六君丸
Ingredients: Common Aucklandia Root, Villous Amomum Fruit, Tangshen, Largehead Atractylodes Rhizome (stir-baked), Indian Bread, Prepared Liquorice Root, Dried Tangerine Peel, Pinellia Tuber (processed with Ginger).
Indication: indigestion, less food intake with belching, sloppy stool, tightness and fullness in the epigastrium and abdomen.
Administration and dosage: 6-9 g per time, twice or three times a day for oral administration.
The specific strength and dosage are according to the medicine instruction.
(The information is only for learning and identification the Chinese Patent Medicine; the specific use of the Medicine please consult the herbalist or health professionals)

Qipi Pills (Mixture) (Qipi Wan (Koufuye))
Chinese phonetic alphabet/pin yin: qǐ pí wán
Chinese characters simplified/traditional:启脾丸(口服液)/啟脾丸(口服液)
Ingredients: Ginseng, Largehead Atractylodes Rhizome (processed with bran), Indian Bread, Liquorice Root, Dried Tangerine Peel, Common Yam Rhizome, Lotus Seed (stir-baked), Hawthorn Fruit (stir-baked), Medicated Leaven, Germinated Barly (stir-baked), Oriental Waterplantain Rhizome.
The content of each ingredients may have a little variety due to different dosage forms.
Indication: indigestion, sloppy stool, abdominal distension and fullness.
Administration and dosage: (for oral administration) pill: 3 g (15 small honeyed pills) or 1 big honeyed pill per time, two or three times a day; mixture: 10 ml pill per time, two or three times a day. Reduce the dosage in children under three years old.
Strength: pill: 3 g per big honeyed pill or 20 g per 100 small honeyed pills; mixture: 10, 100 or 120 ml per bottle.
The specific strength and dosage are according to the medicine instruction.

Precaution and warning: avoid raw, cold and greasy food.
(The information is only for learning and identification the Chinese Patent Medicine; the specific use of the Medicine please consult the herbalist or health professionals)

Yougui Pills (Yougui Wan)

Chinese phonetic alphabet/pin yin: yòu guī wán
Chinese characters simplified/traditional:右归丸/右歸丸
Ingredients: Prepared Rehmannia Root, Prepared Common Monkshood Daughter Root (baked with sand), Cassia Bark, Common Yam Rhizome, Asiatic Cornelian Cherry Fruit (processed with wine), Dodder Seed, Deerhorn Glue, Barbary Wolfberry Fruit, Chinese Angelica, Eucommia Bark (processed with salt).
Indication: soreness and weakness in waist and knee, lassitude, fear of cold, impotence, seminal emission, loose stool and frequent urination.
Administration and dosage: 9 g small honeyed pills or 1 big honeyed pill per time, three times a day for oral administration.
Strength: 1.8 g per ten small honeyed pill, or 9 g per big honeyed pill.
The specific strength and dosage are according to the medicine instruction.
(The information is only for learning and identification the Chinese Patent Medicine; the specific use of the Medicine please consult the herbalist or health professionals)

Wuzi Yanzong Pills (Tablets) (Wuzi Yanzong Wan (Pian))

Chinese phonetic alphabet/pin yin: wǔ zǐ yǎn zhōng wán
Chinese characters simplified/traditional:五子衍宗丸(片)/五子衍宗丸(片)
Ingredients: Barbary Wolfberry Fruit, Dodder Seed (stir-baked), Palmleaf Raspberry Fruit, Chinese Magnoliavine Fruit (steam), Plantain Seed (stir-baked with salt).
The content of each ingredients may have a little variety due to different dosage forms.
Indication: impotence, infertility, seminal emission, premature ejaculation and endless of urination.
Administration and dosage: (for oral administration) pill: 6 g water-honeyed pills, 9 g small honeyed pills, or 1 big honeyed pill per time, twice or three times a day; tablet: 6 tablet per time, three times a day.
Strength: 9 g per big honeyed pill; core weight 0.3 g per sugar-coated tablet.
The specific strength and dosage are according to the medicine instruction.
(The information is only for learning and identification the Chinese Patent Medicine; the specific use of the Medicine please consult the herbalist or health professionals)

Jisheng Shenqi Pills (Jisheng Shenqi Wan)

Chinese phonetic alphabet/pin yin: jì shēng shèn qì wán
Chinese characters simplified/traditional:济生肾气丸/濟生腎氣丸
Ingredients: Prepared Rehmannia Root, Asiatic Cornelian Cherry Fruit, Tree Peony Bark, Common Yam Rhizome, Indian Bread, Oriental Waterplantain Rhizome, Cassia Bark, Prepared Common Monkshood Daugher Root, Twotoothed Achyranthes Root, Plantain Seed.
Indication: difficulty in micturition, soreness and heaviness in waist and knees.
Administration and dosage: 6 g water-honeyed pills, 9 g small honeyed pills, or 1 big honeyed pill per time, twice or three times a day for oral administration.
Strength: 9 g per big honeyed pill.
The specific strength and dosage are according to the medicine instruction.
(The information is only for learning and identification the Chinese Patent Medicine;

the specific use of the Medicine please consult the herbalist or health professionals)

Qing'e Pills (Qing'e Wan)
Chinese phonetic alphabet/pin yin: qīng é wán
Chinese characters simplified/traditional:青娥丸/青娥丸
Ingredients: Eucommia Bark (stir-baked with salt), Malaytea Scurfpea Fruit (stir-baked), Walnut Seed (stir-baked), Garlic Bulb.
Indication: difficulty in movement and weakness in knees.
Administration and dosage: 6-9 g water-honeyed pills or 1 big honeyed pill per time, twice or three times a day for oral administration.
Strength: 9 g per big honeyed pill.
The specific strength and dosage are according to the medicine instruction.
(The information is only for learning and identification the Chinese Patent Medicine; the specific use of the Medicine please consult the herbalist or health professionals)

Danggui Buxue Mixture (Danggui Buxue Koufuye)
Chinese phonetic alphabet/pin yin: dāng guī bǔ xuě kǒu fú yè
Chinese characters simplified/traditional:当归补血口服液/當歸補血口服液
Ingredients: Chinese Angelica, Milkvetch Root.
Indication: easy to fatigue, night sweating, dizziness, palpitation, pale or sallow complexion.
Administration and dosage: 10 ml per time, twice a day for oral administration.
Strength: 10 ml per phial.
The specific strength and dosage are according to the medicine instruction.
(The information is only for learning and identification the Chinese Patent Medicine; the specific use of the Medicine please consult the herbalist or health professionals)

Siwu Mixture (Granules) (Siwu Heji (Keli))
Chinese phonetic alphabet/pin yin: sì wù hé jì
Chinese characters simplified/traditional:四物合剂(颗粒)/四物合劑(顆粒)
Ingredients: Chinese Angelica, Szechwan Lovage Rhizome, White Peony Root, Prepared Rehmannia Root.
The content of each ingredients may have a little variety due to different dosage forms.
Indication: sallow complexion, dizziness, palpitation, shortness of breath and menstrual disorders.
Administration and dosage: (for oral administration) mixture: 10-15 ml per time, three times a day; granule: mixing it with warm boiled water before usage, 5 g per time, three times a day.
Strength: mixture: 10 ml per phial, 100 ml per bottle; granule: 5 g per pack.
The specific strength and dosage are according to the medicine instruction.
(The information is only for learning and identification the Chinese Patent Medicine; the specific use of the Medicine please consult the herbalist or health professionals)

Liuwei Dihuang Pills (Concentrated Pills/Capsules/Soft Capsules/Granules) (Liuwei Dihuang Wan (Nongsuo Wan/Jiaonang/ Ruanjiaonang/Keli))
Chinese phonetic alphabet/pin yin: liù wèi dì huáng wán
Chinese characters simplified/traditional:六味地黄丸(浓缩丸/胶囊/软胶囊/颗粒)/六味地黄丸(濃縮丸/膠囊/軟膠囊/顆粒)

Ingredients: Prepared Rehmannia Root, Asiatic Cornelian Cherry Fruit (processed with wine), Tree Peony Bark, Common Yam Rhizome, Indian Bread, Oriental Waterplantain Rhizome.

The content of each ingredients may have a little variety due to different dosage forms.

Indication: dizziness, tinnitus, soreness and weakness in waist and knees, tidal fever, night sweating, seminal emission and wasting thirst.

Administration and dosage: (for oral administration) pill: 5 g water-honeyed pill or 9 g small honeyed pill, or 1 big honeyed pill per time, twice a day; concentrated pill: 8 pills per time, three times a day; capsule: 0.5-0.6 g per time, twice a day; soft capsule: 3 capsules per time, twice a day; granule: mixing it with hot water before usage, 1 pack per time, twice a day

Strength: pill: 9 g per big honeyed pill, 5 g per pack for watered pill; concentrated pill: 1.44 g per 8 pills (equivalent to 2.1 g of prepared slices), capsule: 0.3 g or 0.5 g per capsule; soft capsule: 0.38 g per capsule; granule: 5 g per pack.

The specific strength and dosage are according to the medicine instruction.

(The information is only for learning and identification the Chinese Patent Medicine; the specific use of the Medicine please consult the herbalist or health professionals)

Zuogui Pills (Zuogui Wan)

Chinese phonetic alphabet/pin yin: zuǒ guī wán

Chinese characters simplified/traditional:左归丸/左歸丸

Ingredients: Prepared Rehmannia Root, Dodder Seed, Twotoothed Achyranthes Root, Glue of Tortoise Shell, Deerhorn Glue, Common Yam Rhizome, Asiatic Cornelian Cherry Fruit, Barbary Wolfberry Fruit.

Indication: soreness and weakness in waist and knee, fatigue and night sweating.

Administration and dosage: 9 g per time, twice a day for oral administration.

Strength: 1 g per ten pills.

The specific strength and dosage are according to the medicine instruction.

Precaution and warning: contraindicated in children, use with caution during pregnancy.

(The information is only for learning and identification the Chinese Patent Medicine; the specific use of the Medicine please consult the herbalist or health professionals)

Dabuyin Pills (Dabuyin Wan)

Chinese phonetic alphabet/pin yin: dà bǔ yīn wán

Chinese characters simplified/traditional:大补阴丸/大補陰丸

Ingredients: Prepared Rehmannia Root, Common Anemarrhena Rhizome (stir-baked with salt), Chinese Cork-tree (stir-baked with salt), Tortoise Carapace and Plastron (stir-baked with vinegar), Pig Spinal Cord.

Indication: tidal fever, spontaneous and night sweating, cough, hemoptysis, tinnitus and seminal emission.

Administration and dosage: 6 g water-honeyed pill per time or 1 big honey pill per time, twice or three times a day for oral administration.

Strength: 9 g per big honeyed pill.

The specific strength and dosage are according to the medicine instruction.

(The information is only for learning and identification the Chinese Patent Medicine; the specific use of the Medicine please consult the herbalist or health professionals)

Yuquan Capsules (Granules) (Yuquan Jiaonang (Keli))

Chinese phonetic alphabet/pin yin: yù quán jiāo náng

Chinese characters simplified/traditional:玉泉胶囊(颗粒)/玉泉膠囊(顆粒)

Ingredients: Snakegourd Root, Kudzuvine Root, Dwarf Lilyturf Tuber, Ginseng, Indian Bread, Smoked Plum, Milkvetch Root, Liquorice Root, Rehmannia Root, Chinese Magnoliavine Fruit.

The content of each ingredients may have a little variety due to different dosage forms.

Indication: thirst, increased water intake and diabetes.

Administration and dosage: capsule: 5 capsules per time, four times a day for oral administration; granules: take the medicine orally after mixing it with hot water, one pack per time, four times a day.

Strength: capsule: 0.5 g per capsule; granule: 5 g per pack.

The specific strength and dosage are according to the medicine instruction.

Precaution and warning: contraindicated during pregnancy.

(The information is only for learning and identification the Chinese Patent Medicine; the specific use of the Medicine please consult the herbalist or health professionals)

Bazhen Granules (Pills) (Bazhen Keli (Wan))

Chinese phonetic alphabet/pin yin: bā zhēn kē lì

Chinese characters simplified/traditional:八珍颗粒(丸)/八珍顆粒(丸)

Ingredients: Tangshen, Largehead Atractylodes Rhizome (stir-baked), Indian Bread, Prepared Liquorice Root, Chinese Angelica, White Peony Root (stir-baked), Szechwan Lovage Rhizome, Prepared Rehmannia Root.

The content of each ingredients may have a little variety due to different dosage forms.

Indication: sallow complexion, poor appetite, weakness of limbs and heavy menstruation.

Administration and dosage: granules: take the medicine orally after mixing it with hot water, one pack per time, twice a day; pills: 6 g water-honeyed pill or 1 big honey pill per time, twice a day.

Strength: 8 g per pack or 3.5 g per pack (without sugar), 9 g per big honeyed pill.

The specific strength and dosage are according to the medicine instruction.

(The information is only for learning and identification the Chinese Patent Medicine; the specific use of the Medicine please consult the herbalist or health professionals)

Guipi Pills (Concentrated Pill/Granules/Mixture) (Guipi Wan (Nongsuo Wan/ Keli/ Heji))

Chinese phonetic alphabet/pin yin: guī pí wán

Chinese characters simplified/traditional:归脾丸(浓缩丸/颗粒/合剂)/歸脾丸(濃縮丸/ 顆粒/合劑)

Ingredients: Tangshen, Largehead Atractylodes Rhizome (processed with bran), Prepared Milkvetch Root, Prepared Liquorice Root, Indian Bread, Thinleaf Milkwort Root (processed), Spine Date Seed (stir-baked), Longan Aril, Chinese Angelica, Common Aucklandia Root, Chinese Date (kernel removed).

The content of each ingredients may have a little variety due to different dosage forms.

Indication: shortness of breath, palpitation, insomnia, dizziness, fatigue, menstrual flooding and spotting.

Administration and dosage: pill: take the medicine orally with ginger tea or warm boiled water. 6 g water-honeyed pills, 9 g small honeyed pills, or 1 big honeyed pill per time, three times a day; concentrated pill: 8-10 pills per time, three times a day; granule: take the medicine orally after mixing it with hot water, 1 pack per time, three times a day; mixture: 10 ml per time, three times a day for oral administration. Shake fully prior to use.

Strength: pill: 9 g per big honeyed pill; concentrated pill: 8 pills correspond to 3 g slice; granule: 3 g per pack; mixture: 10 ml, 100 ml or 120 ml per phial.

The specific strength and dosage are according to the medicine instruction.

(The information is only for learning and identification the Chinese Patent Medicine; the specific use of the Medicine please consult the herbalist or health professionals)

Renshen Yangrong Pills (Renshen Yangrong Wan)

Chinese phonetic alphabet/pin yin: rén shēn yǎng róng wán

Chinese characters simplified/traditional:人参养荣丸/人參養榮丸

Ingredients: Ginseng, Largehead Atractylodes Rhizome (stir with terra), Indian Bread, Prepared Liquorice Root, Chinese Angelica, Prepared Rehmannia Root, White Peony Root (stir-baked with bran), Prepared Milkvetch Root, Dried Tangerine Peel, Thinleaf Milkwort Root (processed), Cassia Bark, Chinese Magnoliavine Fruit (steamed with wine).

Indication: emaciation, nerve weakness, poor appetite, sloppy stool, and weakness after disease.

Administration and dosage: 6 water-honeyed pills or 1 big honeyed pill per time, one or two times a day.

Strength: 9 g per big honeyed pill.

The specific strength and dosage are according to the medicine instruction.

(The information is only for learning and identification the Chinese Patent Medicine; the specific use of the Medicine please consult the herbalist or health professionals)

Shiquan Dabu Pills (Shiquan Dabu Wan)

Chinese phonetic alphabet/pin yin: shí quán bà bǔ wán

Chinese characters simplified/traditional:十全大补丸/十全大補丸

Ingredients: Tangshen, Largehead Atractylodes Rhizome (stir-baked), Indian Bread, Prepared Liquorice Root, Chinese Angelica, Szechwan Lovage Rhizome, White Peony Root (stir-baked with wine), Prepared Rehmannia Root, Prepared Milkvetch Root, Cassia Bark.

Indication: pale complexion, shortness of breath, palpitation, dizziness, night sweating, fatigue, lack of strength, cold limbs and menorrhagia.

Administration and dosage: 6 g water-honeyed pills, 9 g small honeyed pills per time or 1 big honeyed pill per time, two or three times a day.

Strength: 20 g per 100 small honeyed pills, 9 g per big honeyed pill.

The specific strength and dosage are according to the medicine instruction.

(The information is only for learning and identification the Chinese Patent Medicine; the specific use of the Medicine please consult the herbalist or health professionals)

Jianpi Shengxue Granules (Tablets) (Jianpi Shengxue Keli (Pian))

Chinese phonetic alphabet/pin yin: jiàn pí shēng xuě kē lì

Chinese characters simplified/traditional:健脾生血颗粒(片)/健脾生血顆粒(片)

Ingredients: Tangshen, Indian Bread, Largehead Atractylodes Rhizome (stir-baked with bran), Liquorice Root, Milkvetch Root, Common Yam Rhizome, Chicken's Gizzard-sink (stir-baked), Tortoise Carapace and Plastron (processed with vinegar), Liriope Root Tuber, Southern Magnoliavine Fruit (processed with vinegar), Skeleton

Fossil, Oysters Shell (calcined), Chinese Date, Ferrous sulfate ($FeSO_4 \cdot 7H_2O$).
The content of each ingredients may have a little variety due to different dosage forms.

Indication: iron-deficiencey anemia (IDA), reduce or torpid food intake, abdominal complexion, epigastric, bowel movement disorder, vexation, fatigue and lack of strength.

Administration and dosage: granule: take the medicine orally after mixing it with hot water, 15 g for adult, 2.5 g for children under 1 year old, 5 g for between 1 and 3, 7.5 g for between 3 and 5, 10 g for between 5 and 12, per time, three times a day; tablet: 3 tablets for adult, 0.5 tablets for children under 1 year old, 1 tablets for between 1 and 3, 1.5 tablets for between 3 and 5, 2 tablets for between 5 and 12, per time, three times a day, four weeks is one treatment course.

Strength: granule: 5 g per pack; tablet: 0.6 g per tablet.

The specific strength and dosage are according to the medicine instruction.

Precaution and warning: avoid drinking tea. Concomitant drug containing acidum tannicum should be avoided. Teeth color may turn dark in children, which will disappear gradually when the medication is discontinued. Poor appetite, nausea, vomiting, and light diarrhea might occur during medication, it will mostly disappear spontaneously.

(The information is only for learning and identification the Chinese Patent Medicine; the specific use of the Medicine please consult the herbalist or health professionals)

Shengmai Oral Liquid (Capsules) (Shengmai Yin (Jiaonang))
Chinese phonetic alphabet/pin yin: shēng mài yǐn
Chinese characters simplified/traditional:生脉饮(胶囊)/生脈飲(膠囊)
Ingredients: Red Ginseng, Dwarf Lilyturf Tuber, Chinese Magnoliavine Fruit.
The content of each ingredients may have a little variety due to different dosage forms.

Indication: palpitations, shortness of breath, weak pulse and night sweating.

Administration and dosage: (for oral administration) oral liquid: 10 ml per time, three times a day; capsule: 3 capsules per time, three times a day.

Strength: oral liquid: 10 ml per phial; capsule: 0.3 or 0.35 g per capsule.

The specific strength and dosage are according to the medicine instruction.

(The information is only for learning and identification the Chinese Patent Medicine; the specific use of the Medicine please consult the herbalist or health professionals)

Xiaoke Pills (Xiaoke Wan)
Chinese phonetic alphabet/pin yin: xiǎo kě wán
Chinese characters simplified/traditional:消渴丸/消渴丸
Ingredients: Kudzuvine Root, Rehmannia Root, Milkvetch Root, Snakegourd Root, Corn Silk, Southern Magnoliavine Fruit, Common Yam Rhizome, Glibenclamide.
Indication: increase of food, water intake and urination combine with weight loss, fatigue, lack of strength, and type II diabetes.

Administration and dosage: 5-10 pills per time, two or three times a day. Take the medicine with warm boiled water before meals or as advised by health professionals.

Strength: 2.5 g per 10 pills (containing 2.5 mg of glibenclamide).

The specific strength and dosage are according to medicine instruction.

Precaution and warning: this medicine contains glibenclamide. Please strictly follow the instruction of this medicine as prescription drug. Monitoring serum glucose level is recommended.

(The information is only for learning and identification the Chinese Patent Medicine; the specific use of the Medicine please consult the herbalist or health professionals)

Guilu Erxian Concentrated Decoction (Guilu Erxian Gao)
Chinese phonetic alphabet/pin yin: guī lù èr xiān gāo
Chinese characters simplified/traditional:龟鹿二仙膏/龜鹿二仙膏
Ingredients: Tortoise Carapace and Plastron, Pilose Antler, Tangshen, Barbary Wolfberry.
Indication: soreness and weakness in waist and knees, seminal emission, impotence.
Administration and dosage: 15-20 g per time, three times a day.
Strength: 200 g per bottle.
The specific strength and dosage are according to the medicine instruction.
Precaution and warning: use with caution in patients with dyspepsia.
(The information is only for learning and identification the Chinese Patent Medicine; the specific use of the Medicine please consult the herbalist or health professionals)

Qibao Meiran Granules (Qibao Meiran Keli)
Chinese phonetic alphabet/pin yin: qī bǎo měi rán kē lì
Chinese characters simplified/traditional:七宝美髯颗粒/七寶美髯顆粒
Ingredients: Prepared Fleeceflower Root, Chinese Angelica, Malaytea Scurfpea Fruit (stir-baked with Black Sesame), Chinese Wolfberry Fruit (steamed with wine), Dodder Seed (stir-baked), Indian Bread, Twotoothed Achyranthes Root (steamed with wine).
Indication: premature hair graying, seminal emission, premature ejaculation, dizziness, tinnitus, waist and back pain.
Administration and dosage: take the medicine orally after mixing it with hot water, 1 pack per time, twice a day.
Strength: 8 g per pack.
The specific strength and dosage are according to the medicine instruction.
(The information is only for learning and identification the Chinese Patent Medicine; the specific use of the Medicine please consult the herbalist or health professionals)

Tranquilizer(安神药)
Tranquilizer is a kind of medicines, their major functions are to tranquilize and treat epilepsy, convulsion.

Tianwang Buxin Pills (Tianwang Buxin Wan)
Chinese phonetic alphabet/pin yin: tiān wáng bǔ xīn wán
Chinese characters simplified/traditional:天王补心丸/天王補心丸
Ingredients: Danshen Root, Chinese Angelica, Grassleaf Sweetflag Rhizome, Tangshen, Indian Bread, Chinese Magnoliavine Fruit, Dwarf Lilyturf Tuber, Cochinchinese Asparagus Root, Rehmannia Root, Figwort, Thinleaf Milkwort Root (processed), Spine Date Seed (stir-baked), Chinese Arbovitae Kernel, Platycodon Root, Liquorice Root, Cinnabar.
Indication: palpitations, insomnia, constipation and forgetfulness.
Administration and dosage: 8 pills concentrated pill, 6 g water-honeyed pill, 9 g small honeyed pill, or 1 big honeyed pill per time, twice a day.
Strength: 8 pills equivalent to 3 g of prepared slice for concentrated pill, 9 g per big honeyed pill.
The specific strength and dosage are according to the medicine instruction.

Precaution and warning: long-term administration is not advisable.
(The information is only for learning and identification the Chinese Patent Medicine; the specific use of the Medicine please consult the herbalist or health professionals)

Baizi Yangxin Pills (Tablets) (Baizi Yangxin Wan (Pian))
Chinese phonetic alphabet/pin yin: bǎi zǐ yǎng xīn wán
Chinese characters simplified/traditional:柏子养心丸(片)/柏子養心丸(片)
Ingredients: Chinese Arbovitae Kernel, Tangshen, prepared Milkvetch Root, Szechwan Lovage Rhizome, Chinese Angelica, Indian Bread, Processing Thinleaf Milkwort Root, Spine Date Seed, Cassia Bark, Chinese Magnoliavine Fruit (processed with vinegar), Pinellia Rhizome Fermented Mass, Prepared Liquorice Root, Cinnabar.
The content of each ingredients may have a little variety due to different dosage forms.
Indication: palpitations, insomnia, and forgetfulness.
Administration and dosage: (for oral administration) tablets: 3-4 pills per time, twice a day; pills: 6 g water-honeyed pills, or 9 g small honeyed pills, or 1 big honeyed pill per time, twice a day.
Strength: 0.3 g for suger coated tablet core; 9 g per big honeyed pill.
The specific strength and dosage are according to the medicine instruction.
Precaution and warning: long-term administration is not advisable.
Attachment: Pinellia Rhizome Fermented Mass (半夏曲, Latin name: Medicated Pinellia Tuber Leaven) is the fermented product which contains Pinellia Tuber powder, Prepared Pinellia Tuber powder, Ginger juice and Wheat.
(The information is only for learning and identification the Chinese Patent Medicine; the specific use of the Medicine please consult the herbalist or health professionals)

Zaoren Anshen Capsules (Granules) (Zaoren Anshen Jiaonang (Keli))
Chinese phonetic alphabet/pin yin: zǎo rén ān shén jiāo náng
Chinese characters simplified/traditional:枣仁安神胶囊(颗粒)/棗仁安神膠囊(顆粒)
Ingredients: Spine Date Seed (stir-baked), Danshen Root, Chinese Magnoliavine Fruit (processes with vinegar).
The content of each ingredients may have a little variety due to different dosage forms.
Indication: insomnia, vexation, forgetfulness, dizziness and nerve weakness.
Administration and dosage: capsule: 5 capsules per time, once a day before sleep; granule: take the medicine orally after mixing it with hot water. 1 pack per time, once a day before sleep.
Strength: capsule: 0.45 g per capsule; granule: 5 g per pack.
The specific strength and dosage are according to medicine instruction.
Precaution and warning: use with caution during pregnancy.
(The information is only for learning and identification the Chinese Patent Medicine; the specific use of the Medicine please consult the herbalist or health professionals)

Jieyu Anshen Granules (Jieyu Anshen Keli)
Chinese phonetic alphabet/pin yin: jiě yū ān shén kē lì
Chinese characters simplified/traditional:解郁安神颗粒/解郁安神顆粒
Ingredients: Chinese Thorowax Root, Chinese Date, Grassleaf Sweetflag Rhizome, Prepared Pinellia Tuber (processed with Ginger and Alum), Largehead Atractylodes Rhizome (stir-baked), Wizened Wheat, Thinleaf Milkwort Root (processed), Prepared

Liquorice Root, Cape Jasmine Fruit (stir-baked), Lily Bulb, Bile Arisaema, Turmeric Root Tuber, Teeth Fossil, Spine Date Seed (stir-baked), Indian Bread, Chinese Angelica.

Indication: insomnia, vexation, forgetfulness, neurosis and menopausal syndrome.

Administration and dosage: take the medicine orally after mixing it with hot water. 1 pack per time, twice a day.

Strength: 5 g per pack, 2 g per pack (without sucrose).

The specific strength and dosage are according to the medicine instruction.

Attachment: Teeth Fossil (龙齿, Latin name: Draconis Dens) is the teeth fossil of ancient animal. **Attention:** It is illegal for some kinds of skeleton fossil's trade and destroying, use it abide by the law.

(The information is only for learning and identification the Chinese Patent Medicine; the specific use of the Medicine please consult the herbalist or health professionals)

Reconciliation agent(和解剂)

Reconciliation agent is a kind of medicines, which are usually used to treat tide cold and heat, bitter tasted in mouth, nausea, anorexia and distending pain in hypochondrium caused by disorder of visceral organs.

Xiaochaihu Granules (Capsules/Tablets/Effervescent Tablets) (Xiaochaihu Keli (Jiaonang/Pian/Paotengpian))

Chinese phonetic alphabet/pin yin: xiǎo chái hú kē lì

Chinese characters simplified/traditional:小柴胡颗粒(胶囊/片/泡腾片)/小柴胡顆粒(膠囊/片/泡騰片)

Ingredients: Chinese Thorowax Root, Baical Skullcap Root, Prepared Pinellia Tuber (processed with ginger and Alum), Tangshen, Fresh Ginger, Liquorice Root, Chinese Date.

The content of each ingredients may have a little variety due to different dosage forms.

Indication: chills feeling and fever, fullness in chest and hypochondrium, poor appetite, vexation, vomiting, bitter taste in the mouth and dry throat.

Administration and dosage: (for oral administration) granule: 1-2 packs per time, three times a day; capsule: 4 capsules per time, three times a day; tablet: 4-6 tablets per time, three times a day; effervescent tablet: mixing medicine with hot water before usage, 1-2 tablets per time, three times a day.

Strength: granule: 10 g per pack, 4 g per pack (without sucrose), 2.5 g per pack (without sucrose); capsule: 0.4 g per capsule; tablet: 0.4 g per tablet; effervescent tablet: 2.5 g per tablet.

The specific strength and dosage are according to the medicine instruction.

Precaution and warning: not suitable for patients with wind-cold exterior pattern.

(The information is only for learning and identification the Chinese Patent Medicine; the specific use of the Medicine please consult the herbalist or health professionals)

Xiaoyao Pills (Tablets/Capsules/Granules) (Xiaoyao Wan (Pian/Jiaonang/Keli))

Chinese phonetic alphabet/pin yin: xiāo yáo wán

Chinese characters simplified/traditional:逍遥丸(片/胶囊/颗粒)/逍遙丸(片/膠囊/顆粒)

Ingredients: Chinese Thorowax Root, Chinese Angelica, White Peony Root, Largehead Atractylodes Rhizome (stir-baked), Indian Bread, Prepared Liquorice Root,

Peppermint.

The content of each ingredients may have a little variety due to different dosage forms.

Indication: distending pain in chest and hypochondrium, dizziness, poor appetite and menstrual irregulation.

Administration and dosage: (for oral administration) pill: 6-9 g watered pill, 8 pills concentrated pill, 9 g small honeyed pill, or 1 big honeyed pill per time, twice a day; tablet: 4 tablets per time, twice a day; capsule: 1.7-2.0 g per time, twice a day; granule: mixing the medicine with water before usage, 1 pack per time, twice a day.

Strength: pill: 8 pills equal to 3 g of crude drug for concentrated pill, 20 g per 100 pills for small honeyed pill, 9 g per pill for big honeyed pill; tablet: 0.35 g per tablet; capsule: 0.4 or 0.34 g per capsule; granule: 4 g, 5 g, 6 g or 15 g per pack.

The specific strength and dosage are according to the medicine instruction.

(The information is only for learning and identification the Chinese Patent Medicine; the specific use of the Medicine please consult the herbalist or health professionals)

Formula for regulating *QI*(理气药)

Formula for regulating *QI* is a kind of medicines, their major functions are to treat distention and fullness, some of them can treat colic or hernia, amenorrhea and dysmenorrhea, vomit, acid regurgitation.

Sini Powder (Sini San)

Chinese phonetic alphabet/pin yin: sì nì sǎng

Chinese characters simplified/traditional:四逆散/四逆散

Ingredients: Chinese Thorowax Root, White Peony Root, Orange Fruit (stir-baked with bran), Liquorice Root.

Indication: stomach and epigastria distention and pain, limbs cold, diarrhea and dysentery.

Administration and dosage: 9 g per time, twice a day mixing in boiled water for oral taking.

Strength: 9 g per pack.

The specific strength and dosage are according to the medicine instruction.

Precaution and warning: use with caution during pregnancy.

(The information is only for learning and identification the Chinese Patent Medicine; the specific use of the Medicine please consult the herbalist or health professionals)

Zuojin Pills (Capsules) (Zuojin Wan (Jiaonang))

Chinese phonetic alphabet/pin yin: zuǒ jīn wán

Chinese characters simplified/traditional:左金丸(胶囊)/左金丸(膠囊)

Ingredients: Golden Thread, Medicinal Evodia Fruit.

The content of each ingredients may have a little variety due to different dosage forms.

Indication: epigastria and hypochondriac pain, bitter taste in mouth, gastric upset, vomiting, acid reflux and aversion to hot drinks.

Administration and dosage: (for oral administration) pill: 3-6 g per time, twice a day, capsule: 2-4 g per time, twice a day. Take the medicine after meals. For 15 days as one treatment course.

Strength: capsule: 0.35 g per capsule.

The specific strength and dosage are according to the medicine instruction.

(The information is only for learning and identification the Chinese Patent Medicine;

the specific use of the Medicine please consult the herbalist or health professionals)

Shugan Pills (Shugan Wan)
Chinese phonetic alphabet/pin yin: shū gān wán
Chinese characters simplified/traditional:舒肝丸/舒肝丸
Ingredients: Szechwan Chinaberry Fruit, Yanhusuo (processed with vinegar), White Peony Root (stir-baked with wine), Wenyujin Concise Rhizome, Common Aucklandia Root, Chinese Eaglewood Wood, Round Cardamon Fruit, Villous Amomum Fruit, Officinal Magnolia Bark (processed with ginger), Dried Tangerine Peel, Orange Fruit (stir-baked), Indian Bread, Cinnabar.
Indication: distention and fullness in chest and hypochondrium, epigastric pain, gastric upset and vomiting, belching and acid reflux.
Administration and dosage: 4 g water-honeyed pill, 6 g small honeyed or 1 big honey pill per time, two or three times a day for oral administration.
Strength: 20 g per 100 pills for wather-honeyed pills, 20 g per 100 pills for small honeyed pills, 6 g per pill for big honeyed pills, 2.3 g per 20 pills for watered pill.
The specific strength and dosage are according to the medicine instruction.
Precaution and warning: use with caution during pregnancy. Long-term usage of the medicine is not advisable.
(The information is only for learning and identification the Chinese Patent Medicine; the specific use of the Medicine please consult the herbalist or health professionals)

Chaihu Shugan Pills (Chaihu Shuan Wan)
Chinese phonetic alphabet/pin yin: chái hú shū gān wán
Chinese characters simplified/traditional:柴胡舒肝丸/柴胡舒肝丸
Ingredients: Indian Bread, Orange Fruit (stir-baked), Round Cardamon Fruit, White Peony Root (stir-baked with wine), Liquorice Root, Nutgrass Galingale Rhizome (processed with vinegar), Dried Tangerine Peel, Platycodon Root, Officinal Magnolia Bark (processed with vinegar), Hawthorn Fruit (stir-baked), Divaricate Saposhnikovia Root, Medicated Leaven (stir-baked), Chinese Thorowax Root, Baical Skullcap Root, Peppermint, Perilla stem, Common Aucklandia Root, Areca Seed (stir-baked), Common Burreed Tuber (processed with vinegar), Rhubarb (stir-baked with the wine), Dried Immaturity Tangerines Peel (stir-baked), Chinese Angelica, Pinellia Tuber (processed with ginger), Combined Spicebush Root, Zedoray Rhizome (processed with vinegar).
Indication: distention and oppression in the chest and hypochondrium, food retention and vomiting.
Administration and dosage: 10 g small honeyed pill per time or 1 big honey pill per time, twice ar day for oral administration.
Strength: 20 g per 100 pills for small honeyed pills, 10 g per pill for big honeyed pills.
The specific strength and dosage are according to the medicine instruction.
(The information is only for learning and identification the Chinese Patent Medicine; the specific use of the Medicine please consult the herbalist or health professionals)

Qizhi Weitong Granules (Tablets) (Qizhi Weitong Keli (Pian))
Chinese phonetic alphabet/pin yin: qì zhì wèi tòng kē lì
Chinese characters simplified/traditional:气滞胃痛颗粒(片)/氣滯胃痛顆粒(片)
Ingredients: Chinese Thorowax Root, Yanhusuo (baking), Orange Fruit, Nutgrass Galingale Rhizome (processed with vinegar), White Peony Root, Prepared Liquorice Root.

The content of each ingredients may have a little variety due to different dosage forms.

Indication: stuffiness and fullness in the chest with epigstric pain.

Administration and dosage: (for oral administration) granule: mixing it with hot water before usage, 1 pack per time, three times a day; tablet: 3 tablets for thin film-coated one or 6 tablets for sugar-coated one per time, three times a day.

Strength: granule: 5 g per pack; tablet: 0.5 g per tablet for thin file-coated tablet, 0.25 g of the core for sugar-coated tablet.

The specific strength and dosage are according to the medicine instruction.

Precaution and warning: use with caution in pregnant woman.

(The information is only for learning and identification the Chinese Patent Medicine; the specific use of the Medicine please consult the herbalist or health professionals)

Weisu Granules (Weisu Keli)

Chinese phonetic alphabet/pin yin: wèi sū kē lì

Chinese characters simplified/traditional:胃苏颗粒/胃蘇顆粒

Ingredients: Perilla Stem, Nutgrass Galingale Rhizome, Dried Tangerine Peel, Citron Fruit, Finger Citron, Orange Fruit, Areca Seed, Chicken's Gizzard-sink (stir-baked).

Indication: distension pain in the epigstric and hypochondrium, less food intake, constipation and chronic gastritis.

Administration and dosage: mixing it with hot water before usage, 1 pack per time, three times a day for oral administration. One treatment course last for 15 days, 1-3 courses can be offered.

Strength: 15 g per pack, 5 g per pack (without sucrose).

The specific strength and dosage are according to the medicine instruction.

(The information is only for learning and identification the Chinese Patent Medicine; the specific use of the Medicine please consult the herbalist or health professionals)

Muxiang Shunqi Pills (Muxiang Shunqi Wan)

Chinese phonetic alphabet/pin yin: mù xiāng shùn qì wán

Chinese characters simplified/traditional:木香顺气丸/木香順氣丸

Ingredients: Common Aucklandia Root, Villous Amomum Fruit, Nutgrass Galingale Rhizome (processed with vinegar), Areca Seed, Liquorice Root, Dried Tangerine Peel, Officinal Magnolia Bark, Orange Fruit (stir-baked with bran), Atractylodes Rhizome (stir-baked with bran), Dried Immaturity Tangerines Peel (stir-baked with vinegar), Fresh Ginger.

Indication: fullness and oppression in the chest and diaphragm, distending pain in epigastrium and abdomen, vomiting and nausea, belching and loss appetite.

Administration and dosage: 6-9 g per time, twice or three times a day for oral administration.

Strength: 6 g per 100 pills.

The specific strength and dosage are according to the medicine instruction.

Precaution and warning: use with caution in pregnant woman.

(The information is only for learning and identification the Chinese Patent Medicine; the specific use of the Medicine please consult the herbalist or health professionals)

Yueju Pills (Yueju Wan)

Chinese phonetic alphabet/pin yin: yuè jú wán

Chinese characters simplified/traditional:越鞠丸/越鞠丸

Ingredients: Nutgrass Galingale Rhizome (processed with vinegar), Szechwan Lovage

Rhizome, Cape Jasmine Fruit (stir-baked), Atractylodes Rhizome (stir-baked), Medicated Leaven (stir-baked).

Indication: distention and oppression in the chest and diaphragm, abdominal fullness, food retention, belching and acid regurgitation.

Administration and dosage: 6-9 g per time, twice times a day for oral administration. The specific strength and dosage are according to the medicine instruction.

(The information is only for learning and identification the Chinese Patent Medicine; the specific use of the Medicine please consult the herbalist or health professionals)

Hemorheologic medicine(活血药)

Hemorheologic medicine is a kind of medicines, their major functions are to stimulate the circulation of blood and disperse blood stasis, they usually treat cardio-thoraco-algia, sequelae of apoplexy and short of breath.

Fufang Danshen Tablets (Pills/Dripping Pills/ Granules/ Capsules/ Spray/ Aerosol) (Fufang Danshen Pian (Wan/ Diwan/ Keli/ Jiaonang/ Penwuji/ Qiwuji))

Chinese phonetic alphabet/pin yin: fù fāng dān shēn piàn

Chinese characters simplified/traditional:复方丹参片(丸/滴丸/颗粒/胶囊/喷雾剂/气雾剂)/複方丹參片(丸/滴丸/顆粒/膠囊/噴霧劑/氣霧劑)

Ingredients: Danshen Root, Sanchi, Borneol.

The content of each ingredients may have a little variety due to different dosage forms.

Indication: oppression in the chest, stabbing pain in the precordium and heart, angina pectoris in coronary heart disease.

Administration and dosage:(for oral administration) tablet: 3 tablets [tablet strength (1) and (3)], or 1 tablet [tablet strength (2)] per time, three times a day; pill: 1 g per time for [pill strength (1)] or 0.7 g per time for [pill strength (2)], three times a day; dripping pill: for oral or sublingual administration, 10 pills per time, three times a day for 28 days as one treatment course; granules: 1 pack per time, three times a day; capsule: 3 capsules per time, three times a day; spray and aerosol: oral spray and inhalation, 1 to 2 sprays per time, three times a day.

Strength: tablet: (1) 0.32 g per file coated small tablet (equivalent to 0.6 g of prepared slices), (2) 0.8 g per file coated big tablet (equivalent to 1.8 g of prepared slices), (3) suger coated tablet (equivalent to 0.6 g of prepared slices); pill: (1) 1 g of pills is equivalent to 1.8 g of crude drug, (2) 1 g of pills is equivalent to 2.57 g of crude drug; dripping pill: 25 mg per dripping pill or 27 mg per film coated dripping pill; granule: 1 g per pack; capsule: 0.3 g per capsule; spray and aerosol: 8 or 10 ml per phial.

The specific strength and dosage are according to the medicine instruction.

Precaution and warning: use with caution during pregnancy.

(The information is only for learning and identification the Chinese Patent Medicine; the specific use of the Medicine please consult the herbalist or health professionals)

Danqi Tablets (Danqi Pian)

Chinese phonetic alphabet/pin yin: dān qī piàn

Chinese characters simplified/traditional:丹七片/丹七片

Ingredients: Danshen Root, Sanchi.

Indication: heart pain, dizziness, oppression in the chest, headache and abdominal pain during menstruation.

Administration and dosage: 3 to 5 pills per time, three times a day for oral administration.

Strength: uncoated tablets, 0.3 g per tablet; 0.32 g per film coated tablet; 0.3 g per core (sugar-coated) tablet.

The specific strength and dosage are according to the medicine instruction.

Precaution and warning: use with caution during pregnancy.

(The information is only for learning and identification the Chinese Patent Medicine; the specific use of the Medicine please consult the herbalist or health professionals)

Xiaoshuan Tongluo Capsules (Tablets/Granules) (Xiaoshuan Tongluo Jiaonang (Pian/Keli))

Chinese phonetic alphabet/pin yin: xiāo shuān tōng luò jiāo náng

Chinese characters simplified/traditional:消栓通络胶囊(片/颗粒)/消栓通絡膠囊(片/顆粒)

Ingredients: Szechwan Lovage Rhizome, Danshen Root, Milkvetch Root, Oriental Waterplantain Rhizome, Sanchi, Pagoda Tree Flower, Cassia Twig, Turmeric Root Tuber, Common Aucklandia Root, Borneol, Hawthorn Fruit.

The content of each ingredients may have a little variety due to different dosage forms.

Indication: sluggish and stony expression, cold limbs, aching limbs, ischemic stroke and hyperlipidaemia.

Administration and dosage: (for oral administration) capsule: 6 capsules per time, three times a day; tablet: 6 tablets per time, three times a day; granule: 1 pack per time, three times a day.

Strength: capsule: 0.37 g per capsule; tablet: 0.38 g per tablet; 6 g per pack (without sucrose), 12 g per pack.

The specific strength and dosage are according to the medicine instruction.

Precaution and warning: use with caution in pregnant woman. Avoid raw, cold, spicy and greasy food.

(The information is only for learning and identification the Chinese Patent Medicine; the specific use of the Medicine please consult the herbalist or health professionals)

Xuefu Zhuyu Pills (Mixture/Capsules) (Xuefu Zhuyu Wan (Koufuye/ Jiaonang))

Chinese phonetic alphabet/pin yin: xuě fǔ zhú yū wán

Chinese characters simplified/traditional:血府逐瘀丸(口服液/胶囊)/血府逐瘀丸(口服液/膠囊)

Ingredients: Chinese Thorowax Root, Chinese Angelica, Rehmannia Root, Red Peony Root, Safflower, Peach Seed, Orange Fruit (stir-baked with bran), Liquorice Root, Szechwan Lovage Rhizome, Twotoothed Achyranthes Root, Platycodon Root.

The content of each ingredients may have a little variety due to different dosage forms.

Indication: protracted stinging localized headache, vexation, agitation, palpitations and insomnia.

Administration and dosage: (for oral administration) pill: take the medicine with brown sugar water on an empty stomach, 1-2 pills per time, twice a day; mixture: take the medicine on an empty stomach, 20 ml per time, three times a day; capsule: 6 capsule per time, twice a day. For one month a one treatment course.

Strength: pill: 9 g per pill; mixture: 10 ml per phial; capsule: 0.4 g per capsule.

The specific strength and dosage are according to the medicine instruction.

Precaution and warning: contraindicated during pregnancy. Avoid pungent and cold food.

(The information is only for learning and identification the Chinese Patent Medicine;

the specific use of the Medicine please consult the herbalist or health professionals)

Yuanhu Zhitong Tablets (Capsules/Soft Capsules/Dripping Pills/Granules/ Mixture) (Yuanhu Zhitong Pian (Jiaonang/Ruanjiaonang/Diwan/Keli/Koufuye))
Chinese phonetic alphabet/pin yin: yuán hú zhǐ tòng piàn
Chinese characters simplified/traditional:元胡止痛片(胶囊/软胶囊/滴丸/颗粒/口服液)/元胡止痛片(膠囊/軟膠囊/滴丸/顆粒/口服液)
Ingredients: Yanhusuo (processed with vinegar), Dahurian Angelica Root.
The content of each ingredients may have a little variety due to different dosage forms.
Indication: stomachache, hypochondriac pain, headache, and dysmenorrhea.
Administration and dosage: (for oral administration) tablet: 4-6 tablets per time, three times a day; capsule: 4-6 capsules (for 0.25 g per capsule) or 2-3 capsules (for 0.45 g per capsule) per time, three times a day; soft capsule: 2 capsules per time, three times a day; dripping pill: 20-30 pills per time, three times a day; granule: mixing the medicine with hot water before usage, 1 pack per time, three times a day; mixture: 10 ml per time, three times a day. Or take the medicine as advised of health professionals.
Strength: tablet: 0.26 g per film-coated tablet, 0.31 g per film-coated tablet, 0.25 g per core for sugar coated tablet, or 0.3 g per core for sugar coated tablet; capsule: 0.25 g or 0.45 g per capsule; soft capsule: 0.5 g per capsule; dripping pill: 0.5 g per 10 pills; granule: 5 g per pack; mixture: 10 ml per phial.
The specific strength and dosage are according to the medicine instruction.
(The information is only for learning and identification the Chinese Patent Medicine; the specific use of the Medicine please consult the herbalist or health professionals)

Suxiao Jiuxin Pills (Suxiao Jiuxin Wan)
Chinese phonetic alphabet/pin yin: sù xiào jiù xīn wán
Chinese characters simplified/traditional:速效救心丸/速效救心丸
Ingredients: Szechwan Lovage Rhizome, Borneol.
Indication: angina pectorisin coronary heart disease.
Administration and dosage: for sublingual administration, 4-6 pills per time, three times a day; a single dose of 10-15 pills can be offered during acute attack.
Strength: 40 mg per pill.
The specific strength and dosage are according to the medicine instruction.
Precaution and warning: contraindicated during pregnancy. Avoid using alone in patients with chest *bi* disorder and heart pain due to congealing cold, blood stasis and *yin* deficiency. Use with caution in patients with prior allergy. Use with caution in myocardial ischemia with moderate to severe heart failure. During medication, if attacks of angina pectoris become frequent during medication, nitrates (such as glyceryl trinitrate) should be added.
(The information is only for learning and identification the Chinese Patent Medicine; the specific use of the Medicine please consult the herbalist or health professionals)

Guanxin Suhe Pills (Capsules) (Guanxin Suhe Wan (Jiaonang))
Chinese phonetic alphabet/pin yin: guàn xīn sū hé wán
Chinese characters simplified/traditional:冠心苏合丸(胶囊)/冠心蘇合丸(膠囊)
Ingredients: Storax, Borneol, Olibanum (processed), Sandalwood, Inula Root.
The content of each ingredients may have a little variety due to different dosage forms.

Indication: oppression in the chest, precordial pain, angina pectoris in coronary heart disease.

Administration and dosage: pill: take the medicine orally after chewing it into smaller pieces, 1 pill per time, one to three times a day; capsule: 2 capsules per time, three times a day for oral administration. Reduce the dosage in children, or as advised by health professionals.

Strength: 0.35 g per capsule.

The specific strength and dosage are according to the medicine instruction.

Precaution and warning: use with caution in pregnant woman.

(The information is only for learning and identification the Chinese Patent Medicine; the specific use of the Medicine please consult the herbalist or health professionals)

Xinkeshu Tablets (Xinkeshu Pian)

Chinese phonetic alphabet/pin yin: xīn kě shū piàn

Chinese characters simplified/traditional:心可舒片/心可舒片

Ingredients: Danshen Root, Kudzuvine Root, Sanchi, Hawthorn Fruit, Common Aucklandia Root.

Indication: oppression in the chest, palpitation, dizziness, headache, pain in the neck, angina pectoris in coronary heart disease, hyperlipidemia, hypertension and arrhythmia.

Administration and dosage: 4 small tablets or 2 big tablets per time, three times a day for oral administration.

Strength: 0.31 or 0.62 g per tablet.

The specific strength and dosage are according to medicine instruction.

Precaution and warning: use with caution in pregnant woman.

(The information is only for learning and identification the Chinese Patent Medicine; the specific use of the Medicine please consult the herbalist or health professionals)

Jiuqi Niantong Pills (Jiuqi Niantong Wan)

Chinese phonetic alphabet/pin yin: jiǔ qì niān tòng wán

Chinese characters simplified/traditional:九气拈痛丸/九氣拈痛丸

Ingredients: Nutgrass Galingale Rhizome (processed with vinegar), Common Aucklandia Root, Lesser Galangal Rhizome, Dried Tangerine Peel, Turmeric Root Tuber, Zedoray Rhizome (processed with vinegar), Yanhusuo (processed with vinegar), Areca Seed, Liquorice Root, Flying Squirrel's Faeces (stir-baked with vinegar).

Indication: dysmenorrheal, heart pain, distension and fullness in the chest and abdomen.

Administration and dosage: 6-9 g per time, twice a day.

The specific strength and dosage are according to the medicine instruction.

Precaution and warning: use with caution during pregnancy.

(The information is only for learning and identification the Chinese Patent Medicine; the specific use of the Medicine please consult the herbalist or health professionals)

Shexiang Baoxin Pills (Shexiang Baoxin Wan)

Chinese phonetic alphabet/pin yin: shè xiāng bǎo xīn wán

Chinese characters simplified/traditional:麝香保心丸/麝香保心丸

Ingredients: Artificial Musk, Artificial Cow-bezoan, Storax, Toad Venom, Borneol, etc.

Indication: pain in precardium, angina pectoris and myocardial infarction due to myocardial ischemia.

Administration and dosage: 1-2 pills per time, three times a day for oral administration. Or take the medicine at the presence of symptoms.

Strength: 22.5 mg per pill.

The specific strength and dosage are according to the medicine instruction.

Precaution and warning: contraindicated in pregnant woman.

(The information is only for learning and identification the Chinese Patent Medicine; the specific use of the Medicine please consult the herbalist or health professionals)

Xiaoshuan Granules (Mixture) (Xiaoshuan Keli (Koufuye))

Chinese phonetic alphabet/pin yin: xiāo shuān kē lì

Chinese characters simplified/traditional:消栓颗粒(口服液)/消栓顆粒(口服液)

Ingredients: Milkvetch Root, Chinese Angelica, Red Peony Root, Earthworm, Safflower, Szechwan Lovage Rhizome, Peach Seed.

The content of each ingredients may have a little variety due to different dosage forms.

Indication: hemiplegia, deviated tongue and mouth, pale complexion, weakness, shortness of breath and ischemic stroke.

Administration and dosage: granule: take the medicine after mixing it with hot water, 1 pack per time, three times a day; mixture: 10 ml per time, three times a day.

Strength: granule: 4 g per pack; mixture: 10 ml per bottle.

The specific strength and dosage are according to the medicine instruction.

Precaution and warning: contraindicated during pregnancy. Contraindicated in patients with *yin* deficiency and *yang* hyperactivity, wind-fire harassing upwards, and phlegm turbidity clouding the mind.

(The information is only for learning and identification the Chinese Patent Medicine; the specific use of the Medicine please consult the herbalist or health professionals)

Tongxinluo Capsules (Tongxinluo Jiaonang)

Chinese phonetic alphabet/pin yin: tōng xīn luò jiāo náng

Chinese characters simplified/traditional:通心络胶囊/通心絡膠囊

Ingredients: Ginseng, Leech, Scorpion, Red Peony Root, Cicada Slough, Ground Beetle, Centipede, Sandalwood, Rosewood, Olibanum (processed), Spine Date Seed (stir-baked), Borneol.

Indication: angina pectoris of coronary heart and apoplexy, hemiplegia and hemianethesia.

Administration and dosage: 2-4 pills per time, three times a day for oral administration.

Strength: 0.26 g per capsule.

The specific strength and dosage are according to the medicine instruction.

Precaution and warning: contraindicated during pregnancy or menstruation, patients with hemorrhagic ulcer or apoplexy due to *yin* deficiency.

(The information is only for learning and identification the Chinese Patent Medicine; the specific use of the Medicine please consult the herbalist or health professionals)

Wenxin Granules (Tablets) (Wenxin Keli (Pian))

Chinese phonetic alphabet/pin yin: wěn xīn kē lì

Chinese characters simplified/traditional:稳心颗粒(片)/穩心顆粒(片)

Ingredients: Tangshen, Solomonseal Rhizome, Sanchi, Lamber, Nardostachys Root.

The content of each ingredients may have a little variety due to different dosage forms.

Indication: palpitation, shortness of breath, oppression and pain in the chest or heart, Premature Ventricular Contraction (PVC) or atrial premature beat.

Administration and dosage: (for oral administration) granule: mixing the medicine with hot water before usage, 1 pack per time, three times a day; tablet: 4 pills per time, three times a day. Or as advised by health professionals.

Strength: granule: 9 g per pack, 5 g per pack (without sucrose); tablet: 0.5 g per tablet. The specific strength and dosage are according to the medicine instruction.

Precaution and warning: use with caution during pregnancy, contraindicated in patients with arrhythmia.

(The information is only for learning and identification the Chinese Patent Medicine; the specific use of the Medicine please consult the herbalist or health professionals)

Yixinshu Pills (Tablets/Capsules/Granules) (Yixinshu Wan (Pian/Jiaonang/Keli))

Chinese phonetic alphabet/pin yin: yì xīn shū wán

Chinese characters simplified/traditional:益心舒丸(片/胶囊/颗粒)/益心舒丸(片/膠囊/顆粒)

Ingredients: Ginseng, Dwarf Lilyturf Tuber, Milkvetch Root, Chinese Magnoliavine Fruit, Danshen Root, Szechwan Lovage Rhizome, Hawthorn Fruit.

The content of each ingredients may have a little variety due to different dosage forms.

Indication: pain and oppression in chest, palpitation, shortness of breath, intermittent pulses and angina pectoris in coronary heart disease.

Administration and dosage: (for oral administration) pill: 1 pack per time, three times a day; tablet: 2 tablets per time, three times a day; capsule: 3 capsules per time, three times a day.

Strength: granule: 9 g per pack, 5 g per pack (without sucrose); tablet: 0.5 g per tablet. The specific strength and dosage are according to the medicine instruction.

(The information is only for learning and identification the Chinese Patent Medicine; the specific use of the Medicine please consult the herbalist or health professionals)

Styptic(止血药)

Styptic is a kind of medicines, their major functions are to treat trauma hemorrhage and nontraumatic bleeding.

Huaijiao Pills (Huaijiao Wan)

Chinese phonetic alphabet/pin yin: huái jiǎo wán

Chinese characters simplified/traditional:槐角丸/槐角丸

Ingredients: Japanese Pagodatree Pod (simple stir-baking), Garden Burnet Root (carbonized), Baical Skullcap Root, Orange Fruit (stir-frying with bran), Chinese Angelica, Divaricate Saposhnikovia Root.

Indication: bloody stool, swollen and painful hemorrhoid.

Administration and dosage: (for oral administration) 6 g water-honeyed pill, 9 g small honeyed pills, or 1 big honeyed pill per time, twice a day.

Strength: 9 g per big honeyed pill.

The specific strength and dosage are according to the medicine instruction.

(The information is only for learning and identification the Chinese Patent Medicine; the specific use of the Medicine please consult the herbalist or health professionals)

Sanqi Tablets (Sanqi Pian)

Chinese phonetic alphabet/pin yin: sān qī piàn

Chinese characters simplified/traditional:三七片/三七片

Ingredients: Sanchi.

Indication: hemoptysis, hemtemesis, epitaxis, hematochezia, menstrual flooding and spotting, traumatic bleeding and injuries.

Administration and dosage: 4-12 small pills, or 2-6 big pills per time, three times a day for oral administration.

Strength: 0.25 g of crude drug per small tablet, 0.5 g of crude drug per big tablet.

The specific strength and dosage are according to the medicine instruction.

Precaution and warning: contraindicated during pregnancy.

(The information is only for learning and identification the Chinese Patent Medicine; the specific use of the Medicine please consult the herbalist or health professionals)

Zhixue Dingtong Tablets (Zhixue Dingtong Pian)

Chinese phonetic alphabet/pin yin: zhǐ xuě dìng tòng piàn

Chinese characters simplified/traditional:止血定痛片/止血定痛片

Ingredients: Sanchi, Ophicalcite (calcined), Cuttlebone, Liquorice Root.

Indication: pain in duodenal ulcer, gastric hyperacidity, and hemorrhage.

Administration and dosage: 6 tablets per time, three times a day for oral administration.

Strength: 0.43 g per small tablet.

The specific strength and dosage are according to the medicine instruction.

(The information is only for learning and identification the Chinese Patent Medicine; the specific use of the Medicine please consult the herbalist or health professionals)

Prescriptions for resolving food stagnancy(消导剂)

Prescriptions for resolving food stagnancy is a kind of medicines which are usually used to treat stagnation of food, indigestion and bowel movement disorder.

Baohe Pills (Granules/Tablets) (Baohe Wan (Keli/Pian))

Chinese phonetic alphabet/pin yin: bǎo hé wán

Chinese characters simplified/traditional:保和丸(颗粒/片)/保和丸(顆粒/片)

Ingredients: Hawthorn Fruit (charred), Medicated Leaven (stir-baked), Pinellia Tuber (processed), Indian Bread, Dried Tangerine Peel, Weeping Forsythia Capsule, Radish Seed (stir-baked), Germinated Barly (stir-baked).

The content of each ingredients may have a little variety due to different dosage forms.

Indication: food retention, distension and fullness in epigastrium and abdomen, fetid belching, acid regurgitation and no desire for food and drink.

Administration and dosage: (for oral administration) pill: 9-18 g small honeyed pill per time or 1-2 big honeyed pills per time, twice a day; watered pill: 6-9 g per time, twice a day; granules: take the medicine orally after mixing it with hot water, 4.5 g per time, twice a day; tablet: 4 tablets per time, three times a day. Reduce the dosage in children.

Strength: pill: 20 g per 100 pills of small honeyed, 9 g per big honeyed pill; granule: 4.5 g per pack; tablet: film coated tablets 0.4 g per tablet.

The specific strength and dosage are according to the medicine instruction.

(The information is only for learning and identification the Chinese Patent Medicine; the specific use of the Medicine please consult the herbalist or health professionals)

Zhishi Daozhi Pills (Zhishi Daozhi Wan)
Chinese phonetic alphabet/pin yin: zhì shí dǎo zhì wán
Chinese characters simplified/traditional:枳实导滞丸/枳實導滯丸
Ingredients: Immature Orange Fruit (stir-bake), Rhubarb, Golden Thread (stir-baked with ginger juice), Baical Skullcap Root, Medicated Leaven (stir-baked), Largehead Atractylodes Rhizome (stir-baked), Indian Bread, Oriental Waterplantain Rhizome.
Indication: distending pain in the epigastrium and abdomen, poor appetite, constipation, dysentery with tenesmus and indigestion.
Administration and dosage: 6-9 g per time, twice a day for oral administration.
The specific strength and dosage are according to the medicine instruction.
(The information is only for learning and identification the Chinese Patent Medicine; the specific use of the Medicine please consult the herbalist or health professionals)

Liuwei Anxiao Powder (Liuwei Anxiao San)
Chinese phonetic alphabet/pin yin: liù wèi ān xiāo sǎn
Chinese characters simplified/traditional:六味安消散/六味安消散
Ingredients: Inula Root, Rhubarb, Galanga Resurrectionlily Rhizome, Calcitum (calcined), Medicine Terminalia Fruit, Trona.
Indication: indigestion, constipation and dysmenorrheal.
Administration and dosage: 1.5-3 g per time, two or three times a day for oral administration.
Strength: 1.5 g, 3 g, 18 g per pack.
The specific strength and dosage are according to the medicine instruction.
Precaution and warning: contraindicated during pregnancy.
(The information is only for learning and identification the Chinese Patent Medicine; the specific use of the Medicine please consult the herbalist or health professionals)

Kaiwei Jianpi Pills (Kaiwei Jianpi Wan)
Chinese phonetic alphabet/pin yin: kāi wèi jiān pí wán
Chinese characters simplified/traditional:开胃健脾丸/開胃健脾丸
Ingredients: Largehead Atractylodes Rhizome, Tangshen, Indian Bread, Common Aucklandia Root, Golden Thread, Medicated Leaven (stir-baked), Dried Tangerine Peel, Villous Amomum Fruit, Germinated Barly (stir-baked), Hawthorn Fruit, Common Yam Rhizome, Nutmeg (stir-baked with gentle heat), Prepared Liquorice Root.
Indication: indigestion, belching and acid regurgitation, diarrhea and dyspepsia.
Administration and dosage: 6-9 g per time, twice a day.
Strength: 1 g per 10 pills.
The specific strength and dosage are according to the medicine instruction.
(The information is only for learning and identification the Chinese Patent Medicine; the specific use of the Medicine please consult the herbalist or health professionals)

Medicine for the treatment of *Wind*(治风药)
Medicine for the treatment of *Wind* is a kind of medicines, which are usually used to treat aversion to wind, headache, dizziness, hypertension, stroke, hemiplegia.

Chuanxiong Chatiao Powder (Pills/Granules/Tablets/Tea Bag) (Chuanxiong Chatiao San (Wan/Keli/Pian/Daipaocha))
Chinese phonetic alphabet/pin yin: chuān xiōng chá tiáo sǎn

Chinese characters simplified/traditional:川芎茶调散(丸/颗粒/片/袋泡茶)/川芎茶調散(丸/顆粒/片/袋泡茶)

Ingredients: Szechwan Lovage Rhizome, Dahurian Angelica Root, Incised Notopterygium Rhizome and Root, Manchurian Wildginger Root, Divaricate Saposhnikovia Root, Fineleaf Schizonepeta Herb, Peppermint, Liquorice Root.

The content of each ingredients may have a little variety due to different dosage forms.

Indication: headache, chills feeling, fever and stuffy nose.

Administration and dosage: powder and pill: take the medicine orally after mixing it with light tea. 3-6 g per time, twice a day; concentrated pill: take the medicine orally after mixing it with light tea, 8 pills per time, three times a day; granule: take the medicine after mixing it with warm water or light tea, 1 pack per time, twice a day; tablet: take the medicine orally after mixing it with light tea, 4 to 6 pills per time, three times a day; tea bag: take the medicine orally after soaking it in hot water 20-40 min, 2 packs per time, twice to three times a day.

Strength: concentrated pill: 8 pills equivalent to 3 g of prepared slice; granule: 7.8 g per pack, 4 g per pack (without sucrose); tea bag: 1.6 g per pack.

The specific strength and dosage are according to the medicine instruction.

Precaution and warning: use with caution during pregnancy.

(The information is only for learning and identification the Chinese Patent Medicine; the specific use of the Medicine please consult the herbalist or health professionals)

Xiongju Shangqing Pills (Tablets) (Xiongju Shangqing Wan (Pian))

Chinese phonetic alphabet/pin yin: xiōng jú shàng qīng wán

Chinese characters simplified/traditional:芎菊上清丸(片)/芎菊上清丸(片)

Ingredients: Szechwan Lovage Rhizome, Chrysanthemum Flower, Baical Skullcap Root, Cape Jasmine Fruit, Shrub Chastetree Fruit (stir-baked), Golden Thread, Peppermint, Weeping Forsythia Capsule, Fineleaf Schizonepeta Spike, Incised Notopterygium Rhizome and Root, Chinese Lovage, Platycodon Root, Divaricate Saposhnikovia Root, Liquorice Root, Dahurian Angelica Root.

The content of each ingredients may have a little variety due to different dosage forms.

Indication: chills feeling, fever, migraine, general headache, runny nose, toothache and sore throat.

Administration and dosage: (for oral administration) pill: 6 g watered pills or 1 big honeyed pill per time, twice a day; tablet: 4 tablets per time, twice a day.

Strength: pill: 9 g per big honeyed pill; tablet: 0.25 g or 0.3 g per core of sugar coated tablet.

The specific strength and dosage are according to the medicine instruction.

Precaution and warning: use with caution in patients of weak constitution.

(The information is only for learning and identification the Chinese Patent Medicine; the specific use of the Medicine please consult the herbalist or health professionals)

Zhengtian Pills (Capsules) (Zhengtian Wan (Jiaonang))

Chinese phonetic alphabet/pin yin: zhèng tiān wán

Chinese characters simplified/traditional:正天丸(胶囊)/正天丸(膠囊)

Ingredients: Gambir Plant, White Peony Root, Szechwan Lovage Rhizome, Chinese Angelica, Rehmannia Root, Dahurian Angelica Root, Divaricate Saposhnikovia Root, Incised Notopterygium Rhizome and Root, Peach Seed, Safflower, Manchurian Wildginger Root, Doubleteeth Pubescent Angelica Root, Ephedra, Common

Monkshood Daughter Root (heifupian), Suberect Spatholobus Stem.
The content of each ingredients may have a little variety due to different dosage forms.

Indication: migraine, tension headache, neuropathic headache, cervical spondylosis, headache and premenstrual headache.

Administration and dosage: pill: 6 g per time, two or three times a day; capsule: 2 capsules per time, three times a day. Take the medicine orally after meal. One treatment course lasts for fifteen days.

Strength: pill: 60 g per bottle or 6 g per pack; capsule: 0.45 g per pack.

The specific strength and dosage are according to the medicine instruction.

Precaution and warning: blood pressure should be monitored during medication; use with caution during pregnancy; it is suggested to take the medicine after meals; in patients with heart disease, heart rhythm should be monitored.

(The information is only for learning and identification the Chinese Patent Medicine; the specific use of the Medicine please consult the herbalist or health professionals)

Tianma Gouteng Granules (Tianma Gouteng Keli)

Chinese phonetic alphabet/pin yin: tiān má gōu téng kē lì

Chinese characters simplified/traditional:天麻钩藤颗粒/天麻鈎藤顆粒

Ingredients: Tall Gastrodia Tuber, Gambir Plant, Abalone Shell, Cape Jasmine Fruit, Baical Skullcap Root, Twotoothed Achyranthes Root, Eucommia Bark (stir-baked with salt), Motherwort Herb, Chinese Taxillus Herb, Tuber Fleeceflower Stem, Indian Bread.

Indication: headache, dizziness, tinnitus, blurred vision, tremor, insomnia and hypertension.

Administration and dosage: take the medicine orally after mixing it with hot water, 1 pack per time, three times a day.

Strength: 5 g per pack (without sucrose), 10 g per pack.

The specific strength and dosage are according to the medicine instruction.

(The information is only for learning and identification the Chinese Patent Medicine; the specific use of the Medicine please consult the herbalist or health professionals)

Naoliqing Pills (Capsules) (Naoliqing Wan (Jiaonang))

Chinese phonetic alphabet/pin yin: nǎo lì qīng wán

Chinese characters simplified/traditional:脑立清丸(胶囊)/腦立清丸(膠囊)

Ingredients: Magnetite, Hematite, Nacre, Prepared Pinellia Tuber (processed with alum), Chinese Distiller's Yeast, Chinese Distiller's Yeast (stir-baked), Twotoothed Achyranthes Root, Menthol, Borneol, Pig-bile (or Pig Gall Powder).

The content of each ingredients may have a little variety due to different dosage forms.

Indication: hypertension, dizziness and vertigo, tinnitus and bitter taste in the mouth, insomnia and vexation.

Administration and dosage: (for oral administration) pill: 10 pills per time, twice a day; capsule: 3 capsules per time, twice a day.

Strength: 1.1 g per 10 pills, 0.33 g per capsule.

The specific strength and dosage are according to the medicine instruction.

Precaution and warning: contraindicated with pregnant woman and patients with weak and deficiency cold constitution.

Attachment: Chinese Distiller's Yeast (酒曲, Latin name: Saccharomyces Cerevisiae Fermentata) is stemed rice add the *Aspergillus conidia*, then fermented.

Songling Xuemaikang Capsules (Songling Xuemaikang Jiaonang)
Chinese phonetic alphabet/pin yin: sōng líng xuě mài kāng jiāo náng
Chinese characters simplified/traditional:松龄血脉康胶囊/松齡血脈康膠囊
Ingredients: Fresh Pine Needle, Kudzuvine Root, Pearl Powder.
Indication: headache, dizziness, palpitation, insomnia, hypertension and primary hyperlipidemia.
Administration and dosage: 3 capsules per time, three times a day for oral administration.
Strength: 0.5 g per capsule.
The specific strength and dosage are according to the medicine instruction.
Attachment: Fresh Pine Needle (鲜松叶, Latin name: Pinus Folium Recence (Song Leaf Recence)) is the fresh leaf of *Pinus armandi* Franch., *Pinus taiwanensis* Hayata. or other species of pine.

Dampness medicine(祛湿药)
Dampness medicine is a kind of medicines, which are usually used to treat edema, urinary pain, urinary frequency, difficulty in micturition and other urinary diseases.

Shenyan Siwei Tablets (Shenyan Siwei Pian)
Chinese phonetic alphabet/pin yin: shèn yán sì wèi piàn
Chinese characters simplified/traditional:肾炎四味片/腎炎四味片
Ingredients: Thin Peduncle Lespedeza, Baical Skullcap Root, Shearer's Pyrrosia Leaf, Milkvetch Root.
Indication: edema, puffy swelling, lumbago, difficulty in micturition and chronic nephritis.
Administration and dosage: 2.8-2.88 g per time, three times a day for oral administration.
Strength: 0.35 g per core for sugar-coated tablet, 0.36 g per tablet or 0.70 g per tablet.
The specific strength and dosage are according to the medicine instruction.
Attachment: Thin Peduncle Lespedeza (细梗胡枝子, Latin name: Lespedeza Herba) is the dried whole herb of *Lespedeza virgata* (Thunb.) DC.

Shenyan Kangfu Tablets (Shenyan Kangfu Pian)
Chinese phonetic alphabet/pin yin: shèn yán kāng fù piàn
Chinese characters simplified/traditional:肾炎康复片/腎炎康復片
Ingredients: American Ginseng, Ginseng, Rehmannia Root, Eucommia Bark (processed with salt), Common Yam Rhizome, Spreading Hedvotis Herb, Black Bean, Glabrous Greenbrier Rhizome, Motherwort Herb, Danshen Root, Oriental Waterplantain Rhizome, Lalang Grass Rhizome, Platycodon Root.
Indication: lassitude and lack of strength, soreness and weakness in waist and knees, edema in face and limbs, chronic nephritis, proteinuria and hematuria.
Administration and dosage: 8 sugar-coated tablets or 5 film-coated tablets per time,

three times a day. Reduce the dosage in pediatric patients.

Strength: 0.3 g per core for sugar-coated tablet, 0.48 g per film-coated tablet.

The specific strength and dosage are according to the medicine instruction.

Precaution and warning: contraindicated during pregnancy or in patient with acute nephritic edema.

(The information is only for learning and identification the Chinese Patent Medicine; the specific use of the Medicine please consult the herbalist or health professionals)

Bazheng Mixture (Bazheng Heji)

Chinese phonetic alphabet/pin yin: bā zhèng hé jì

Chinese characters simplified/traditional:八正合剂/八正合劑

Ingredients: Lilac Pink Herb, Plantain Seed (stir-baked), Common Knotgrass Herb, Rhubarb, Talc, Armand Clematis Stem, Cape Jasmine Fruit, Liquorice Root, Common Rush.

Indication: scanty, deep-colored urine, difficult and painful urination, dry mouth and throat.

Administration and dosage: 15-20 ml per time, three times a day, shake well before use for oral administration.

Strength: 100-200 ml per bottle.

The specific strength and dosage are according to the medicine instruction.

(The information is only for learning and identification the Chinese Patent Medicine; the specific use of the Medicine please consult the herbalist or health professionals)

Longbishu Capsules (Longbishu Jiaonang)

Chinese phonetic alphabet/pin yin: lóng bì shū jiāo náng

Chinese characters simplified/traditional:癃闭舒胶囊/癃閉舒膠囊

Ingredients: Malaytea Scurfpea Fruit, Motherwort Herb, Christina Loosestrife, Japanese Climbing Fern Spore, Lamber, Appendiculate Cremastra Pseudobulb.

Indication: difficulty in micturition, soreness and weakness in waist and knees, frequent, urgent, painful and thread urination and hyperplasia of prostate.

Administration and dosage: 3 capsules per time, twice a day for oral administration.

Strength: 0.3 g per capsule.

The specific strength and dosage are according to the medicine instruction.

(The information is only for learning and identification the Chinese Patent Medicine; the specific use of the Medicine please consult the herbalist or health professionals)

Sanjin Tablets (Sanjin Pian)

Chinese phonetic alphabet/pin yin: sān jīn piàn

Chinese characters simplified/traditional:三金片/三金片

Ingredients: Cherokee Rose root, Chinaroot Greenbrier Rhizome, Melastoma Normale Root, Japanese Climbing Fern Herb, Asiatic Pennywort Herb.

Indication: pyretic stranguria, dysuria with pain, acute and chronic pyelonephritis, cystitis and urinary infection.

Administration and dosage: 5 small tablets or 3 big tablets per time, three or four times a day for oral administration.

Strength: 0.18 g per tablet (small film-coated tablets, equal to 2.1 g of prepared slices), 0.29 g per tablet (big film-coated tablets, equal to 3.5 g of prepared slices), small sugar-coated tablet (0.17 g core weight, equal to 2.1 g of prepared slices), big sugar-coated tablet (0.28 g core weight, equal to 3.5 g of prepared slices).

The specific strength and dosage are according to the medicine instruction.

Attachment: Melastoma Normale Root (羊开口, Latin name: Melastomae Normalis Radix) is the dried root of *Melastoma normale* D. Don.
(The information is only for learning and identification the Chinese Patent Medicine; the specific use of the Medicine please consult the herbalist or health professionals)

Paishi Granules (Paishi Keli)
Chinese phonetic alphabet/pin yin: pái shí kē lì
Chinese characters simplified/traditional:排石颗粒/排石顆粒
Ingredients: Longtube Ground Ivy Herb, Plantain Seed (stir-baked with salt water), Akebiae Stem, Paniculate Swallowwort Root, Shearer's Pyrrosia Leaf, Lilac Pink Herb, Honeysuckle Stem, Talc, Chingma Abutilon Seed, Liquorice Root.
Indication: lumbo and abdominal pain, urinary stoppage or haematuria, and urolithiasis.
Administration and dosage: take the medicine after mixing it with hot water, 1 pack per time, three times a day.
Strength: 20 g per pack, 5 g per pack (without sucrose).
The specific strength and dosage are according to the medicine instruction.
(The information is only for learning and identification the Chinese Patent Medicine; the specific use of the Medicine please consult the herbalist or health professionals)

Yinzhihuang Mixture (Granules/Capsules/Effervescent Tablets) (Yinzhihuang Koufuye (Keli/Jiaonang/Paotengpian))
Chinese phonetic alphabet/pin yin: yīn zhī huáng kǒu fú yè
Chinese characters simplified/traditional:茵栀黄口服液(颗粒/胶囊/泡腾片)/茵栀黄口服液(顆粒/膠囊/泡騰片)
Ingredients: Gapillary Wormwood Extract, Cape Jasmine Fruit Extract, Baical Skullcap Root Extract (calculated with baicalin), Japanese Honeysuckle Flower Extract.
The content of each ingredients may have a little variety due to different dosage forms.
Indication: distending pain in chest and hypochondrium, nausea, vomiting, dark colored urine, acute and chronic hepatitis.
Administration and dosage: (for oral administration) mixture: 10 ml per time, three times a day; granule: mixing the medicine with hot water before usage, 6 g per time, three times a day; capsule: 0.66-0.78 g per time, three times a day; effervescent tablet: drink the liquid after dissolving the medicine in warm boiled water, 2 tablets per time, three times a day.
Strength: mixture: 10 ml per ampule (containing 0.4 g of baicalin); granule: 3 g per pack; capsule: 0.33 g or 0.26 g per capsule; effervescent tablet: 0.6 g per tablet (with 0.2 g of baicalin).
The specific strength and dosage are according to the medicine instruction.
Precaution and warning: avoid alcohol and spicy food.
(The information is only for learning and identification the Chinese Patent Medicine; the specific use of the Medicine please consult the herbalist or health professionals)

Xiaoyan Lidan Tablets (Xiaoyan Lidan Pian)
Chinese phonetic alphabet/pin yin: xiāo yán lì dǎn piàn
Chinese characters simplified/traditional:消炎利胆片/消炎利膽片
Ingredients: Common Andrographis Herb, Serrate Rabdosia Herb, Indian

Quassiawood.

Indication: hypochondriac pain, bitter taste in the mouth, acute cholecystitis or angiocholitis.

Administration and dosage: 6 tablets of small film-coated tablets, or 6 tablets of sugar-coated tablet, or 3 big film-coated tablets per time, three times a day.

Strength: small film-coated tablet (0.26 g, equivalent to 2.6 g of prepared slice of crude drugs), big file-coated tablet (0.52 g equivalent to 5.2 g of prepared slice of crude drugs), sugar-coated tablet (0.25 g for each core, equivalent to 2.6 g of prepared slice of crude drugs).

The specific strength and dosage are according to the medicine instruction.

Precaution and warning: avoid smoking, alcohol, greasy and heavy food.

Attachment: Serrate Rabdosia Herb (溪黄草, Latin name: Isodi Lophanthoidis Herba) is the dried whole herb of *Rabdosia serra* (Maxim.) Hara.

(The information is only for learning and identification the Chinese Patent Medicine; the specific use of the Medicine please consult the herbalist or health professionals)

Xianglian Pills (Tablets) (Xianglian Wan (Pian))

Chinese phonetic alphabet/pin yin: xiāng lián wán

Chinese characters simplified/traditional:香连丸(片)/香連丸(片)

Ingredients: Golden Thread (processed with Medicinal Evodia Fruit), Common Aucklandia Root.

The content of each ingredients may have a little variety due to different dosage forms.

Indication: purulent, hemafecia, tenesmus, fever, abdominal pain, enteritis and bacillary dysentery.

Administration and dosage: (for oral administration) pill: 3-6 g honeyed pill, or 6-12 concentrated pills per time, two or three times a day; tablet: 5 big file-coated tablets or sugar-coated tablets for adult per time, three times a day, 2-3 small film-coated tablets or small sugar-coated tablets for children per time, three times a day.

Strength: concentrated pill: 1.7 g per 10 pills or 2 g per 10 pills; tablet: (1) 0.1 g per small film-coated tablet (equivalent to 0.35 g of the ingredient), (2) 0.3 g per big film-coated tablet tablet (equivalent to 1 g of the ingredients), (3) small sugar-coated tablet (0.1 g per core, equivalent to 0.35 g of the ingredients), (4) sugar-coated tablets (0.3 g per core, equivalent to 1 g of the ingredients).

The specific strength and dosage are according to the medicine instruction.

(The information is only for learning and identification the Chinese Patent Medicine; the specific use of the Medicine please consult the herbalist or health professionals)

Xianglian Huazhi Pills (Xianglian Huazhi Wan)

Chinese phonetic alphabet/pin yin: xiāng lián huà zhì wán

Chinese characters simplified/traditional:香连化滞丸/香連化滯丸

Ingredients: Golden Thread, Common Aucklandia Root, Baical Skullcap Root, Immature Orange Fruit (stir-baked with bran), Dried Tangerine Peel, Dried Immaturity Tangerines Peel (processed with vinegar), Officinal Magnolia Bark (processed with ginger), Areca Seed (stir-baked), Talc, White Peony Root (stir-baked), Chinese Angelica, Liquorice Root.

Indication: pus and bloody stool, tenesmus, fever and abdominal pain.

Administration and dosage: 5 g watered pills, 8 g water-honeyed pills, or 2 big honeyed pills per time, twice a day for oral administration.

Strength: 0.3 g per 10 watered pills, 10g per 100 water-honeyed pills, 6 g per big

honeyed pill.
The specific strength and dosage are according to the medicine instruction.
Precaution and warning: avoid row, cold and greasy food. Contraindicated during pregnancy.
(The information is only for learning and identification the Chinese Patent Medicine; the specific use of the Medicine please consult the herbalist or health professionals)

Wuling Powder (Capsules) (Wuling San (Jiaonang))
Chinese phonetic alphabet/pin yin: wǔ líng sǎn
Chinese characters simplified/traditional:五苓散(胶囊)/五苓散(膠囊)
Ingredients: Indian Bread, Oriental Waterplantain Rhizome, Chuling, Cassia Bark, Largehead Atractylodes Rhizome (stir-baked).
The content of each ingredients may have a little variety due to different dosage forms.
Indication: anuresis, edema, abdominal distension, vomiting, diarrhea and thirst with no desire for drink.
Administration and dosage: (for oral administration) powder: 6-9 g per time, twice a day; capsule; 3 capsules per time, twice a day.
Strength: powder: 6 or 9 g per pack; capsule; 0.45 g per capsule.
The specific strength and dosage are according to the medicine instruction.
(The information is only for learning and identification the Chinese Patent Medicine; the specific use of the Medicine please consult the herbalist or health professionals)

Bixie Fenqing Pill (Bixie Fenqing Wan)
Chinese phonetic alphabet/pin yin: bì xiè fēn qīng wán
Chinese characters simplified/traditional:萆薢分清丸/萆薢分清丸
Ingredients: Hypoglaucous Collett Yam Rhizome, Grassleaf Sweetflag Rhizome, Liquorice Root, Combined Spicebush Root, Sharpleaf Glangal Fruit (stir-baked with salt).
Indication: turbidity and frequent urination.
Administration and dosage: 6-9 g per time, twice a day for oral administration.
Strength: 1 g per 20 pills.
The specific strength and dosage are according to the medicine instruction.
Precaution and warning: avoid greasy, spicy food, tea and vinegar.
(The information is only for learning and identification the Chinese Patent Medicine; the specific use of the Medicine please consult the herbalist or health professionals)

Juanbi medicine(蠲痹药)
Juanbi medicine is a kind of medicines, which are usually used to treat Joint swelling and pain, unfavourable flexion and extension, numbness in the limbs and rheumatoid arthritis diseases.

Xiaohuoluo Pills (Xiaohuoluo Wan)
Chinese phonetic alphabet/pin yin: xiǎo huó luò wán
Chinese characters simplified/traditional:小活络丸/小活絡丸
Ingredients: Bile Arisaema, Prepared Common Monkshood Mother Root, Prepared Kusnezoff Monkshood Root, Earthworm, Olibanum (processed), Myrrh (processed).
Indication: pain in the joints and limbs, cold pain, stabbing pain, or pain worsening at night, sluggishness of joint movement, numbness and convulsions of joints.
Administration and dosage: 3 g (15 pills) small honeyed pills or 1 big honeyed pill per

time, twice a day. Take the medicine orally with warm boiled water or yellow wine.
Strength: 20 g per 100 pills for small honeyed pill, 3 g per pill for big honeyed pill.
The specific strength and dosage are according to the medicine instruction.
Precaution and warning: contraindicated with pregnant women.
(The information is only for learning and identification the Chinese Patent Medicine;
the specific use of the Medicine please consult the herbalist or health professionals)

Mugua Pills (Mugua Wan)
Chinese phonetic alphabet/pin yin: mù guā wán
Chinese characters simplified/traditional:木瓜丸/木瓜丸
Ingredients: Papaya, Chinese Angelica, Szechwan Lovage Rhizome, Dahurian
Angelica Root, Chinese Clematis Root, Cibot Rhizome (processed), Twotoothed
Achyranthes Root, Suberect Spatholobus Stem, Kadsura Pepper Stem, Ginseng,
Prepared Common Monkshood Mother Root, Prepared Kusnezoff Monkshood Root.
Indication: joint pain, swelling, inhibited of joint bending and stretch, numbness of
limbs.
Administration and dosage: 30 pills per time, twice a day for oral administration.
The specific strength and dosage are according to the medicine instruction.
Precaution and warning: contraindicated with pregnant women.
(The information is only for learning and identification the Chinese Patent Medicine;
the specific use of the Medicine please consult the herbalist or health professionals)

Fengshi Gutong Capsules (Pills) (Fengshi Gutong Jiaonang (Wan))
Chinese phonetic alphabet/pin yin: fēng shī gǔ tòng jiāo náng
Chinese characters simplified/traditional:风湿骨痛胶囊(丸)/風濕骨痛膠囊(丸)
Ingredients: Prepared Common Monkshood Mother Root, Prepared Kusnezoff
Monkshood Root, Safflower, Liquorice Root, Papaya, Smoked Plum, Ephedra.
The content of each ingredients may have a little variety due to different dosage
forms.
Indication: lumbar vertebrae pain, cold pain in the joints of the limbs and rheumatic
arthritis.
Administration and dosage :(for oral administration) capsule: 2-4 capsules per time,
twice a day; pill: 10-15 water-honeyed pills per time, twice a day.
Strength: 0.3 g per capsule, 1.5 g per 10 water-honeyed pills.
The specific strength and dosage are according to the medicine instruction.
Precaution and warning: contraindicated with pregnant women. It contains toxic
ingredients, avoid overdose.
(The information is only for learning and identification the Chinese Patent Medicine;
the specific use of the Medicine please consult the herbalist or health professionals)

Simiao Pills (Simiao Wan)
Chinese phonetic alphabet/pin yin: sì miào wán
Chinese characters simplified/traditional:四妙丸/四妙丸
Ingredients: Atractylodes Rhizome, Twotoothed Achyranthes Root, Chinese
Cork-tree (processed with salt), Coix Seed.
Indication: swelling and redness of feet and knees, pain in sinews and bones.
Administration and dosage: 6 g per time, twice a day for oral administration.
Strength: 1 g per 15 pills.
The specific strength and dosage are according to the medicine instruction.
Precaution and warning: use with caution during pregnancy.

(The information is only for learning and identification the Chinese Patent Medicine; the specific use of the Medicine please consult the herbalist or health professionals)

Tongfengding Capsules (Tongfengding Jiaonang)
Chinese phonetic alphabet/pin yin: tòng fēng dìng jiāo náng
Chinese characters simplified/traditional:痛风定胶囊/痛風定膠囊
Ingredients: Largeleaf Gentian Root, Chinese Cork-tree, Yanhusuo, Red Peony Root, Medicinal Cyathula Root, Oriental Waterplantain Rhizome, Plantain Seed, Glabrous Greenbrier Rhizome.
Indication: painful *bi* disorder, heat and pain in joints accompanied with fever, persistent sweating, thirst and vexation, slippery and rapid pulse, and gout.
Administration and dosage: 4 capsules per time, three times a day for oral administration.
Strength: 0.4 g per capsule.
The specific strength and dosage are according to the medicine instruction.
Precaution and warning: use with caution during pregnancy. Avoid drinking tea right after taking the medicine.
(The information is only for learning and identification the Chinese Patent Medicine; the specific use of the Medicine please consult the herbalist or health professionals)

Qufeng Zhitong Pills (Tablets/Capsules) (Qufeng Zhitong Wan (Pian/Jiaonang))
Chinese phonetic alphabet/pin yin: qū fēng zhǐ tòng wán
Chinese characters simplified/traditional:祛风止痛丸(片/胶囊)/祛風止痛丸(片/膠囊)
Ingredients: Common Heron's Bill Herb, Coloured Mistletoe Herb, Himalayan Teasel Root, Chinese Clematis Root, Doubleteeth Pubescent Angelica Root, Prepared Kusnezoff Monkshood Root, Safflower.
The content of each ingredients may have a little variety due to different dosage forms.
Indication: swollen joints, numbness of the limbs, pain in waist and knees.
Administration and dosage: (for oral administration) pill: 2.2 g per time, twice a day; tablet: 6 tablets per time, twice a day; capsule: 6 capsule per time, twice a day.
Strength: pill: 2.2 g per bag (1.1 g per 10 pills); capsule: 0.3 g per capsule.
The specific strength and dosage are according to the medicine instruction.
Precaution and warning: contraindicated during pregnancy.
(The information is only for learning and identification the Chinese Patent Medicine; the specific use of the Medicine please consult the herbalist or health professionals)

Jingfukang Granules (Jingfukang Keli)
Chinese phonetic alphabet/pin yin: jǐng fù kāng kē lì
Chinese characters simplified/traditional:颈复康颗粒/頸復康顆粒
Ingredients: Incised Notopterygium Rhizome and Root, Szechwan Lovage Rhizome, Kudzuvine Root, Largeleaf Gentian Root, Chinese Clematis Root, Atractylodes Rhizome, Danshen Root, White Peony Root, Earthworm (stir-baked with wine), Safflower, Olibanum (processed), Milkvetch Root, Tangshen, Rehmannia Root, Abalone Shell, Ophicalcite (calcined), Amur Cork-tree, Cowherb Seed (stir-baked), Peach Seed (baked), Myrrh (processed), Ground Beetle (stir-baked with wine).
Indication: dizziness, stiff nape and neck, numbness of arms, sore pain in the shoulder and back.
Administration and dosage: 1-2 pack per time, twice a day after meals. Take the

medicine orally after mixing it with hot water.

Strength: 5 g per pack.

The specific strength and dosage are according to the medicine instruction.

Precaution and warning: use with caution during pregnancy. Patients with peptic ulcer or renal hypertension should be use with caution. Discontinue the medication when common cold, fever so sore nose and throat occurs.

(The information is only for learning and identification the Chinese Patent Medicine; the specific use of the Medicine please consult the herbalist or health professionals)

Duhuo Jisheng Mixture (Pills) (Duhuo Jisheng Heji (Wan))

Chinese phonetic alphabet/pin yin: dú huó jì shēng hé jì

Chinese characters simplified/traditional:独活寄生合剂(丸)/獨活寄生合劑(丸)

Ingredients: Doubleteeth Pubescent Angelica Root, Chinese Taxillus Herb, Largeleaf Gentian Root, Saposhnikovia Root, Manchurian Wildginger Root, Chinese Angelica, White Peony Root, Szechwan Lovage Rhizome, Prepared Rehmannia Root, Eucommia Bark (processed with salt water), Medicinal Cyathula Root, Tangshen, Indian Bread, Liquorice Root, Cassia Twig.

The content of each ingredients may have a little variety due to different dosage forms.

Indication: cold pain in the waist and knees, sluggishness of joint movement, numbness of limbs.

Administration and dosage:(for oral administration) mixture: 15-20 ml, three times a day, shaking fully before use; pill: 6 g water-honeyed pills or 1 big honeyed pill per time, twice a day.

Strength: mixture: 20 or 100 ml per bottle; pill: 9 g per big honeyed pill, 6 g per pack for water-honeyed pills.

The specific strength and dosage are according to the medicine instruction.

Precaution and warning: use with caution during pregnancy.

(The information is only for learning and identification the Chinese Patent Medicine; the specific use of the Medicine please consult the herbalist or health professionals)

Tianma Pills (Tianma Wan)

Chinese phonetic alphabet/pin yin: tiān má wán

Chinese characters simplified/traditional:天麻丸/天麻丸

Ingredients: Tall Gastrodia Tuber, Incised Notopterygium Rhizome and Root, Doubleteeth Pubescent Angelica Root, Eucommia Bark (stir-baked with salt), Twotoothed Achyranthes Root, Hypoglaucous Collett Yam Rhizome, Prepared Common Monkshood Daugher Root (processed), Chinese Angelica, Rehmannia Root, Figwort.

Indication: spasm of limbs, numbness of extremities, soreness and weakness in waist and knees.

Administration and dosage: 6 g water-honeyed pills, 9 g small honeyed pills, or 1 big honeyed pill per time, two or three times a day for oral administration.

Strength: 20 g per 100 pills for small honeyed pill, 9 g per big honeyed pill.

The specific strength and dosage are according to the medicine instruction.

Precaution and warning: use with caution during pregnancy.

(The information is only for learning and identification the Chinese Patent Medicine; the specific use of the Medicine please consult the herbalist or health professionals)

Wangbi Granules (Wangbi Keli)

Chinese phonetic alphabet/pin yin: wāng bì kē lì

Chinese characters simplified/traditional:尪痹颗粒/尪痹顆粒

Ingredients: Rehmannia Root, Prepared Rehmannia Root, Himalayan Teasel Root, Prepared Common Monkshood Daugher Root (heifupian), Doubleteeth Pubescent Angelica Root, Fortune's Drynaria Rhizome, Cassia twig, Epimedium Leaf, Divaricate Saposhnikovia Root, Chinese Clematis Root, Chinese Honeylocust Spine, Sheep Bone, White Peony Root, Cibot Rhizome (processed), Common Anemarrhena Rhizome, Common Clubmoss Herb, Safflower.

Indication: muscle and joint pain, stiff and deformed joint with inhibited bending and stretching, fear of cold and rheumatoid arthritis.

Administration and dosage: mixed in boiled water for oral taking, 6 g per time, three times a day.

Strength: 3 g or 6 g per pack.

The specific strength and dosage are according to the medicine instruction.

Precaution and warning: contraindicated during pregnancy. Avoid raw or cold food.

(The information is only for learning and identification the Chinese Patent Medicine; the specific use of the Medicine please consult the herbalist or health professionals)

Surgical and dermatological medicine(外科、皮肤科用药)

Surgical and dermatological medicine is a kind of medicines which are usually used to treat erysipelas, sores, skin ulcers, acne, burn, scald and other kinds of skin disease.

Ruyi Jinhuang Powder (Ruyi Jinhuang San)

Chinese phonetic alphabet/pin yin: rú yì jīn huáng sǎn

Chinese characters simplified/traditional:如意金黄散/如意金黄散

Ingredients: Turmeric, Rhubarb, Chinese Cork-tree, Atractylodes Rhizome, Officinal Magnolia Bark, Dried Tangerine Peel, Liquorice Root, Jackinthepulpit Tuber, Dahurian Angelica Root, Snakegourd Root.

Indication: painful swelling of sore, ulcer, traumatic injuries and erysipelas node.

Administration and dosage: apply it to the *pars affecta* (redness and swelling, heat, pain) after mixing it with green tea, vegetable oil or honey, several times a day for external usage.

The specific strength and dosage are according to the medicine instruction.

Precaution and warning: for topical application only. Oral administration is prohibited.

(The information is only for learning and identification the Chinese Patent Medicine; the specific use of the Medicine please consult the herbalist or health professionals)

Zicao Ointment (Zicao Gao)

Chinese phonetic alphabet/pin yin: zǐ cǎo gāo

Chinese characters simplified/traditional:紫草膏/紫草膏

Ingredients: Arnebia Root, Chinese Angelica, Rehmannia Root, Divaricate Saposhnikovia Root, Dahurian Angelica Root, Olibanum, Myrrh.

Indication: pain in bright-colored wounds with purulent, or sore with abscess to be drained off.

Administration and dosage: apply it to the *pars affecta* after strapping it to the gauze, change dressing once a day or every other day for topical application.

The specific strength and dosage are according to the medicine instruction.

(The information is only for learning and identification the Chinese Patent Medicine; the specific use of the Medicine please consult the herbalist or health professionals)

Jingwanhong Ointment (Jingwanhong Ruangao)
Chinese phonetic alphabet/pin yin: jīng wàn hóng ruǎn gāo
Chinese characters simplified/traditional:京万红软膏/京萬紅軟膏
Ingredients: Garden Burnet Root, Rehmannia Root, Chinese Angelica, Peach Seed, Golden Thread, Cochinchina Momordica Seed, Poppy Capsule, Carbonized Hair, Fortune Windmillpalm Petiole, Chinese Lobelia Herb, Ground Beetle, Japanese Ampelopsis Root, Chinese Cork-tree, Arnebia Root, Japanese Honeysuckle Flower, Safflower, Rhubarb, Lightyellow Sophora Root, Chinese Gall, Pagoda Tree Flower, Papaya, Atractylodes Rhizome, Dahurian Angelica Root, Red Peony Root, Baical Skullcap Root, Figwortflower Picrorhiza Rhizome, Szechwan Lovage Rhizome, Cape Jasmine Fruit, Smoked Plum, Borneol, Dragon's Blood, Olibanumm, Myrrh.
Indication: scald and burn, skin damage, wound ulceration, sore and ulcer.
Administration and dosage: cleaning the wound with normal saline then apply the ointment to the *pars affecta*, or apply it to the sterilized gauze first and then cover the wound with gauze, and bind it up, once a day.
Strength: 10 or 20 g per branch, 30 or 50 g per bottle.
The specific strength and dosage are according to the medicine instruction.
Precaution and warning: use with caution during pregnancy.
(The information is only for learning and identification the Chinese Patent Medicine; the specific use of the Medicine please consult the herbalist or health professionals)

Neixiao Luoli Tablets (Neixiao Luoli Pian)
Chinese phonetic alphabet/pin yin: nèi xiāo luó lì piàn
Chinese characters simplified/traditional:内消瘰疬片/內消瘰癧片
Ingredients: Common Selfheal Fruit-Spike, Thunberg Fritillary Bulb, Seaweed, Japanese Ampelopsis Root, Snakegourd Root, Weeping Forsythia Capsule, Rhubarb (prepared), Exsiccated Sodium Sulfate, Clam Shell (calcined), Helite, Orange Fruit, Platycodon Root, Menthol, Rehmannia Root, Chinese Angelica, Figwort, Liquorice Root .
Indication: scrofula, lump under skin without heat or pain.
Administration and dosage: 4-8 tablets per time, once or twice a day for oral administration.
Strength: 0.6 g per tablet.
The specific strength and dosage are according to the medicine instruction.
(The information is only for learning and identification the Chinese Patent Medicine; the specific use of the Medicine please consult the herbalist or health professionals)

Xiaojin Pills (Tablets/Capsules) (Xiaojin Wan (Pian/Jiaonang))
Chinese phonetic alphabet/pin yin: xiǎo jīn wán
Chinese characters simplified/traditional:小金丸(片/胶囊)/小金丸(片/膠囊)
Ingredients: Musk (or Artificial Musk), Cochinchina Momordica Seed (removed from shell and oil), Prepared Kusnezoff Monkshood Root, Beautiful Sweetgum Resin, Olibanum (processed), Myrrh (processed), Flying Squirrel's Faeces (stir-baked with vinegar), Chinese Angelica (stir-baked with wine), Earthworm, Aromatic Ink.
The content of each ingredients may have a little variety due to different dosage forms.
Indication: one or more palpable movable mass under the skin, or hard, painful swollen bones and joints with normal skin color, scrofula, goiter, tumor, rocky mass in the breast and mammary hyperplasia.

Administration and dosage: (for oral administration) pill: grind into small piece before oral administration, 1.2-3 g per time, twice a day; tablet: 2-3 tablets per time, twice a day; capsule: 1.05-3 g per time, twice a day. Reduce the dosage in children.

Strength: pill: 3 g per 100 pills, 6 g per 100 pills, 6 g per 10 pills, or 0.6 g per bottle (bag); tablet: 0.36 g per tablet; capsule: 0.3 g or 0.35 g per capsule.

The specific strength and dosage are according to the medicine instruction.

Precaution and warning: contraindicated during pregnancy.

Attachment: Aromatic Ink (香墨) is a kind of solid ink which is made of pine smoke, gum and perfumes.

(The information is only for learning and identification the Chinese Patent Medicine; the specific use of the Medicine please consult the herbalist or health professionals)

Yanghe Jiening Plaster (Yanghe Jiening Gao)

Chinese phonetic alphabet/pin yin: yáng hé jiě níng gāo

Chinese characters simplified/traditional:阳和解凝膏/陽和解凝膏

Ingredients: Fresh Great Burdock Achene (or Great Burdock Achene), Fresh Garden Balsam Stem (or Garden Balsam Stem), Common Monkshood Mother Root, Cassia Twig, Rhubarb, Chinese Angelica, Kusnezoff Monkshood Root, Common Monkshood Daughter Root, Earthworm, Stiff Silkworm, Red Peony Root, Dahurian Angelica Root, Japanese Ampelopsis Root, Common Bletilla Tuber, Szechwan Lovage Rhizome, Himalayan Teasel Root, Divaricate Saposhnikovia Root, Fineleaf Schizonepeta Herb, Flying Squirrel's Faeces, Common Aucklandia Root, Citron Fruit, Dried Tangerine Peel, Cassia Bark, Olibanum, Myrrh, Storax, Artificial Musk.

Indication: scrofula, painful *bi* disorder and phlegm.

Administration and dosage: for topical administration, warm the paste with heat before applying the paste onto the *pars affecta*.

Strength: 1.5 g, 3 g, 6 g, or 9 g net weight per piece.

The specific strength and dosage are according to the medicine instruction.

Attachment: Garden Balsam Stem (凤仙透骨草, Latin name: Impatientis Balsaminae Caulis) is the processed stem of *Impatiens balsamina* L.

(The information is only for learning and identification the Chinese Patent Medicine; the specific use of the Medicine please consult the herbalist or health professionals)

Rupixiao Tablets (Capsules/Granules) (Rupixiao Pian (Jiaonang/ Keli))

Chinese phonetic alphabet/pin yin: rǔ pì xiāo piàn

Chinese characters simplified/traditional:乳癖消片(胶囊/颗粒)/乳癖消片(膠囊/顆粒)

Ingredients: Pilose Antler, Dandelion, Kelp, Snakegourd Root, Suberect Spatholobus Stem, Sanchi, Red Peony Root, Seaweed, Uniflower Swisscentaury Rood, Common Aucklandia Root, Figwort, Tree Peony Bark, Common Selfheal Fruit-Spike, Weeping Forsythia Capsule, Safflower.

The content of each ingredients may have a little variety due to different dosage forms.

Indication: hyperplasia of mammary gland and early mastitis.

Administration and dosage: (for oral administration) tablet: 5-6 tablets for 0.34 g per tablet, or 3 tablets for 0.67 g per tablet per time, three times a day; capsule: 5-6 capsules per time, three times a day; granules: mixing the medicine with hot water before usage, 8 g per time, three times a day.

Strength: tablet: 0.34 g per film coated tablet, 0.67 g per film coated tablet, 0.34 g per

sugar-coated tablet core; capsule: 0.32 g per capsule; granule: 8 g per pack.
The specific strength and dosage are according to the medicine instruction.
Precaution and warning: use with caution during pregnancy.
(The information is only for learning and identification the Chinese Patent Medicine; the specific use of the Medicine please consult the herbalist or health professionals)

Mayinglong Shexiang Ointment (Mayinglong Shexiang Gao)
Chinese phonetic alphabet/pin yin: mǎ yīng lóng shè xiāng gāo
Chinese characters simplified/traditional:马应龙麝香膏/馬應龍麝香膏
Ingredients: Artificial Musk, Artificial Cow-bezoan, Pearl, Calamine (calcined), Borax, Synthesis Borneol, Lamber.
Indication: hemorrhoids, perianal eczema, fecal pain or bearing-down sensation.
Administration and dosage: apply the paste onto the *pars affecta* for topical application.
The specific strength and dosage are according to the medicine instruction.
Precaution and warning: contraindicated with pregnant woman.
(The information is only for learning and identification the Chinese Patent Medicine; the specific use of the Medicine please consult the herbalist or health professionals)

Xiaoyin Tablets (Capsules) (Xiaoyin Pian (Jiaonang))
Chinese phonetic alphabet/pin yin: xiāo yín piàn
Chinese characters simplified/traditional:消银片(胶囊)/消銀片(膠囊)
Ingredients: Rehmannia Root, Tree Peony Bark, Red Peony Root, Chinese Angelica, Lightyellow Sophora Root, Japanese Honeysuckle Flower, Figwort, Great Burdock Achene, Cicada Slough, Densefruit Pittany Root-bark, Divaricate Saposhnikovia Root, Dyers Woad Leaf, Safflower.
The content of each ingredients may have a little variety due to different dosage forms.
Indication: psoriasis guttata skin rash with bright red base and covered with silver scale or dry skin rash with thick silver scale, light red base and heavy itching.
Administration and dosage: (for oral administration) tablet: 5-7 tablets per time, three times a day; capsule: 5-7 capsules per time, three times a day. One treatment course last for one month.
Strength: tablet: 0.32 g per tablet for film coating tablets, 0.3 g per core for sugar coating tablet; capsule: 0.3 g per capsule.
The specific strength and dosage are according to the medicine instruction.
(The information is only for learning and identification the Chinese Patent Medicine; the specific use of the Medicine please consult the herbalist or health professionals)

Gynecologic medicine(妇科药)
Gynecologic medicine is a kind of medicines which are mainly used to treat Gynecologic diseases.

Dahuang Zhechong Pills (Dahuang Zhechong Wan)
Chinese phonetic alphabet/pin yin: dà huáng zhè chóng wán
Chinese characters simplified/traditional:大黄䗪虫丸/大黃䗪蟲丸
Ingredients: Rhubarb (processed), Ground Beetle (stir-baked), Leech (processed), Gadfly (removed wings and feet, stir-baked), Grub (stir-baked), Dried Lacquer (calcined), Peach Seed, Bitter Apricot (stir-baked), Baical Skullcap Root, Rehmannia Root, White Peony Root, Liquorice Root.

Indication: abdominal masses, scaly dry skin, dark complexion, tidal fever, emaciation and amenorrhea.

Administration and dosage: 3 g water-honeyed pill per time, 3-6 g small honeyed pills per time, or 1 big honey pill per time, once or twice a day for oral administration.

Strength: 3 g per big honeyed pill.

The specific strength and dosage are according to the medicine instruction.

Precaution and warning: contraindicated during pregnancy. It should be discontinued when skin allergy is present. Long-term administration is not advisable.

Attachment: Grub (蛴螬, Latin name: Holotrichia Diomphalia) is the larva of *Holotrichia diomphalia* Bates.

(The information is only for learning and identification the Chinese Patent Medicine; the specific use of the Medicine please consult the herbalist or health professionals)

Motherwort Herb Concentrated Decoction (Granules/Mixture/Capsules) (Yimucao Gao (Keli/Koufuye/Jiaonang))

Chinese phonetic alphabet/pin yin: yì mǔ cǎo gāo

Chinese characters simplified/traditional:益母草膏(颗粒/口服液/胶囊)/益母草膏(顆粒/口服液/膠囊)

Ingredients: Motherwort Herb.

The content of each ingredients may have a little variety due to different dosage forms.

Indication: menoxenia, scanty menstruation, extended cycles, prolonged postpartum hemorrhage and postpartum subinvolution of uterus.

Administration and dosage: (for oral administration) concentrated decoction: 10 g per time, once or twice a day; granule: mixing the medicine with warm boiled water, 15 g or 5 g (without sucrose) per time, twice a day; mixture: 10-20 ml per time, three times a day; capsule: 2-4 capsules per time, three times a day.

Strength: concentrated decoction: 125 g or 250 g per bottle; granule: 15 g per pack or 5 g (without sucrose) per pack; mixture: 10 ml per phial; capsule: 0.36 g per capsule (equivalent to 2.5 g prepared slice of crude drugs).

The specific strength and dosage are according to the medicine instruction.

Precaution and warning: contraindicated during pregnancy.

(The information is only for learning and identification the Chinese Patent Medicine; the specific use of the Medicine please consult the herbalist or health professionals)

Fuke Shiwei Tablets (Fuke Shiwei Pian)

Chinese phonetic alphabet/pin yin: fù kē shí wèi piàn

Chinese characters simplified/traditional:妇科十味片/婦科十味片

Ingredients: Nutgrass Galingale Rhizome (processed with vinegar), Szechwan Lovage Rhizome, Chinese Angelica, Yanhusuo (processed with vinegar), Largehead Atractylodes Rhizome, Liquorice Root, Chinese Date, White Peony Root, Prepared Rehmannia Root, Red Peony Root, Calcium Carbonate.

Indication: menoxenia, dysmenorrhea, delayed menstruation, scanty menses with clot, pain in lesser abdomen during menstruation, breast distending pain, vexation and restlessness.

Administration and dosage: 4 pills per time, three times a day.

Strength: 0.3 g per tablet, or 0.33 g per film-coated tablet.

The specific strength and dosage are according to the medicine instruction.

(The information is only for learning and identification the Chinese Patent Medicine; the specific use of the Medicine please consult the herbalist or health professionals)

Qizhi Xiangfu Pills (Qizhi Xiangfu Wan)

Chinese phonetic alphabet/pin yin: qī zhì xiāng fù wán

Chinese characters simplified/traditional:七制香附丸/七制香附丸

Ingredients: Nutgrass Galingale Rhizome (processed with vinegar), Rehmannia Root, Indian Bread, Chinese Angelica, Prepared Rehmannia Root, Szechwan Lovage Rhizome, Largehead Atractylodes Rhizome (stir-baked), White Peony Root, Motherwort Herb, Argy Wormwood (carbonized), Baical Skullcap Root, Pulp of Asiatic Cornelian Cherry Fruit (processed with wine), Cochinchinese Asparagus Root, Donkey-Hide Glue, Spine Date Seed (stir-baked), Villous Amomum Fruit, Yanhusuo (processed with vinegar), Argy Wormwood Leaf, Rice Grain, Fennel (processed with salt), Ginseng, Liquorice Root.

Indication: distending pain in the chest and hypochondrium, scanty menstruation, swoller pain in the lower abdomen during menstruation or before menstruation and menstruation delay.

Administration and dosage: 6 g per time, two times a day for oral administration.

Strength: 6 g per pack.

The specific strength and dosage are according to the medicine instruction.

(The information is only for learning and identification the Chinese Patent Medicine; the specific use of the Medicine please consult the herbalist or health professionals)

Wuji Baifeng Pills (Tablets/Granules) (Wuji Baifeng Wan (Pian/Keli))

Chinese phonetic alphabet/pin yin: wū jī bái fèng wán

Chinese characters simplified/traditional:乌鸡白凤丸(颗粒)/烏雞白鳳丸(顆粒)

Ingredients: Silkie-chicken (removed form feather, claw and intestine)，Deerhorn Glue, Turtle Carapace (processed with vinegar), Oysters Shell (calcined), Mantis Egg-case, Ginseng, Milkvetch Root, Chinese Angelica, White Peony Root, Nutgrass Galingale Rhizome (processed with vinegar), Cochinchinese Asparagus Root, Liquorice Root, Rehmannia Root, Prepared Rehmannia Root, Szechwan Lovage Rhizome, Starwort Root, Danshen Root, Common Yam Rhizome, Gordon Euryale Seed (stir-baked), Degelatined Deer-horn.

The content of each ingredients may have a little variety due to different dosage forms.

Indication: thin-built physique with weak constitution, menstrual irregularities, menstrual flooding and spotting and abnormal vaginal discharge.

Administration and dosage: (for oral administration) pill: 6 g small water-honeyed pill, 9 g small water-honeyed pills, or 1 big honey pill per time, twice a day; tablet: 2 tablets per time, twice a day; granule: mixing it with hot water before usage, 1 pack per time, twice a day.

Strength: pill: 9 g per big honeyed pill; tablet: 0.5 g per tablet; granule: 2 g per pack.

The specific strength and dosage are according to the medicine instruction.

Attachment: silkie-chicken (or black-chicken) (乌鸡, Latin name: Pullus Cum Osse Nigko) is *Gallus domesticlus* brisson. **Attention**: to protect the rare wild animals, don't use it from wild animal.

(The information is only for learning and identification the Chinese Patent Medicine; the specific use of the Medicine please consult the herbalist or health professionals)

Nyujin Pills (Nüjin Wan)

Chinese phonetic alphabet/pin yin: nǚ jīn wán

Chinese characters simplified/traditional:女金丸/女金丸

Ingredients: Chinese Angelica, White Peony Root, Szechwan Lovage Rhizome, Prepared Rehmannia Root, Tangshen, Largehead Atractylodes Rhizome (stir-baked), Indian Bread, Liquorice Root, Cassia Bark, Motherwort Herb, Tree Peony Bark, Myrrh (processed), Yanhusuo (processed with vinegar), Chinese Lovage, Dahurian Angelica Root, Baical Skullcap Root, Blackend Swallowwort Root, Nutgrass Galingale Rhizome (processed with vinegar), Villous Amomum Fruit, Dried Tangerine Peel, Red Halloysite (calcined), Degelatined Deer-horn, Donkey-Hide Glue .

Indication: advanced, delayed or heavy menstruation, prolonged flow of menses and dysmenorrheal.

Administration and dosage: 5 g small water-honeyed pill, 9 g small honeyed pills, or 1 big honey pill per time, twice a day for oral administration.

Strength: 2 g per 10 water-honeyed pill, 20 g per 100 small honeyed pills, 9 g per big honeyed pill.

The specific strength and dosage are according to the medicine instruction.

Precaution and warning: use with caution in pregnant woman.

(The information is only for learning and identification the Chinese Patent Medicine; the specific use of the Medicine please consult the herbalist or health professionals)

Shaofu Zhuyu Pills (Shaofu Zhuyu Wan)

Chinese phonetic alphabet/pin yin: shào fǔ zhú yū wán

Chinese characters simplified/traditional:少腹逐瘀丸/少腹逐瘀丸

Ingredients: Chinese Angelica, Cattail Pollen, Flying Squirrel's Faeces (stir-baked with vinegar), Red Peony Root, Fennel (stir-baked with salt), Yanhusuo (processed with vinegar), Myrrh (stir-baked), Szechwan Lovage Rhizome, Cassia Bark, Prepared Dried Ginger.

Indication: menstrual irregularities and dysmenorrheal, postpartum pain or tenderness.

Administration and dosage: take the medicine orally with warm yellow wine or boiled water. 1 pill per time, twice or three times a day.

Strength: 9 g per pill.

The specific strength and dosage are according to the medicine instruction.

Precaution and warning: contraindicated during pregnancy.

(The information is only for learning and identification the Chinese Patent Medicine; the specific use of the Medicine please consult the herbalist or health professionals)

Aifu Nuangong Pills (Aifu Nuangong Wan)

Chinese phonetic alphabet/pin yin: ài fù nuǎn gōng wán

Chinese characters simplified/traditional:艾附暖宫丸/艾附暖宫丸

Ingredients: Argy Wormwood Leaf (carbonized), Nutgrass Galingale Rhizome (processed with vinegar), Medicinal Evodia Fruit (processed), Cassia Bark, Chinese Angelica, Szechwan Lovage Rhizome, White Peony Root (stir-baked with wine), Rehmannia Root, prepared Milkvetch Root, Himalayan Teasel Root.

Indication: menstrual irregularities and dysmenorrheal, clot and cold pain in lower abdomen, soreness and weakness in waist and knees during the menstruation.

Administration and dosage: 9 g small honeyed pill per time or 1 big honey pill per time, twice or three times per day for oral administration.

Strength: 9 g per big honeyed pill.

The specific strength and dosage are according to the medicine instruction.

Precaution and warning: contraindicated during pregnancy.

Gujing Pills (Gujing Wan)

Chinese phonetic alphabet/pin yin: gù jīng wán

Chinese characters simplified/traditional:固经丸/固經丸

Ingredients: Amur Cork-tree (stir-baked with salt), Baical Skullcap Root (processed with wine), Tree-of-heaven Bark (stir-baked with bran), Nutgrass Galingale Rhizome (processed with vinegar), White Peony Root (stir-baked), Tortoise Carapace and Plastron (processed with vinegar).

Indication: advanced menstruation, heavy menstruation, dark colored menstruation, red and white vaginal discharge.

Administration and dosage: 6 g per time, twice a day for oral administration.

The specific strength and dosage are according to the medicine instruction.

Gongxuening Capsules (Gongxuening Jiaonang)

Chinese phonetic alphabet/pin yin: gōng xuě níng jiāo náng

Chinese characters simplified/traditional:宫血宁胶囊/宫血寧膠囊

Ingredients: Paris Rhizome.

Indication: flooding and spotting, heavy menstruation, uterine atony bleeding due to postpartum or miscarriage, pain in lower abdomen, lumber and scaral region, and increasing vaginal discharge in chronic pelvic inflammation.

Administration and dosage: for profuse menstruation or uterine bleeding, take 1-2 pills orally per time, three times a day. Discontinue the medication when the bleeding stops. For chronic pelvic inflammation, take 2 pills orally per time, three times a day for four weeks as one treatment course.

Strength: 0.13 g per capsule.

The specific strength and dosage are according to the medicine instruction.

Gengnian'an Pills (Tablets/Capsules) (Gengnian'an Wan (Pian/ Jiaonang))

Chinese phonetic alphabet/pin yin: gēng nián ān wán

Chinese characters simplified/traditional:更年安丸(片/胶囊)/更年安丸(片/膠囊)

Ingredients: Rehmannia Root, Oriental Waterplantain Rhizome, Dwarf Lilyturf Tuber, Prepared Rehmannia Root, Figwort, Indian Bread, Common Curculigo Rhizome, Magnetite, Tree Peony Bark, Nacre, Chinese Magnoliavine Fruit, Tuber Fleeceflower Stem, Prepared Fleeceflower Root, Wizened Wheat, Gambir Plant.

The content of each ingredients may have a little variety due to different dosage forms.

Indication: vexation, sweating, dizziness, tinnitus and other menopausal symptoms.

Administration and dosage: (for oral administration) tablet: 6 tablets per time, twice or three times a day; capsule: 3 capsules per time, three times a day.

Strength: tablet: (1) 0.31 g per thin film coated tablet, (2) 0.3 g of the core per sugar coated tablet; capsule: 0.3 g per capsule.

The specific strength and dosage are according to the medicine instruction.

Kunbao Pills (Kunbao Wan)
Chinese phonetic alphabet/pin yin: kūn bǎo wán
Chinese characters simplified/traditional:坤宝丸/坤寶丸
Ingredients: Glossy Privet Fruit (processed with wine), Palmleaf Raspberry Fruit, Dodder Seed, Barbary Wolfberry Fruit, Prepared Fleeceflower Root (processed), Tortoise Carapace and Plastron, Chinese Wolfberry Root-bark, Fourleaf Ladybell Root, Dwarf Lilyturf Tuber, Spine Date Seed (stir-baked), Rehmannia Root, White Peony Root, Red Peony Root, Chinese Angelica, Suberect Spatholobus Stem, Nacre, Dendrobium, Chrysanthemum Flower, Yerbadetajo Herb, Mulberry Leaf, Blackend Swallowwort Root, Common Anemarrhena Rhizome, Baical Skullcap Root.
Indication: menopausal syndrome, hot flush and sweating, vexation and tantrum, insomnia, forgetfulness, dizziness, tinnitus, sore pain in the limbs.
Administration and dosage: 50 pills per time, twice a day for 2 consecutive months for oral administration.
Strength: 10 g per 100 pills.
The specific strength and dosage are according to the medicine instruction.
(The information is only for learning and identification the Chinese Patent Medicine; the specific use of the Medicine please consult the herbalist or health professionals)

Qianjin Zhidai Pills (Qianjin Zhidai Wan)
Chinese phonetic alphabet/pin yin: qiān jīn zhǐ dài
Chinese characters simplified/traditional:千金止带丸/千金止帶丸
Ingredients: Tangshen, Largehead Atractylodes Rhizome (stir-baked), Chinese Angelica, White Peony Root, Szechwan Lovage Rhizome, Nutgrass Galingale Rhizome (processed with vinegar), Common Aucklandia Root, Villous Amomum Fruit, Fennel (stir-baked with salt), Yanhusuo (processed with vinegar), Eucommia Bark (stir-baked with salt), Himalayan Teasel Root, Malaytea Scurfpea Fruit (stir-baked with salt), Cockcomb Flower, Natural Indigo, Tree-of-heaven Bark (stir-baked), Oysters Shell (calcined).
Indication: irregular menstruation, continuous overflow of menses or dribbling in pale or red color without clot, profuse white thin vaginal discharge and lethargy.
Administration and dosage: 6-9 g for watered pills or 1 big honeyed pill per time, two or three times a day for oral administration.
Strength: 9 g per big honeyed pill.
The specific strength and dosage are according to the medicine instruction.
(The information is only for learning and identification the Chinese Patent Medicine; the specific use of the Medicine please consult the herbalist or health professionals)

Baidai Pills (Baidai Wan)
Chinese phonetic alphabet/pin yin: bái dài wán
Chinese characters simplified/traditional:白带丸/白帶丸
Ingredients: Chinese Cork-tree (stir-baked with wine), Tree-of-heaven Bark, White Peony Root, Chinese Angelica, Nutgrass Galingale Rhizome (processed with vinegar).
Indication: abnormal vaginal, profuse and yellow vaginal discharge.
Administration and dosage: 6 g per time, twice a day for oral administration.
The specific strength and dosage are according to the medicine instruction.
(The information is only for learning and identification the Chinese Patent Medicine; the specific use of the Medicine please consult the herbalist or health professionals)

Fuke (or Gynaecology) Qianjin Tablets (Capsules) (Fuke Qianjin Pian (Jiaonang))

Chinese phonetic alphabet/pin yin: fù kē qiān jīn piàn

Chinese characters simplified/traditional:妇科千金片(胶囊)/婦科千金片(膠囊)

Ingredients: Philippine Flemingia Root，Cherokee Rose Root, Common Andrographis Herb, Chinese Mahonia Stem, Zanthoxyli dissite, Chinese Angelica, Suberect Spatholobus Stem, Tangshen.

The content of each ingredients may have a little variety due to different dosage forms.

Indication: profuse, yellow, thick and foul vaginal discharge, lesser abdominal pain, lumbus and sacrum pain, lassitude and lack of strength, chronic pelvic inflammation, endometritis and chronic cervicitis.

Administration and dosage: tablet: 6 pills per time, three times a day for oral administration; capsule: take it orally with warm boiled water, 2 pills per time, three times a day for 14 days as one treatment course.

Strength: 0.4 g per capsule.

The specific strength and dosage are according to the medicine instruction.

Attachment: Philippine Flemingia Root (千斤拔, Latin name: Moghaniae Radix) is the dried root of *Flemingia philippinensis* Merr. et Rolfe.

Zanthoxyli dissite (单面针, Latin name: Zanthoxylum dissitum Radix et Caulis) is the dried root and stem of *Zanthoxylum echinocarpum* Hemsl.

(The information is only for learning and identification the Chinese Patent Medicine; the specific use of the Medicine please consult the herbalist or health professionals)

Xiaomi Suppositories (Xiaomi Shuan)

Chinese phonetic alphabet/pin yin: xiāo mí shuān

Chinese characters simplified/traditional:消糜栓/消糜栓

Ingredients: Total Ginsenoside of Ginseng stems and leaves (人参茎叶皂苷), Arnebia Root, Chinese Cork-tree, Lightyellow Sophora Root, Alum (calcine and dried), Borneol, Cutch.

Indication: profuse, yellow, thick and fishy vaginal discharge, genital itching, trichomonas vaginitis, nonspecific vaginitis and cervical erosion.

Administration and dosage: for vaginal administration, 1 piece per time, once a day.

Strength: 3 g per suppository.

The specific strength and dosage are according to the medicine instruction.

Precaution and warning: contraindicated during pregnancy.

(The information is only for learning and identification the Chinese Patent Medicine; the specific use of the Medicine please consult the herbalist or health professionals)

Baofukang Suppositories (Baofukang Shuan)

Chinese phonetic alphabet/pin yin: bǎo fù kāng shuān

Chinese characters simplified/traditional:保妇康栓/保婦康栓

Ingredients: Zedoray Oil, Borneol.

Indication: abnormal vaginal discharge, profuse and yellow vaginal discharge, genitalia itching, mycotic vaginitis, senile vaginitis and cervical erosion.

Administration and dosage: insert the suppository deep into the vagina after cleaning the external genitalia, 1 piece per time every night, or as advised by health professions.

Strength: 1.74 g per suppository.

The specific strength and dosage are according to the medicine instruction.

Precaution and warning: contraindicated during pregnancy and used with caution during lactation.

(The information is only for learning and identification the Chinese Patent Medicine; the specific use of the Medicine please consult the herbalist or health professionals)

Chanfukang Granules (Chanfukang Keli)

Chinese phonetic alphabet/pin yin: chǎn fù kāng kē lì

Chinese characters simplified/traditional:产复康颗粒/產復康顆粒

Ingredients: Motherwort Herb, Chinese Angelica, Ginseng, Milkvetch Root, Fleeceflower Root, Peach Seed, Cattail Pollen, Prepared Rehmannia Root, Nutgrass Galingale Rhizome (processed with vinegar), Kelp, Largehead Atractylodes Rhizome, Black Agaric(黑木耳).

Indication: massive bleeding after postpartum, dribbling after urination, lassitude, lack of strength, sore and weakness in waist and legs.

Administration and dosage: take the medicine orally after mixing with hot water, 20 g [strength (1) and (2)] or 5 g [strength (3)] per time, three times a day, for 5-7 days as one treatment course; long time medicine is allowed in puerperium.

Strength: (1) 20 g per pack, (2) 10 g per pack, (3) 5 g per pack (without sugar).

The specific strength and dosage are according to the medicine instruction.

Precaution and warning: use with caution in patient with postpartum massive hemorrhage.

(The information is only for learning and identification the Chinese Patent Medicine; the specific use of the Medicine please consult the herbalist or health professionals)

Tongru Granules (Tongru Keli)

Chinese phonetic alphabet/pin yin: tōng rǔ kē lì

Chinese characters simplified/traditional:通乳颗粒/通乳顆粒

Ingredients: Milkvetch Root, Prepared Rehmannia Root, Ricepaperplant Pith, Lilac Pink Herb, Snakegourd Root, Beautiful Sweetgum Fruit, Uniflower Swisscentaury Rood, Tangshen, Chinese Angelica, Szechwan Lovage Rhizome, White Peony Root (stir-baked with wine), Cowherb Seed, Chinese Thorowax Root, Pangolin Scales (scalded), Degelatined Deer-horn.

Indication: insufficiency or absence of lactation and blocked lactation.

Administration and dosage: 30 g or 10 g (sucrose free) per time, three times a day for oral administration.

Strength: (1) 15 g per bag, (2) 30 g per bag, (3) 5 g per bag (without sugar).

The specific strength and dosage are according to the medicine instruction.

(The information is only for learning and identification the Chinese Patent Medicine; the specific use of the Medicine please consult the herbalist or health professionals)

Guizhi Fuling Pills (Tablets/Capsules) (Guizhi Fuling Wan (Pian/ Jiaonang))

Chinese phonetic alphabet/pin yin: guì zhī fú líng wán

Chinese characters simplified/traditional:桂枝茯苓丸(片/胶囊)/桂枝茯苓丸(片/膠囊)

Ingredients: Cassia Twig, Indian Bread, Tree Peony Bark, Peach Seed, Red Peony Root.

The content of each ingredients may have a little variety due to different dosage forms.

Indication: abdominal masses, amenorrhea, dysmenorrheal, postpartum lochia in women, hysteromyoma, chronic pelvic inflammatory mass, endometriosis and ovarian cysts.

Administration and dosage: (for oral administration) pill: 1 pill per time, once or twice a day; tablet: 3 tablets per time, three times a day after meals, one treatment course lasts for one month; capsule: 3 tablets per time, three times a day after meals, 8 weeks as one treatment course for prostate hyperplasia, 12 weeks for the other indications.

Strength: (1) 20 g per pack, (2) 10 g per pack, (3) 5 g per pack (without sugar).

The specific strength and dosage are according to the medicine instruction.

Precaution and warning: contraindicated during pregnancy, discontinue the medication during menstrual period. Epigastric discomfort or dull pain might occur occasionally, which will disappear spontaneously when the medication is discontinued.

(The information is only for learning and identification the Chinese Patent Medicine; the specific use of the Medicine please consult the herbalist or health professionals)

Pediatric medicine(儿科药)

Pediatric medicine is a kind of medicines which are mainly used to treat children diseases.

Xiao'er Resuqing Syrup (Mixture/Granules) (Xiao'er Resuqing Tangjiang (Koufuye/Keli))

Chinese phonetic alphabet/pin yin: xiǎo ér rè sù qīng táng jiāng

Chinese characters simplified/traditional:小儿热速清糖浆(口服液/颗粒)/小兒熱速清糖漿(口服液/顆粒)

Ingredients: Chinese Thorowax Root, Baical Skullcap Root, Buffalo Horn, Japanese Honeysuckle Flower, Isatis Root, Weeping Forsythia Capsule, Rhubarb, Kudzuvine Root.

The content of each ingredients may have a little variety due to different dosage forms.

Indication: common cold, high fever, headache, swollen sore throat, stuffy and runny nose, cough and dry stool.

Administration and dosage: (for oral administration) syrup: for children under 1 year old, 2.5-5 ml per time, for 1-3 years old, 5-10 ml per time, for 3-7 years old, 10-15 ml per time, for 7-12 years old, 15-20 ml, three or four times a day; mixture: 2.5-5 ml per time for children under 1 year old, 5-10 ml for between 1 and 3, 10-15 ml for between 3 and 7, 15-20 ml for between 7 and 12, three to four times a day; granule: 1.5-3 g [granule strength (1)] or 0.1-1 g [granule strength (2)] per time for children under 1 year old, for 1 between 3, 3-6 g [granule strength (1)] or 1-2 g [granule strength (2)] per time, for 3 between 7, 6-9 g [granule strength (1)] or 2-3 g [granule strength (2)] per time, for 7 between 12, 9-12 g [granule strength (1)] or 3-4 g [granule strength (2)] per time, three or four times a day.

Strength: syrup: 120 ml per bottle or 10 ml per phial; mixture: 10 ml per phial; granule: (1) 6 g per pack, (2) 2 g per pack.

The specific strength and dosage are according to the medicine instruction.

Precaution and warning: the dosage can be increased in severe case of if the medicine show no effects in 24 hours.

(The information is only for learning and identification the Chinese Patent Medicine; the specific use of the Medicine please consult the herbalist or health professionals)

Jieji Ningsou Pills (Jieji Ningsou Wan)
Chinese phonetic alphabet/pin yin: jiě jī níng sòu wán
Chinese characters simplified/traditional:解肌宁嗽丸/解肌寧嗽丸
Ingredients: Perilla leaf, Hogfennel Root, Kudzuvine Root, Bitter Apricot, Platycodon Root, Pinellia Tuber (processed), Dried Tangerine Peel, Thunberg Fritillary Bulb, Snakegourd Root, Orange Fruit, Indian Bread, Common Aucklandia Root, Figwort, Liquorice Root.
Indication: common cold with fever, cough and excessive phlegm in children.
Administration and dosage: 0.5 g pill for children under 1 year old, 1 pill for children between 1 and 3 years per time, twice a day for oral administration.
Strength: 3 g per pill.
The specific strength and dosage are according to the medicine instruction.
(The information is only for learning and identification the Chinese Patent Medicine; the specific use of the Medicine please consult the herbalist or health professionals)

Xiao'er Yanbian Granules (Xiao'er Yanbian Keli)
Chinese phonetic alphabet/pin yin: xiǎo ér yān biǎn kē lì
Chinese characters simplified/traditional:小儿咽扁颗粒/小兒咽扁顆粒
Ingredients: Japanese Honeysuckle Flower, Blackberrylily Rhizome, Tinospora Root, Platycodon Root, Figwort, Dwarf Lilyturf Tuber, Artificial Cow-bezoan, Borneol.
Indication: sore and swollen throat, cough with abundant expectoration, mouth and tongue erosions, acute pharyngitis and acute tonsillitis.
Administration and dosage: 4 g or 2 g (sucrose-free) per time for children between 1 and 2 year-old, twice a day; 4 g or 2 g (sucrose-free) for between 3 and 5 years, three time a day; 8 g or 4 g (sucrose-free) for between 6 and 14 years, two or three times a day; take the medicine orally after mixing it with hot water.
Strength: 8 g per pack or 4 g per pack (sucrose-free).
The specific strength and dosage are according to the medicine instruction.
(The information is only for learning and identification the Chinese Patent Medicine; the specific use of the Medicine please consult the herbalist or health professionals)

Xiao'er Huadu Powder (Xiao'er Huadu San)
Chinese phonetic alphabet/pin yin: xiǎo ér huà dú sǎn
Chinese characters simplified/traditional:小儿化毒散/小兒化毒散
Ingredients: Artificial Cow-bezoan, Pearl, Realgar, Rhubarb, Golden Thread, Liquorice Root, Snakegourd Root, Tendrilleaf Fritilary Bulb, Red Peony Root, Olibanum (processed), Myrrh (processed), Borneol.
Indication: painful swollen mouth sores, or skin wounds, vexation and restlessness, thirst and constipation.
Administration and dosage: 0.6 g pill per time, once or twice a day for oral administration. Reduce the dosage in children under 3 years old. For external application, apply it onto the *pars affecta*.
The specific strength and dosage are according to the medicine instruction.
Precaution and warning: long-term oral administration is not advisable.
(The information is only for learning and identification the Chinese Patent Medicine; the specific use of the Medicine please consult the herbalist or health professionals)

Xiao'er Xiesuting Granules (Xiao'er Xiesuting Keli)
Chinese phonetic alphabet/pin yin: xiǎo ér xiè sù tíng kē lì

Chinese characters simplified/traditional:小儿泻速停颗粒/小兒瀉速停顆粒
Ingredients: Creeping Euphorbia, Cutch, Smoked Plum, Hawthorn Fruit (charred), Indian Bread, White Peony Root, Liquorice Root.
Indication: watery stool, abdominal pain, poor appetite, diarrhea (at autumn), and protracted or chronic diarrhea in children.
Administration and dosage: 1.5-3 g per time for children under 6 months old, 3-6 g per time for between 6 month and 1 year-old, 6-9 g per time for between 1 and 3 years old,10-15 g per time for 3 to 7 years old, 15-20 g per time for between 7 and 12 years old, three to four times a day for oral administration.
Strength: 3 g per pack, 5 g per pack, or 10 g per pack.
The specific strength and dosage are according to the medicine instruction.
Precaution and warning: avoid raw, cold and greasy food. Seek medical care immediately if the diarrhea gets worse and dehydration is present.
(The information is only for learning and identification the Chinese Patent Medicine; the specific use of the Medicine please consult the herbalist or health professionals)

Xiao'er Xiaoshi Tablets (Xiao'er Xiaoshi Pian)
Chinese phonetic alphabet/pin yin: xiǎo ér xiāo shí piàn
Chinese characters simplified/traditional:小儿消食片/小兒消食片
Ingredients: Chicken's Gizzard-sink (stir-baked), Hawthorn Fruit, Medicated Leaven (stir-baked), Germinated Barly (stir-baked), Areca Seed, Dried Tangerine Peel.
Indication: less food intake, constipation, abdominal distension and emaciation with sallow complexion.
Administration and dosage: for tablet, 2-4 tablets per time for children between 1 and 3 years old, 4-6 tablets for between 3 and 7 years old, 6-8 tablets for adults per time, three times a day for oral or chewing administration. For film-coated tablet, 2-3 tablets per time for children between 1 and 3 years old, 3-5 tablets for between 3 and 7 years old, 5-6 tablets for adults per time, three times a day for oral or chewing administration.
Strength: 0.3 g per tablet, 0.4 g per film-coated tablet.
The specific strength and dosage are according to the medicine instruction.
(The information is only for learning and identification the Chinese Patent Medicine; the specific use of the Medicine please consult the herbalist or health professionals)

Xiao'er Huashi Pills (Mixture) (Xiao'er Huashi Wan (Koufuye))
Chinese phonetic alphabet/pin yin: xiǎo ér huà shí wán
Chinese characters simplified/traditional:小儿化食丸(口服液)/小兒化食丸(口服液)
Ingredients: Medicated Leaven (charred by stir-baked), Hawthorn Fruit (charred by stir-baked), Germinated Barly (charred by stir-baked), Areca Seed (charred by stir-baked), Zedoray Rhizome (processed with vinegar), Common Burreed Tuber (processed), Pharbitis Seed (charred by stir-baked), Rhubarb.
The content of each ingredients may have a little variety due to different dosage forms.
Indication: indigestion, anorexia, vexation and restlessness, nausea and vomiting, thirst, abdominal distension and dry stool.
Administration and dosage: (for oral administration) pill: 1pill per time for children under 1 year old, 2 pills for over 1 year old per time, twice a day; mixture: 10 ml per time, twice a day in children above three years old.
Strength: pill: 1.5 g per pill; mixture: 10 ml per phial.
The specific strength and dosage are according to the medicine instruction.

Precaution and warning: avoid spicy, oily, greasy food.

(The information is only for learning and identification the Chinese Patent Medicine; the specific use of the Medicine please consult the herbalist or health professionals)

Yinianjin Powder (Capsule) (Yinianjin (Jiaonang))

Chinese phonetic alphabet/pin yin: yí niàn jīn

Chinese characters simplified/traditional:一捻金(胶囊)/一捻金(膠囊)

Ingredients: Rhubarb, Pharbitis Seed (stir-baked), Areca Seed, Ginseng, Cinnabar.

Indication: less food and milk intake, abdominal distension, constipation, wheezing and coughing with copious sputum.

Administration and dosage: (for oral administration) powder: 0.3 g per time for children under 1 year old, 0.6 g for between 1 and 3, 1 g for between 4 and 6, once or twice a day; capsule: it can be taken orally by mixing its content with warm water, 1 capsule per time for child under 1 year old, 1-2 capsules for 1 to 3 year-old per time, 3 capsules for 4 to 6 years old per time, once or twice a day. Children over 6 years old should take the medicine as advised by health professionals.

Strength: powder: 1.2 g per pack; capsule: 0.3 g per capsule.

The specific strength and dosage are according to the medicine instruction.

Precaution and warning: long-term administration is inadvisable.

(The information is only for learning and identification the Chinese Patent Medicine; the specific use of the Medicine please consult the herbalist or health professionals)

Fei'er Pills (Fei'er Wan)

Chinese phonetic alphabet/pin yin: féi ér wán

Chinese characters simplified/traditional:肥儿丸/肥兒丸

Ingredients: Nutmeg (simmered), Common Aucklandia Root, Medicated Leaven (stir-baked), Germinated Barly (stir-baked), Figwortflower Picrorhiza Rhizome, Areca Seed, Rangooncreeper Fruit.

Indication: indigestion in children, intestinal parasites and diarrhoea.

Administration and dosage: 1-2 pills per time, once or twice a day for oral administration. Reduce the dosage in children under 3 years old.

Strength: 3 g per pill.

The specific strength and dosage are according to the medicine instruction.

(The information is only for learning and identification the Chinese Patent Medicine; the specific use of the Medicine please consult the herbalist or health professionals)

Lusika Pills (Lusika Wan)

Chinese phonetic alphabet/pin yin: lù sī kǎ wán

Chinese characters simplified/traditional:鹭鸶咯丸/鷺鷥喀丸

Ingredients: Ephedra, Bitter Apricot, Gypsum, Liquorice Root, Manchurian Wildginger Root, Perilla Fruit (stir-baked), Mustard Seed (stir-baked), Great Burdock Achene (stir-baked), Snakegourd peel, Blackberrylily Rhizome, Natural Indigo, Clam Shell, Snakegourd root, Cape Jasmine Fruit (stir-baked with ginger), Artificial Cow-bezoan.

Indication: paroxysmal cough, rattling sound in the throat, wheezing, dry throat, hoarse voice and pertusis.

Administration and dosage: take the medicine orally with pear soup or warm boiled water. 1 pill per time, twice a day.

Strength: 1.5 g per pill.

The specific strength and dosage are according to the medicine instruction.

Xiao'er Xiaoji Zhike Mixture (Xiao'er Xiaoji Zhike Koufuye)

Chinese phonetic alphabet/pin yin: xiǎo ér xiāo jī zhǐ ké kǒu fú yè

Chinese characters simplified/traditional:小儿消积止咳口服液/小兒消積止咳口服液

Ingredients: Hawthorn Fruit (charred), Areca Seed, Immature Orange Fruit, Loquat Leaf (stir-baked with honey), Snakegourd Fruit, Radish Seed (stir-baked), Pepperweed Seed (stir-baked), Platycodon Root, Weeping Forsythia Capsule, Cicada Slough.

Indication: cough worsening at night, sputum rattling in the throat, abdominal distention and fetid mouth odour.

Administration and dosage: 5 ml per time for children under 1 year old, 10 ml per time for 1-2 years old, 15 ml per time for 3-4 years old, 20 ml per time for children above 5 years old; three times a day for oral administration. One treatment last for five days.

Strength: 10 ml per phial.

The specific strength and dosage are according to the medicine instruction.

Longmu Zhuanggu Granules (Longmu Zhuanggu Keli)

Chinese phonetic alphabet/pin yin: lóng mǔ zhuàng gǔ kē lì

Chinese characters simplified/traditional:龙牡壮骨颗粒/龍牡壯骨顆粒

Ingredients: Tangshen, Milkvetch Root, Liriope Root Tuber, Tortoise Carapace and Plastron (processed with vinegar), Largehead Atractylodes Rhizome (baked), Common Yam Rhizome, Southern Magnoliavine Fruit (processed with vinegar), Skeleton Fossil, Oysters Shell (calcined), Indian Bread, Chinese Date, Liquorice Root, Calcium Lactate (乳酸钙), Chicken's Gizzard-sink (stir-baked), Vitamine D, Calcium Gluconate (葡萄糖酸钙)

Indication: osteomalacia in children or profuse perspiration, night terrors, poor appetite, indigestion and retarded development.

Administration and dosage: mixing the medicine with water before oral administration, 5 g or 3 g (sucrose free) for children under 2 years, 7.5 g or 4.5 g (sucrose free) for children between 2 to 7, 10 g or 6 g (sucrose free) for children above 7 years per time, three times a day.

Strength: 5 g or 3 g (without sucrose) per pack.

The specific strength and dosage are according to the medicine instruction.

Hupo Baolong Pills (Hupo Baolong Wan)

Chinese phonetic alphabet/pin yin: hǔ pò bào lóng wán

Chinese characters simplified/traditional:琥珀抱龙丸/琥珀抱龍丸

Ingredients: Common Yam Rhizome (stir-baked), Cinnabar, Liquorice Root, Lamber, Tabasheer, Sandalwood, Orange Fruit (stir-baked), Indian Bread, Bile Arisaema, Immature Orange Fruit (stir-baked), Red Ginseng.

Indication: fever, vexation and agitation, wheezing, phlegm, dyspnea, fright and seizure of infantile

Administration and dosage: 1.8 g (9 pills) small honeyed pills, or 1 big honeyed pill per time, twice a day; for infants, 0.6 g (3 pills) small honeyed pills, or 1/3 big honeyed pill per time take it after dissolving for oral administration.

Strength: (1) 20 g per 100 pills for small honeyed pills, (2) 1.8 g per pill for big honeyed pills.

The specific strength and dosage are according to the medicine instruction.

Precaution and warning: contraindicated in patients with chornic infantile convulsion, long-term illness and *qi* deficiency, long-term administration is not advisable.

(The information is only for learning and identification the Chinese Patent Medicine; the specific use of the Medicine please consult the herbalist or health professionals)

Niuhuang Baolong Pills (Niuhuang Baolong Wan)

Chinese phonetic alphabet/pin yin: niú huáng bào lóng wán

Chinese characters simplified/traditional:牛黄抱龙丸/牛黄抱龍丸

Ingredients: Cow-bezoar, Bile Arisaema, Tabasheer, Indian Bread, Lamber, Artificial Musk, Scorpion, Stiff Silkworm (stir-baked), Realgar, Cinnabar.

Indication: infantile convulsion, high fever and coma.

Administration and dosage: 1 pill per time, once or twice a day for oral administration. Reduce the dosage in children.

The specific strength and dosage are according to the medicine instruction.

Precaution and warning: long-term administration is not advisable.

(The information is only for learning and identification the Chinese Patent Medicine; the specific use of the Medicine please consult the herbalist or health professionals)

Ophthalmic remedy(眼科用药)

Ophthalmic remedy is a kind of medicines which are mainly used to treat diseases of eye.

Mingmu Shangqing Tablets (Mingmu Shangqing Pian)

Chinese phonetic alphabet/pin yin: míng mù shàng qīng piàn

Chinese characters simplified/traditional:明目上清片/明目上清片

Ingredients: Platycodon Root, Prepared Rhubarb, Snakegourd Root, Gypsum, Dwarf Lilyturf Tuber, Figwort, Cape Jasmine Fruit, Puncturevine Caltrop Fruit, Cicada Slough, Liquorice Root, Dried Tangerine Peel, Chrysanthemum Flower, Plantain Seed, Chinese Angelica, Baical Skullcap Root, Red Peony Root, Golden Thread, Orange Fruit, *l*-Menthol, Weeping Forsythia Capsule, Fineleaf Schizonepeta Herb Oil.

Indication: red, painful and swelling in eyes, blurry vision, dizziness, vertigo, itchy eyes, dry stool and short voiding of dark-colored urination.

Administration and dosage: 4 tablets per time, twice a day for oral administration.

Strength: 0.6 g per tablet, 0.63 g per film-coated tablet.

The specific strength and dosage are according to the medicine instruction.

Precaution and warning: use with caution during pregnancy.

(The information is only for learning and identification the Chinese Patent Medicine; the specific use of the Medicine please consult the herbalist or health professionals)

Huanglian Yanggan Pills (Huanglian Yanggan Wan)

Chinese phonetic alphabet/pin yin: huáng lián yáng gān wán

Chinese characters simplified/traditional:黄连羊肝丸/黃連羊肝丸

Ingredients: Golden Thread, Figwortflower Picrorhiza Rhizome, Baical Skullcap Root, Chinese Cork-tree, Chinese Gentian, Chinese Thorowax Root, Dried Immaturity Tangerines Peel (stir-baked with vinegar), Common Scouring Rush Herb, Pale Butterflybush Flower, Motherwort fruit, Cassia Seed (stir-baked), Abalone Shell (calcined), Bat Dung, Fresh Sheep Liver (鲜羊肝).

Indication: red, painful, swelling eyes, blurry vision, photophobia and pterygium.

Administration and dosage: 9 g (18 pills) small honeyed pills, or 1 large honeyed pill per time, once or twice a day.

Strength: (1) 20 g per 100 pills for small honeyed pills, (2) 9 g per pill for big honeyed pills.

The specific strength and dosage are according to the medicine instruction.

Attachment: Bat Dung (夜明砂, Latin name: Vespertilionis Faeces) is dried Faeces of *Vespertilio superas* Thomas, *Murina leucogaster* Milne-Edwards, *Pipstrellus abramus*Temminck, *Plecotus auritus* Linnaeus, or other species of bat.

(The information is only for learning and identification the Chinese Patent Medicine; the specific use of the Medicine please consult the herbalist or health professionals)

Shihu Yeguang Pills (Shihu Yeguang Wan)

Chinese phonetic alphabet/pin yin: shí hú yè guāng wán

Chinese characters simplified/traditional:石斛夜光丸/石斛夜光丸

Ingredients: Dendrobium, Ginseng, Common Yam Rhizome, Indian Bread, Liquorice Root, Desertliving Cistanche Herb, Barbary Wolfberry Fruit, Dodder Seed, Rehmannia Root, Prepared Rehmannia Root, Chinese Magnoliavine Fruit, Cochinchinese Asparagus Root, Dwarf Lilyturf Tuber, Bitter Apricot, Divaricate Saposhnikovia Root, Szechwan Lovage Rhizome, Orange Fruit (stir-baked with bran), Golden Thread, Twotoothed Achyranthes Root, Chrysanthemum Flower, Puncturevine Caltrop Fruit (stir-baked with salt), Feather Cockscomb Seed, Cassia Seed, Powdered Buffalo Horn Extract, Goat Horn (山羊角).

Indication: cataract with dim and blurry vision.

Administration and dosage: 7.3 g water-honeyed pill, 11 g small honeyed pills, or 2 large honeyed pill per time, twice a day.

Strength: 5.5 g per big honeyed pill.

The specific strength and dosage are according to the medicine instruction.

(The information is only for learning and identification the Chinese Patent Medicine; the specific use of the Medicine please consult the herbalist or health professionals)

Zhangyanming Tablets (Zhangyanming Pian)

Chinese phonetic alphabet/pin yin: zhàng yǎn míng piàn

Chinese characters simplified/traditional:障眼明片/障眼明片

Ingredients: Grassleaf Sweetflag Rhizome, Cassia Seed, Desertliving Cistanche Herb, Kudzuvine Root, Feather Cockscomb Seed, Tangshen, Shrub Chastetree Fruit, Barbary Wolfberry Fruit, Plantain Seed, White Peony Root, Asiatic Cornelian Cherry Fruit, Liquorice Root, Dodder Seed, Largetrifoliolious Bugbane Rhizome, Hedge Prinsepia Nut (removed the endocarp), Chrysanthemum Flower, Pale Butterflybush Flower, Szechwan Lovage Rhizome, Solomonseal Rhizome (processed with wine), Prepared Rehmannia Root, Amur Cork-tree, Milkvetch Root.

Indication: dry eyes, monocular diplopia, mild impaired vision, incipient cataract and metaphase cataract.

Administration and dosage: 4 tablets [strength (1) and (3)], or 2 tablets [strength (2)] per time, three time a day.

Strength: (1) film coated tablets, 0.21 g per tablet, (2) film coated tablets, 0.42 g per tablet, (3) sugar coated tablets, 0.21 g per tablets core.

The specific strength and dosage are according to the medicine instruction.

Precaution and warning: avoid spicy food.

(The information is only for learning and identification the Chinese Patent Medicine; the specific use of the Medicine please consult the herbalist or health professionals)

Fufang Xueshuantong Capsules (Fufang Xueshuantong Jiaonang)

Chinese phonetic alphabet/pin yin: fù fāng xuě shuān tōng jiāo náng

Chinese characters simplified/traditional:复方血栓通胶囊/複方血栓通膠囊

Ingredients: Sanchi, Milkvetch Root, Danshen Root, Figwort.

Indication: chest and heart pain, palpitations, flusteredness, short of breath, vexation, impaired vision, vision disorder, lassitude, and stable angina pectoris.

Administration and dosage: 3 capsules per time, three times a day for oral administration.

Strength: 0.5 g per capsule.

The specific strength and dosage are according to the medicine instruction.

Precaution and warning: use with caution during pregnancy.

(The information is only for learning and identification the Chinese Patent Medicine; the specific use of the Medicine please consult the herbalist or health professionals)

Otolaryngology and Stomatology medicine(耳鼻喉、口腔科用药)

Otolaryngology and Stomatology medicine is a kind of medicines which are mainly used to treat diseases of ear, nose, throat (E.N.T), or oral cavity.

Erlong Pills (Erlong Wan)

Chinese phonetic alphabet/pin yin: ěr lóng wán

Chinese characters simplified/traditional:耳聋丸/耳聾丸

Ingredients: Chinese Gentian, Baical Skullcap Root, Rehmannia Root, Oriental Waterplantain Rhizome, Akebiae Stem, Cape Jasmine Fruit, Chinese Angelica, Altai Anemone Rhizome, Liquorice Root, Antelope Horn.

Indication: dizziness, headache, deafness, tinnitus and purulent discharge form the ear.

Administration and dosage: 7 g small honeyed pills or 1 big honeyed pill per time, twice a day for oral administration.

Strength: 7 g per 45 pills (small honeyed pills), 7 g per pill (big honeyed pill).

The specific strength and dosage are according to the medicine instruction.

Precaution and warning: Avoid spicy food.

Attachment: Altai Anemone Rhizome (九节菖蒲, Latin name: Anemones Altaicae Rhizoma) is dried root and stem of *Anemone altaica* Fisch. ex C. A. Mey. It is toxic.

(The information is only for learning and identification the Chinese Patent Medicine; the specific use of the Medicine please consult the herbalist or health professionals)

Erlong Zuoci Pills (Erlong Zuoci Wan)

Chinese phonetic alphabet/pin yin: ěr lóng zuǒ cí wán

Chinese characters simplified/traditional:耳聋左慈丸/耳聾左慈丸

Ingredients: Magnetite, Prepared Rehmannia Root, Asiatic Cornelian Cherry Fruit (processed), Tree Peony Bark, Common Yam Rhizome, Indian Bread, Oriental Waterplantain Rhizome, Chinese Thorowax Root.

Indication: deafness, tinnitus, dizziness and vertigo.

Administration and dosage: 6 g water-honeyed pills or 1 big honeyed pill per time, twice a day for oral administration.

Strength: 1 g per 10 water-honeyed pills, 3 g per 15 water-honeyed pills, 9 g per big honeyed pill.

The specific strength and dosage are according to the medicine instruction.

Precaution and warning: Avoid spicy food.

(The information is only for learning and identification the Chinese Patent Medicine; the specific use of the Medicine please consult the herbalist or health professionals)

Biyankang Tablets (Biyankang Pian)

Chinese phonetic alphabet/pin yin: bí yán kāng piàn

Chinese characters simplified/traditional:鼻炎康片/鼻炎康片

Ingredients: Cablin Patchouli Herb, Siberian Cocklebur Seed, Small Centipeda Herb, Ephedra, Wild Chrysanthemum Flower, Chinese Angelica, Baical Skullcap Root, Pig Gall Powder, Peppermint Oil, Chlorphenamine Maleate (马来酸氯苯那敏).

Indication: acute, chronic and allergic rhinitis.

Administration and dosage: 4 tablets per time, three times a day for oral administration.

The specific strength and dosage are according to the medicine instruction.

Precaution and warning: contraindicated in pregnant woman or patients with hypertension. Vehicle driving, machine operating and working at height are not advised during medication. Avoid spicy food. Avoid overdose and prolonged usage.

Strength: 0.37 g per tablet (contains 1 mg of chlorphemamine maleate).

(The information is only for learning and identification the Chinese Patent Medicine; the specific use of the Medicine please consult the herbalist or health professionals)

Qianbai Biyan Tablets (Capsules) (Qianbai Biyan Pian (Jiaonang))

Chinese phonetic alphabet/pin yin: qiān bǎi bí yán piàn

Chinese characters simplified/traditional:千柏鼻炎片(胶囊)/千柏鼻炎片(膠囊)

Ingredients: Climbing Groundsel Herb, Spikemoss, Incised Notopterygium Rhizome and Root, Cassia Seed, Ephedra, Szechwan Lovage Rhizome, Dahurian Angelica Root.

The content of each ingredients may have a little variety due to different dosage forms.

Indication: stuffy and itch nose with purulent nasal mucus and thick sputum, smell reducing, rhinitis and nasal sinusitis.

Administration and dosage: (for oral administration) tablet: 3-4 tablets per time, three times a day; capsule: 2 capsules per time, three times a day; for 15 days as one treatment course. Reduce the dosage when symptoms are relieved.

Strength: 0.44 g per file-coated tablet; 0.5 g per capsule.

The specific strength and dosage are according to the medicine instruction.

(The information is only for learning and identification the Chinese Patent Medicine; the specific use of the Medicine please consult the herbalist or health professionals)

Biyuanshu Capsules (Mixture) (Biyuanshu Jiaonang (Koufuye))

Chinese phonetic alphabet/pin yin: bí yuān shū jiāo náng

Chinese characters simplified/traditional:鼻渊舒胶囊(口服液)/鼻淵舒膠囊(口服液)

Ingredients: Siberian Cocklebur Seed, Biond Magnolia Flower, Peppermint, Dahurian Angelica Root, Baical Skullcap Root, Cape Jasmine Fruit, Chinese Thorowax Root, Manchurian Wildginger Root, Szechwan Lovage Rhizome, Milkvetch Root, Armand Clematis Stem, Platycodon Root, Indian Bread.
The content of each ingredients may have a little variety due to different dosage forms.
Indication: rhinitis and nasosinusitis.
Administration and dosage:(for oral administration) capsule: 3 pills per time, three times a day; mixture: 10 ml per time, twice or three times a day; for seven days as one treatment course.
Strength: 0.3 g per capsule; 10 ml per phial.
The specific strength and dosage are according to the medicine instruction.
(The information is only for learning and identification the Chinese Patent Medicine; the specific use of the Medicine please consult the herbalist or health professionals)

Xinqin Granules (Tablets) (Xinqin Keli (Pian))
Chinese phonetic alphabet/pin yin: xīn qín kē lì
Chinese characters simplified/traditional:辛芩颗粒(片)/辛芩顆粒(片)
Ingredients: Manchurian Wildginger Root, Baical Skullcap Root, Fineleaf Schizonepeta Herb, Divaricate Saposhnikovia Root, Dahurian Angelica Root, Siberian Cocklebur Seed, Milkvetch Root, Largehead Atractylodes Rhizome, Cassia Twig, Grassleaf Sweetflag Rhizome.
The content of each ingredients may have a little variety due to different dosage forms.
Indication: itchy nose, sneezing, thin nasal discharge and allergic rhinitis.
Administration and dosage:(for oral administration) granule: mixing the medicine with hot water before usage, 1 pack per time, three times a day; tablet: 3 tablets per time, three times a day; for 20 days as one treatment course.
Strength: granule: 20 g per pack, 5 g per pack (without sucrose); tablet: 0.8 g per tablet.
The specific strength and dosage are according to the medicine instruction.
Precaution and warning: use with caution in children and the elderly. Contraindicated in pregnant women, infant and patients with renal insufficiency.
(The information is only for learning and identification the Chinese Patent Medicine; the specific use of the Medicine please consult the herbalist or health professionals)

Bingpeng Powder (Bingpeng San)
Chinese phonetic alphabet/pin yin: bīng péng sǎn
Chinese characters simplified/traditional:冰硼散/冰硼散
Ingredients: Borneol, Borax (calcined), Cinnabar, Exsiccated Sodium Sulfate.
Indication: sore throat, swelling and painful gum, mouth and tongue sore.
Administration and dosage: blow the drug to the *pars affecta* with small dosage per time, several times a day.
The specific strength and dosage are according to the medicine instruction.
Precaution and warning: used with caution during pregnancy, long-term administration is not advisable.
(The information is only for learning and identification the Chinese Patent Medicine; the specific use of the Medicine please consult the herbalist or health professionals)

Guilin Xiguashuang (Guilin Xiguashuang)

Chinese phonetic alphabet/pin yin: guì lín xī guā shuāng

Chinese characters simplified/traditional:桂林西瓜霜/桂林西瓜霜

Ingredients: Mirabilite Preparation, Borax (calcined), Chinese Cork-tree, Golden Thread, Vietnamese Sophora Root, Blackberrylily Rhizome, Thunberg Fritillary Bulb, Natural Indigo, Borneol, Soapberry Fruit (charred), Rhubarb, Baical Skullcap Root, Liquorice Root, Menthol.

Indication: swollen sore throat, enlarge tonsils, swelling pain or bleeding of gum, acute or chronic pharyngitis, tonsillitis, stomatitis, mouth ulcer.

Administration and dosage: apply proper amount of medicine for *pars affecta* for topical application several times a day; for severe cases, combined with oral administration, 1-2 g per time, three times a day.

Strength: 1 g, 2 g, 2.5 g or 3 g per bottle.

The specific strength and dosage are according to the medicine instruction.

Attachment: Soapberry Fruit (无患子, Latin name: Sapindi Fructus) is the fruit of *Sapindus mukorossi* Gaertn.

(The information is only for learning and identification the Chinese Patent Medicine; the specific use of the Medicine please consult the herbalist or health professionals)

Fufang Yuxincao Tablets (Fufang Yuxincao Pian)

Chinese phonetic alphabet/pin yin: fù fāng yú xīn cǎo piàn

Chinese characters simplified/traditional:复方鱼腥草片/複方魚腥草片

Ingredients: Heartleaf Houttuynia Herb, Baical Skullcap Root, Isatis Root, Weeping Forsythia Capsule, Japanese Honeysuckle Flower.

Indication: sore throat, acute pharyngitis and acute tonsillitis.

Administration and dosage: 4-6 tablets per time, three times a day for oral administration.

The specific strength and dosage are according to the medicine instruction.

(The information is only for learning and identification the Chinese Patent Medicine; the specific use of the Medicine please consult the herbalist or health professionals)

Liushen Pills (Liushen Wan)

Chinese phonetic alphabet/pin yin: liù shén wán

Chinese characters simplified/traditional:六神丸/六神丸

Ingredients: Artificial Musk, Toad Venom, Realgar, etc.

Indication: swollen, sore throat, carbuncle and swelling.

Administration and dosage: 10 pills per time for adult, three times a day; 1 pill for children in 1 year, 2 pills for 2 years, 3-4 pills for 3 years, 5-6 pills for between 4 and 8 years old, 8-9 pills for between 9 and 10-year-old per time, three times a day for oral administration. Mixing the medicine with cold boiled water or vinegar into paste to apply onto *pars affecta* for external application.

Strength: granule: 3.125 g per 1000 pills.

The specific strength and dosage are according to the medicine instruction.

Precaution and warning: use with caution in pregnant women and infant.

Incompatible with digoxin, atropine and Iodine preparation.

(The information is only for learning and identification the Chinese Patent Medicine; the specific use of the Medicine please consult the herbalist or health professionals)

Xuanmai Ganjie Granules (Capsules/Buccal Tablets) (Xuanmai Ganjie Keli (Jiaonang/Hanpian))

Chinese phonetic alphabet/pin yin: xuán mài gān jú kē lì

Chinese characters simplified/traditional:玄麦甘桔颗粒(胶囊/含片)/玄麥甘桔顆粒(膠囊/含片)

Ingredients: Figwort, Dwarf Lilyturf Tuber, Liquorice Root, Platycodon Root.
The content of each ingredients may have a little variety due to different dosage forms.

Indication: dryness of the mouth and nose, and swollen sore throat.

Administration and dosage: (for oral administration) granule: mixing the medicine with hot water before usage, 1 pack per time, three or four times a day; capsule: 3-4 capsules per time, three times a day; buccal tablet: for sublingual administration, 1-2 tablets per time, 12 tablets a day.

Strength: granule: 10 g per pack, 6 g per pack (low glucose), 5 g per pack (without sucrose); capsule: 0.35 g per capsule; tablet: 1 g per tablet or 1 g per film-coated tablet.

The specific strength and dosage are according to the medicine instruction.

Precaution and warning: use with caution in children and the elderly.

(The information is only for learning and identification the Chinese Patent Medicine; the specific use of the Medicine please consult the herbalist or health professionals)

Qingyin Pills (Qingyin Wan)

Chinese phonetic alphabet/pin yin: qīng yīn wán

Chinese characters simplified/traditional:清音丸/清音丸

Ingredients: Sarcocarp of Medicine Terminalia Fruit, Tendrilleaf Fritillary Bulb, Bai Yao Jian, Pulp of Smoked Plum, Kudzuvine Root, Indian Bread, Liquorice Root, Snakegourd Root.

Indication: discomfort in the throat, dry mouth and tongue, hoarseness and loss of voice.

Administration and dosage: take the medicine orally with warm boiled water or dissolve it in mouth, 2 g water-honeyed pill or 1 big honeyed pill per time, twice a day.

Strength: 10 g per 100 water-honeyed pills, 3 g per big honeyed pill.

The specific strength and dosage are according to the medicine instruction.

Precaution and warning: avoid smoking, alcohol and spicy food.

Attachment: Bai Yao Jian (百药煎, nick name: Chinese Gall Leaven) is the fermented block substance of gallnut and tea.

(The information is only for learning and identification the Chinese Patent Medicine; the specific use of the Medicine please consult the herbalist or health professionals)

Zhuhuang Powder (Zhuhuang San)

Chinese phonetic alphabet/pin yin: zhū huáng sǎn

Chinese characters simplified/traditional:珠黄散/珠黄散

Ingredients: Artificial Cow-bezoan, Pearl.

Indication: sore throat, swollen and eroded throat, and unhealing mouth ulcer.

Administration and dosage: blow small amount of the medicine to the *pars affecta*, two or three times a day

The specific strength and dosage are according to the medicine instruction.

Precaution and warning: avoid spicy, greasy and salty food.

(The information is only for learning and identification the Chinese Patent Medicine; the specific use of the Medicine please consult the herbalist or health professionals)

Huangshi Xiangsheng Pills (Huangshi Xiangsheng Wan)

Chinese phonetic alphabet/pin yin: huáng shì xiǎng shēng wán

Chinese characters simplified/traditional:黄氏响声丸/黄氏響聲丸

Ingredients: Peppermint, Thunberg Fritillary Bulb, Weeping Forsythia Capsule, Cicada Slough, Boat-fruited Sterculia Seed, Rhubarb (stir-baked with wine), Szechwan Lovage Rhizome, Cutch, Platycodon Root, Medicine Terminalia Fruit (without core), Liquorice Root, *l*-Menthol.

Indication: hoarse voice, swollen sore throat, dry and burning sensation in the throat, acute and chronic laryngitis, nodules in the vocal cords and early period of polyp of vocal cord.

Administration and dosage: 8 pills [strength (1)] or 6 pills [strength (2)] per time, or 20 sugar-coated pills [strength (3)] per time, three times a day for oral administration after meals. Reduce the dose in children.

Strength: (1) 0.1 g per pill for charcoal coated pills, (2) 0.133 g per pill for charcoal coated pills, (3) 400 pills per bottle for sugar coated pills.

The specific strength and dosage are according to the medicine instruction.

Precaution and warning: use with caution in patients with stomach coldness and sloppy stool.

(The information is only for learning and identification the Chinese Patent Medicine; the specific use of the Medicine please consult the herbalist or health professionals)

Qingyan Pills (Qingyan Wan)

Chinese phonetic alphabet/pin yin: qīng yān wán

Chinese characters simplified/traditional:清咽丸/清咽丸

Ingredients: Platycodon Root, Calcitum, Peppermint, sarcocarp of Medicine Terminalia Fruit, Liquorice Root, Pulp of Smoked Plum, Natural Indigo, Borax (calcined), Borneol.

Indication: swelling and sore throat, hoarse voice, dry mouth and tongue.

Administration and dosage: 6 g small honeyed pills or 1 big honeyed pill per time, two or three times a day for oral administration.

Strength: 6 g per 30 small honeyed pill, 6 g per big honeyed pill.

The specific strength and dosage are according to the medicine instruction.

Precaution and warning: avoid smoking, alcohol and spicy food.

(The information is only for learning and identification the Chinese Patent Medicine; the specific use of the Medicine please consult the herbalist or health professionals)

Kouyanqing Granules (Kouyanqing Keli)

Chinese phonetic alphabet/pin yin: kǒu yán qīng kē lì

Chinese characters simplified/traditional:口炎清颗粒/口炎清顆粒

Ingredients: Cochinchinese Asparagus Root, Dwarf Lilyturf Tuber, Figwort, Honeysuckle Flower, Liquorice Root.

Indication: inflammation in the mouth.

Administration and dosage: 2 packs per time, once or twice a day for oral administration.

Strength: 10 g per pack, 3 g per pack (without sucrose).

The specific strength and dosage are according to the medicine instruction.

(The information is only for learning and identification the Chinese Patent Medicine; the specific use of the Medicine please consult the herbalist or health professionals)

Orthopedics and Traumatology pharmacy(骨伤科用药)

Orthopedics and Traumatology pharmacy is a kind of medicines which are mainly used to treat diseases such as fractures and muscle injury, traumatic injuries, stasis and distention of pain.

Qili Powder (Qili San)

Chinese phonetic alphabet/pin yin: qī lí sǎn

Chinese characters simplified/traditional:七厘散/七厘散

Ingredients: Dragon's Blood, Olibanum (processed), Myrrh (processed), Safflower, Cutch, Borneol, Artificial Musk, Cinnabar.

Indication: traumatic injuries, blood-stasis pain and wound bleeding.

Administration and dosage: 1-1.5 g per time, one to three times a day for oral administration; apply it on the *pars affecta* for external use.

Strength: 1.5 g or 3 g per bottle.

The specific strength and dosage are according to the medicine instruction.

Precaution and warning: contraindicated during pregnancy, long-term oral administration is not advisable.

(The information is only for learning and identification the Chinese Patent Medicine; the specific use of the Medicine please consult the herbalist or health professionals)

Dieda Pills (Dieda Wan)

Chinese phonetic alphabet/pin yin: diē dǎ wán

Chinese characters simplified/traditional:跌打丸/跌打丸

Ingredients: Sanchi, Chinese Angelica, White Peony Root,Red Peony Root, Peach Seed, Safflower, Dragon's Blood, Chinese Siphonostegia Herb, Fortune's Drynaria Rhizome (scalded), Himalayan Teasel Root, Sappan Wood, Tree Peony Bark, Olibanum (processed), Myrrh (processed), Turmeric, Common Burreed Tuber (processed with vinegar), Divaricate Saposhnikovia Root, Muskmelon Seed, Immature Orange Fruit (stir-baked), Platycodon Root, Liquorice Root, Akebiae Stem, Pyrite (calcined), Ground Beetle .

Indication: traumatic injuries, ruptured sinew, bone fracture, static pain and swelling, sprain of waist and abdominal cramp.

Administration and dosage: 3 g small honeyed pills per time or 1 big honey pill per time, twice a day for oral administration.

Strength: 2 g per 10 pills for small honeyed pills, 3 g per pill for big honeyed pill.

The specific strength and dosage are according to the medicine instruction.

Precaution and warning: contraindicated during pregnancy.

(The information is only for learning and identification the Chinese Patent Medicine; the specific use of the Medicine please consult the herbalist or health professionals)

Huoxue Zhitong Powder (Capsules) (Huoxue Zhitong San (Jiaonang))

Chinese phonetic alphabet/pin yin: huó xuě zhǐ tòng sǎn

Chinese characters simplified/traditional:活血止痛散(胶囊)/活血止痛散(膠囊)

Ingredients: Chinese Angelica, Sanchi, Olibanum (processed), Borneol, Ground Beetle, Pyrite (calcined).

The content of each ingredients may have a little variety due to different dosage forms.

Indication: traumatic injuries with swelling pain.

Administration and dosage: take the medicine with warm yellow wine or warm boiled water. Powder: 1.5 g per time, twice a day; capsule: 3 pills per time for [strength (1)],

4 pills per time for [strength (2)], 6 pills per time for [strength (3)], all of them are twice a day.

Strength: capsule: (1) 0.5 g per capsule, (2) 0.37 g per capsule, (3) 0.25 g per capsule.

The specific strength and dosage are according to the medicine instruction.

Precaution and warning: contraindicated during pregnancy.

(The information is only for learning and identification the Chinese Patent Medicine; the specific use of the Medicine please consult the herbalist or health professionals)

Yao'ai Paper Strip-rolls (Yao'ai Tiao)

Chinese phonetic alphabet/pin yin: yào ài tiáo

Chinese characters simplified/traditional:药艾条/藥艾條

Ingredients: Argy Wormwood Leaf, Cassia Twig, Lesser Galangal Rhizome, Cablin Patchouli Herb, Rosewood, Nutgrass Galingale Rhizome, Dahurian Angelica Root, Dried Tangerine Peel, Danshen Root, Common Monkshood Mother Root.

Indication: muscle aching and numbness, joint and limbs pain, and cold pain in epigastrium and abdomen.

Administration and dosage: use direct moxibustion till skin turns red, once or twice a day.

Strength: 28 g per roll.

The specific strength and dosage are according to the medicine instruction.

Precaution and warning: avoid scald. Please use it under the guidance of the herbalist or health professionals.

(The information is only for learning and identification the Chinese Patent Medicine; the specific use of the Medicine please consult the herbalist or health professionals)

Argy wormwood Leaf Carboniferous Strip-rolls (Wuyan Jiutiao)

Chinese phonetic alphabet/pin yin: wú yān jiū tiáo

Chinese characters simplified/traditional:无烟灸条/無煙灸條

Ingredients: Incised Notopterygium Rhizome and Root, Manchurian Wildginger Root, Dahurian Angelica Root, Nardostachys Root, Common Aucklandia Root, Argy Wormwood Leaf (carbonized and processed with vinegar).

Indication: sore and numbness of muscle, joint and limbs pain, and cold pain in epigastrium and abdomen.

Administration and dosage: use direct moxibustion till skin turns red, once or twice a day.

Strength: 28 g per roll.

The specific strength and dosage are according to the medicine instruction.

Precaution and warning: avoid scald. Please use it under the guidance of the herbalist or health professionals.

(The information is only for learning and identification the Chinese Patent Medicine; the specific use of the Medicine please consult the herbalist or health professionals)

INDEX

Special thanks

Thank the follow websites generous support the pictures for this book:

http://www.tcm166.com (国医在线)

http://www.18ladys.com (中药大全)

https://www.cndzys.com (大众养生网)

http://www.tmyy.net (天马(安徽)国药科技股份有限公司)

http://www.yunyao.net (云药网)

http://www.zgycsc.com (中国药材市场)

http://www.qnong.com.cn (黔农网)

http://zhongyao.aipinkd.com (问药堂)

http://www.zhongyoo.com (中药查询)

http://zhongyibaike.com (中医百科)

https://aglbyc.1688.com (安国冷背药材有限公司)

http://www.xyzyw.cn (信誉藏药网)

Some pictures were bought from http://www.plantphoto.cn(中国植物图像库)

The pictures of this book are proofreaded by Huang Hongying (Chief pharmacist of Qinghai Hospital of Traditional Chinese Medicine, China) and Lu Xue-feng (professor of Northwest Institute of Planteau Biology, China).

Thanks for Ma Mingfang and Zhang Xinyi's (both of Qinghai Province Institute for Food Control, China) help to edit this book.

Appendix

Map of Five Elements

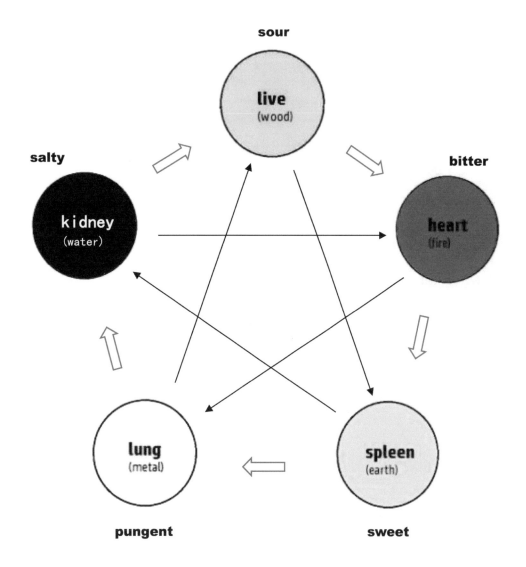

generation among five elements

restriction among five elements

Map of Eight Diagrams

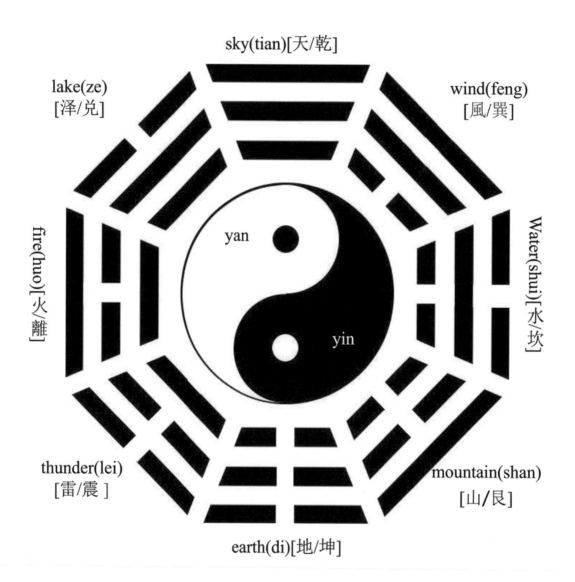

sky(tian)[天/乾]

lake(ze)
[泽/兑]

wind(feng)
[風/巽]

fire(huo)[火/離]

Water(shui)[水/坎]

yan

yin

thunder(lei)
[雷/震]

mountain(shan)
[山/艮]

earth(di)[地/坤]

Map of Main and collateral channels (Meridian tropism)

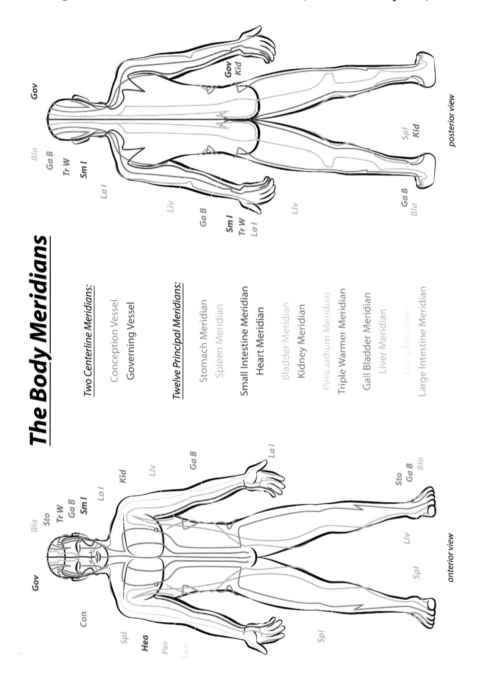

The Body Meridians

Two Centerline Meridians:

Conception Vessel
Governing Vessel

Twelve Principal Meridians:

Stomach Meridian
Spleen Meridian

Small Intestine Meridian
Heart Meridian

Bladder Meridian
Kidney Meridian

Pericardium Meridian
Triple Warmer Meridian

Gall Bladder Meridian
Liver Meridian

Lung Meridian
Large Intestine Meridian

posterior view

anterior view

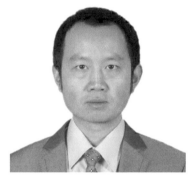

Chen Rui is a senior engineer of food and herb test, pharmacist, and master of botany.